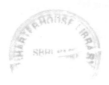

OXFORD MEDICAL PUBLICATIONS

Colour Atlas of Bone, Joint, and Soft Tissue Pathology

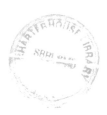

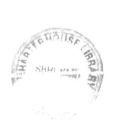

Colour Atlas of Bone, Joint, and Soft Tissue Pathology

Nicholas A. Athanasou

Reader in Orthopaedic Pathology, University of Oxford
Consultant Pathologist, Nuffield Orthopaedic Centre, Oxford

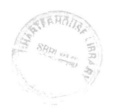

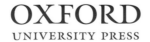

OXFORD

UNIVERSITY PRESS

OXFORD
UNIVERSITY PRESS

Great Clarendon Street, Oxford OX2 6DP

Oxford University Press is a department of the University of Oxford
and furthers the University's aim of excellence in research, scholarship,
and education by publishing worldwide in

Oxford New York

Athens Auckland Bangkok Bogotá Buenos Aires Calcutta
Cape Town Chennai Dar es Salaam Delhi Florence Hong Kong Istanbul
Karachi Kuala Lumpur Madrid Melbourne Mexico City Mumbai
Nairobi Paris São Paulo Singapore Taipei Tokyo Toronto Warsaw
and associated companies in Berlin Ibadan

Oxford is a registered trade mark of Oxford University Press

Published in the United States
by Oxford University Press Inc., New York

British Library Cataloguing in Publication Data
Data available

Library of Congress Cataloging in Publication Data

ISBN 0 19 262792 9

Typeset by EXPO Holdings, Malaysia
Printed in China

Preface

The purpose of this atlas is to provide an illustrated guide to the histopathology of bone, joint, and soft tissue lesions. Although primarily directed towards diagnostic histopathologists, many of whom do not regularly encounter this type of pathology, it is hoped that this atlas will also be of use to physicians, surgeons, radiologists, and others involved in the diagnosis and treatment of pathological conditions of bone, joint, and soft tissues. As histopathologists and their clinical colleagues are expected to have knowledge of the full range of conditions which occur in orthopaedic pathology, this atlas differs from other works of this nature, most of which deal separately with the pathology (particularly that of the diverse range of neoplasms) encountered in one or other of these tissues, by aiming to present in a single volume the features of both non-neoplastic and neoplastic conditions that arise in bone, joint, and soft tissue.

The photomicrographs in this atlas provide representative appearances of the (often highly variable) morphological features of pathological lesions occurring in bone, joint, and soft tissue. Where possible, the histopathology is shown at both low and high power in order to demonstrate both the overall architecture and cytological detail of the lesion. Most of the figures are of haematoxylin and eosin stained preparations but illustrations of the use of special stains and immunohistochemistry to show specific pathological features have also been included. As examination of the gross specimen may provide useful diagnostic information, the macroscopic appearance of some lesions has also been illustrated. The captions which accompany the figures not only describe the histological findings but also the typical clinical background in which the lesion develops, as this often provides essential diagnostic information. The typical radiographic appearances of bone and joint lesions are also illustrated and described as, not uncommonly, osteoarticular pathologists are called upon to base their diagnosis as much on the radiological appearances as on the histological findings. In a work of this nature, only the main, clinical, radiological, and pathological features of each lesion can be described and the reader is referred to the articles and books listed in the bibliography to obtain more detailed information and additional references on a particular condition.

In the preparation of this atlas, I have drawn upon material collected by many of my colleagues at the Nuffield Orthopaedic Centre and John Radcliffe Hospital, Oxford. I am very grateful for their courtesy and assistance. I am particularly indebted to Dr Colin Woods who allowed me access to his diagnostic files and illustrations. I am also grateful to Dr Roger Smith, Dr Simon Ostlere, Mr Andrew Carr, Mr Michael Benson, Professor Margaret Esiri and Dr Stephen Gould who helped me to track down the radiology and histology of a number of uncommon lesions. I am especially indebted to my secretary, Mrs Margaret Pearce, who uncomplainingly typed the many revised versions of the manuscript for this atlas and Mr Paul Cooper of the Photographic Department of the Nuffield Orthopaedic Centre for his patience and helpful advice. I also wish to thank the staff of Oxford University Press, in particular Esther Hunt, Helen Liepman and John Harrison for their help in producing this atlas. I am grateful to Blackwell Scientific Publications for permission to use several illustrations from *Diagnostic Orthopaedic Pathology* by C. G. Woods and to BMJ Publishing for permission to reproduce Figures 7.67a and b.

Oxford   N. A. A.
July 1998

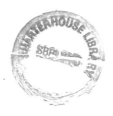

Abbreviations

AA	amyloid A protein
AL	amyloid L protein
AS	ankylosing spondylitis
CDH	congenital dislocation of hip
COMP	cartilage oligomeric matrix protein
CPPD	calcium pyrophosphate dihydrate
CREST	calcinosis, Raynaud's phenomenon, oesophageal dysfunction, sclerodactyly, telangirctasia
CT	computed tomography
DFSP	dermatofibrosarcoma protuberans
DISH	diffuse idiopathic skeletal hyperostosis
FGFR	fibroblast growth factor receptor
FIO	fibrogenesis imperfecta ossium
FOP	fibrodysplasia (myositis) ossificans progressiva
HAP	hydroxyapatite
MFH	malignant fibrous histiocytoma
MPNST	malignant peripheral nerve sheath tumour
MPS	mucopolysaccharidoses
MRI	magnetic resonance imaging
NF-1	neurofibromatosis
NSE	neurone-specific enolase
OA	osteoarthritis
OI	osteogenesis imperfecta
PAS	periodic acid-Schiff (stain)
PMMA	polymethylmethacrylate
PNET	primitive neuroectodermal tumour
POH	progressive osseous heteroplasia
PSC	primary synovial chondromatosis
PTH	parathyroid hormone
PVNS	pigmented villonodular synovitis
RA	rheumatoid arthritis
SEDC	spondyloepiphyseal dysplasia congenita
UHMWP	ultra-high molecular weight polyethylene
VDDR	vitamin D-dependent rickets

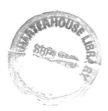

Contents

1 Normal skeletal structure and development page 1

2 Repair, necrosis, and reactive changes in skeletal tissue page 17

3 Infections of bone and joint page 37

4 Disorders of skeletal development page 53

5 Metabolic and endocrine disorders of the skeleton page 71

6 Diseases of joints and periarticular tissues page 87

7 Bone tumours and tumour-like lesions page 115

8 Soft tissue tumours and tumour-like lesions page 165

Bibliography page 231

Index page 233

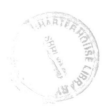

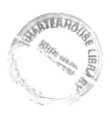

1

Normal skeletal structure and development

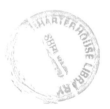

Bone structure

Figure 1.1 Bone: gross structure The skeleton provides the framework of the body. It is divided into the axial skeleton, which includes the vertebrae, skull, ribs, sternum, and hyoid bone, and the appendicular skeleton, which includes the bones of the upper and lower limbs and the pelvis. Grossly, each bone is enclosed by a bone cortex composed of compact (dense) bone; this surrounds a medullary cavity containing cancellous (trabecular, spongy) bone. A dense fibrous tissue membrane (periosteum) covers the cortex except over the articular surfaces which are covered by cartilage. Adipocytes and haematopoietic tissue fill the marrow spaces between bone trabeculae. Both cortical and cancellous bone contain an extensive vascular network. In a long bone the following regions are described: (1) the epiphysis, the expanded end of the bone which is covered by articular cartilage; (2) diaphysis or shaft; (3) metaphysis, which is the junctional zone between the epiphysis and the diaphysis; (4) growth plate (physis), a cartilaginous structure that separates the epiphysis from the metaphysis and is the zone of endochondral ossification in an actively growing bone. These terms are useful in describing the location of a pathological lesion in bone and are shown schematically in this figure of the lower femur.

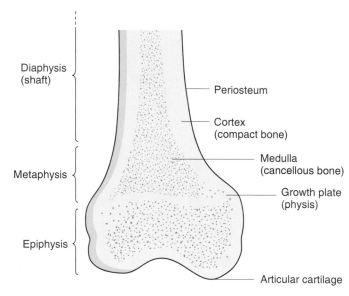

Figure 1.1

Figure 1.2 Bone composition Bone is a specialized connective tissue in which bone cells lie within an extracellular matrix that has organic and inorganic components. The organic component, which comprises 35 per cent of the bone matrix, is composed mainly (95 per cent) of type I collagen fibres, the remainder consisting of non-collagen proteins of bone (e.g. osteocalcin, osteonectin, osteopontin), plasma proteins, lipids, and glycosaminoglycans. 65 per cent of the bone matrix consists of an inorganic mineral component made up of crystalline salts, mainly calcium and phosphate, in the form of calcium hydroxyapatite $[(Ca)_{10}(PO_4)_6(OH)_2)]$. Bone matrix that is unmineralized is termed osteoid. As bone specimens are usually decalcified, the mineral and organic phases cannot be distinguished histologically in routine sections. For this purpose it is necessary to stain sections of undecalcified bone. This figure shows undecalcified trabecular bone stained with Goldner trichrome. The central mineralized portion of the bone trabeculae (stained green) is distinguished from unmineralized matrix covering the bone surface (arrow). The thickness of this osteoid seam reflects the extent of bone mineralization.

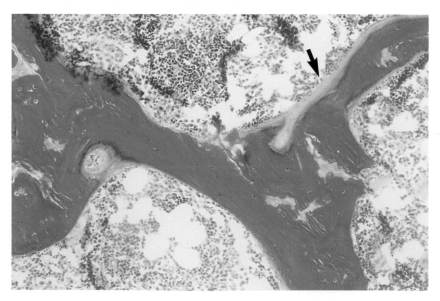

Figure 1.2

Figure 1.3 **Lamellar bone** In histological terms, bone is distinguished on the basis of its matrix organization. In lamellar (mature) bone, the matrix is composed of bundles of thin collagen fibres. Each bundle is laid down approximately at right angles to adjacent bundles, producing the characteristic parallel arrangement of alternating light and dark bands seen on polarization microscopy. This structural organization provides the highest density of collagen per unit volume of tissue. The normal mature skeleton (both cortical and cancellous bone) is composed almost entirely of lamellar bone. 1.3a shows the normal bone cortex and underlying medullary cavity containing bone trabeculae separated by haematopoietic and fatty marrow. 1.3b shows the appearance of the bone under polarized light to indicate the lamellar arrangement of collagen fibres.

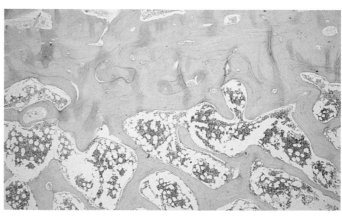
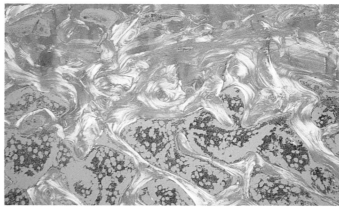

Figure 1.3

a

b

Figure 1.4 **Woven bone** Woven (immature) bone is the type of bone that is first formed in the developing skeleton. It is also formed in a variety of pathological conditions where there is rapid bone formation. Woven bone is less strong than lamellar bone. The osteocytes in woven bone lie in large round lacunae and are more closely packed than in lamellar bone (a). Woven bone is characterized by the presence of bundles of randomly arranged short, thick collagen fibres, a feature best appreciated by examination under polarized light (b). The difference in the histological appearance and matrix organization of lamellar and woven bone is clearly evident when the two types of bone lie in apposition (c, d).

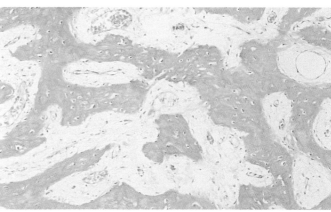
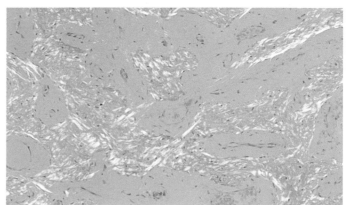

Figure 1.4

a

b

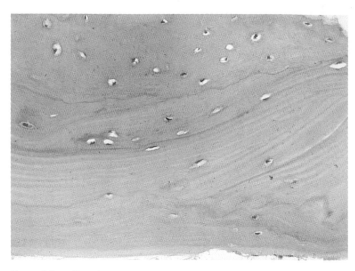

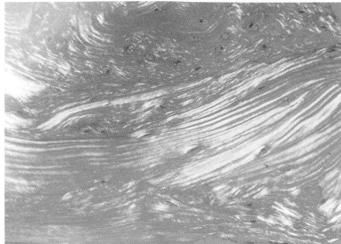

Figure 1.4 continued

| c | d |

Figure 1.5 **Cortical bone** The normal bone cortex is composed almost entirely of lamellar compact bone (a). 1.5b shows the arrangement of bone lamellae in compact bone under polarized light. Most of the lamellae are concentrically arranged around a central Haversian canal which is lined by osteoblastic cells and contains blood vessels. These concentric lamellae are oriented in the long axis of the bone, forming long cylindrical columns which are termed Haversian systems or osteons. Haversian canals often appear larger in newly-formed Haversian systems. Small segments of lamellar bone (interstitial lamellae) fill the spaces between individual Haversian systems. In addition, on the periosteal and endosteal surfaces there are circumferential lamellae which are oriented around the long axis of the bone.

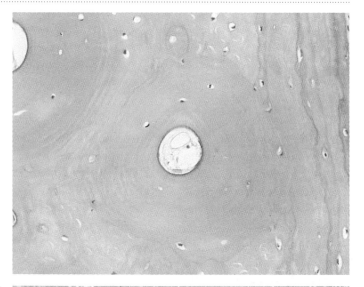

Figure 1.5

| a |

| b |

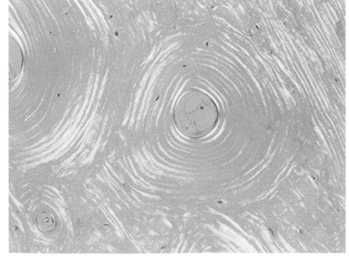

Figure 1.6 **Periosteum** The periosteum is a layer of dense fibrous tissue which covers the outer surface of most bones (a). It is thick and loosely attached to the cortex in children but thinner and more adherent in adults. It consists of an outer fibrous layer and an inner cellular (cambium) layer of osteo-progenitor cells; these cells are flattened and spindle-shaped when inactive (a), but, during growth or repair, are capable of differentiating into osteoblasts which lay down bone matrix on the underlying cortical bone surface (b). Collagen fibres in the outer layer of the periosteum are continuous with those of the joint capsule, ligaments, and tendons.

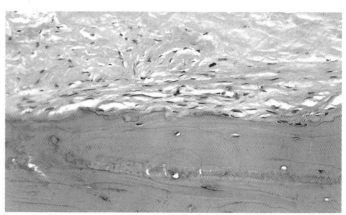

Figure 1.6

a

b

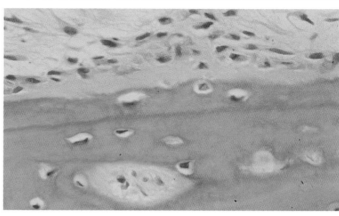

Figure 1.7 **Cancellous bone** Cancellous bone is found in the medulla and is made up of a trabecular network of plates and bars of bone (bone trabeculae) (a). In the mature skeleton, these are composed of lamellar bone with lamellae of mineralized collagen fibres oriented in parallel along the long axis of a bone trabecula. Cancellous bone trabeculae are relatively thin and do not usually contain Haversian systems; they are nourished by surrounding vessels within haematopoietic or fatty marrow. Bone trabeculae are lined by a continuous layer of flattened bone lining cells or plump osteoblasts and separated by fatty or haematopoietic marrow (b). This cellular lining of bone comprises the endosteum which covers the surface of bone trabeculae, the inner (medullary) surface of the cortex, and Haversian canals in bone.

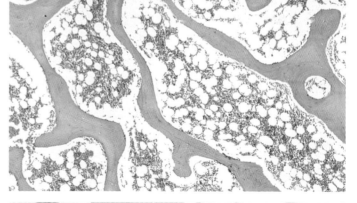

Figure 1.7

a

b

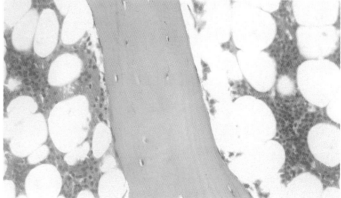

Figure 1.8 **Cement lines** Basophilic cement lines are found in both cortical and cancellous bone. These lines effectively mark the boundary between discrete areas of bone remodelling. This figure shows several prominent cement lines (arrow) in a bone trabecula. Uninterrupted straight cement lines are associated with normal remodelling whereas cement lines which are indented (reversal lines) are seen where new bone formation has occurred after extensive osteoclastic resorption. An increase in the number and prominence of cement lines in cortical or cancellous bone is indicative of increased bone remodelling activity that may be related to a pathological process.

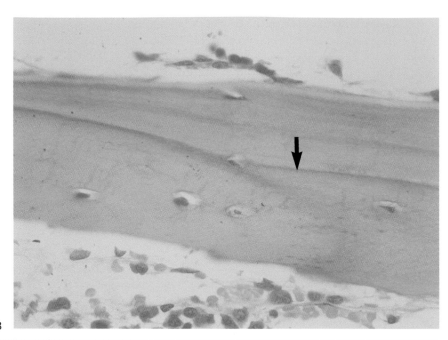

Figure 1.8

Bone cells

Cells of the osteoblast lineage (osteoblasts, bone lining cells, osteocytes) are responsible for bone formation; they are derived from a mesenchymal stromal stem cell of bone from which not only osteoprogenitor cells but also progenitors for the other connective tissue cells in bone (e.g. adipocytes, chondrocytes, fibroblasts) are derived. In contrast, osteoclasts, which carry out bone resorption, are derived from the pluripotential haematopoietic stem cell from which other peripheral blood cells are also formed. The osteoclast lineage is closely related to that of monocytes and macrophages. The activity and formation of cells of the osteoblast and osteoclast lineage in bone are closely coupled; in general, where there is prominent bone-remodelling activity, both osteoblasts and osteoclasts are present.

Figure 1.9 **Osteoblasts and bone lining cells** Osteoblasts are plump, round, or polygonal mononuclear cells which produce the organic matrix of bone and play a role in its subsequent mineralization. 1.9a shows osteoblasts (arrow) laying down matrix along a bone surface (appositional new bone formation). Osteoblasts have a basophilic or amphophilic cytoplasm and a large hyperchromatic ovoid nucleus which is often polarized away from the bone surface. Osteoblasts contain large amounts of alkaline phosphatase and in normal bone do not show mitotic activity. A layer of flattened and elongated cells (arrow) with little cytoplasm and a thin central basophilic nucleus (bone lining cells) covers areas of mature or resting bone (b).

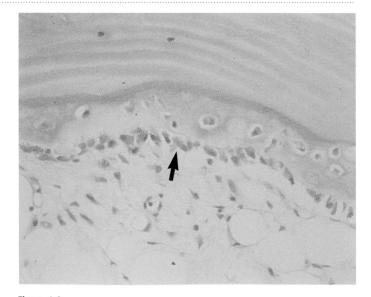

Figure 1.9

a

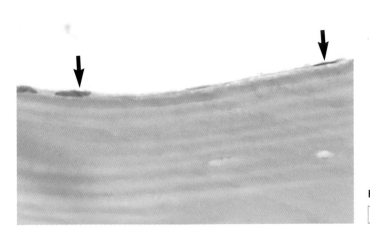

Figure 1.9 continued

b

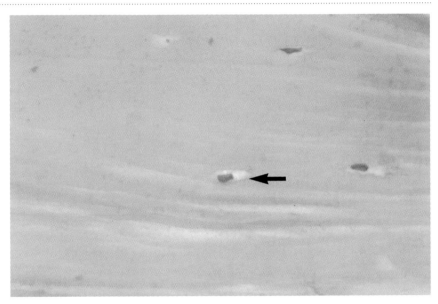

Figure 1.10 Osteocytes Osteocytes are effectively osteoblasts that have become entombed in the mineralized matrix which they have formed. This figure shows osteocytes in mature cortical bone. The osteocytes (arrow) lie in lacunae and have densely stained nuclei and indistinct cytoplasm. Osteocytes in lamellar bone lie in oval or flattened lacunae which are generally oriented in the direction of collagen fibres whereas osteocytes in immature bone are found in large round lacunae (see 1.4a). Osteocytes retain continuity with each other, osteoprogenitor cells on the external bone surface, and osteoblasts/bone lining cells of the endosteum by means of fine cytoplasmic processes which lie in canaliculi, tiny hollow channels that lie within the bone matrix. This system is likely to be important in the transduction of strain-generated signals in response to mechanical stimuli throughout bone tissue.

Figure 1.10

Figure 1.11 Osteoclasts Osteoclasts (arrow) are large multinucleated cells ranging in size from 20 to over 100 μm in diameter. These cells are responsible for bone resorption and are uncommonly seen in normal mature bone but, in areas of active bone remodelling, are found within or near cavities on the bone surface termed Howship's lacunae (a). Osteoclasts have rounded vesicular nuclei which contain prominent nucleoli. The cytoplasm is strongly acidophilic and contains abundant (tartrate-resistant) acid phosphatase. Osteoclasts can be identified immunohistochemically (even in sections of decalcified tissue) by the expression of leucocyte common antigen (b, immunoperoxidase) and macrophage antigens such as CD68 (c, immunoperoxidase).

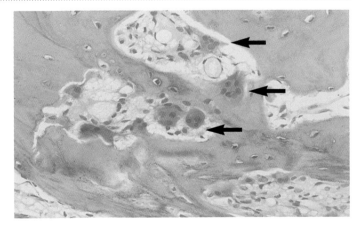

Figure 1.11

a

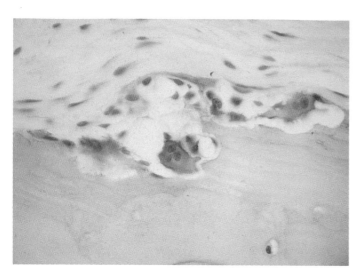

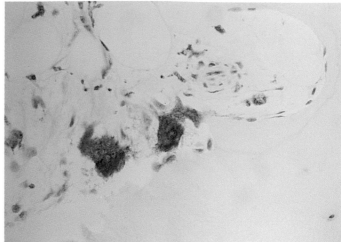

Figure 1.11 continued

b   c

Bone development, growth, and remodelling

In the embryonic and growing skeleton, bone development involves ossification of a pre-existing connective tissue model which is composed of either mesenchymal fibroblastic tissue (intramembranous ossification) or cartilage (endochondral ossification). In both types of bone development, woven bone is first laid down and then subsequently remodelled to form the lamellar bone of the mature skeleton. Bone growth occurs by apposition, that is the deposition of bone matrix by osteoblasts on the surface of a pre-existing substrate, such as bone itself (see 1.9a). Bone growth in width occurs by means of appositional deposition of newly formed bone on the surface of the underlying cortex by osteoprogenitor cells in the periosteum (see 1.6b). Appositional bone formation on the surface of pre-existing bone also occurs in the process of bone remodelling, the continuous turnover of bone which takes place in the mature skeleton throughout life.

Figure 1.12 **Bone development by intramembranous ossification** In intramembranous ossification, bone is directly formed within primitive mesenchymal connective tissue. Mesenchymal cells proliferate and differentiate into osteoblasts that form osteoid which is then rapidly mineralized to woven bone. 1.12a shows an area of woven bone formation by osteoblasts within cellular mesenchymal connective tissue of the developing calvarium. This bone formation occurs at several points within the membrane, each focus of ossification enlarging and then fusing with its neighbours. This event-ually results in the formation of a continuous mass of woven bone which is subsequently remodelled to lamellar bone. Intramembranous ossification occurs in the flat bones of the skull vault, facial bones, and shaft of the clavicle. Intramembranous ossification may also be seen in the mature skeleton when osteoprogenitor cells in the bone marrow or in fibrous tissue are stimulated to undergo osteoblastic differentiation. 1.12b shows bone formation within the marrow of an osteoarthritic femoral head in which considerable remodelling is seen in the subchondral bone.

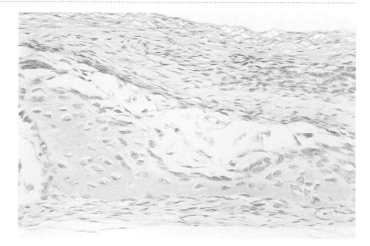

Figure 1.12

a

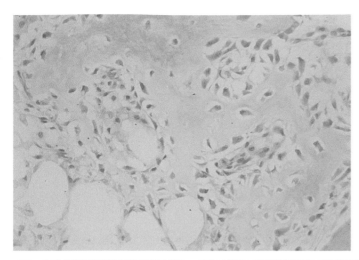

Figure 1.12 continued

b

Figure 1.13 **Bone development by endo-chondral ossification** Endochondral ossification is the process whereby bone formation occurs on the basis of a continuously enlarging cartilage model. The long bones, pelvis, vertebrae, and bones of the base of the skull are formed by endochondral ossification. In the embryonic skeleton, at about the 8th week of intrauterine life, primary centres of ossification appear within the cartilage anlage of bones. In long bones, cartilage cells in the centre of the bone shaft become hypertrophied and later necrotic as the intervening cartilage matrix calcifies (a). Mesenchymal cells in the overlying perichondrium also proliferate and become vascularized, and are thus converted into a periosteum from which osteoblast differentiation and formation of osteoid and woven bone proceeds. There is extension of this vascularized bone-forming tissue into the central cartilaginous area and deposition of bony matrix on the scaffold of calcified cartilage. In fetal long bones, continuing endochondral ossification of the cartilage model results in the bone shaft being converted into bone with only the epiphyseal bone ends being formed of cartilage. At varying time intervals after birth, secondary centres of ossification appear within the cartilaginous epiphysis of bone. 1.13b shows a developing secondary centre of ossification (marked by differential trichrome staining) within the lower femur of a $5\frac{1}{2}$ month old child. Secondary centres of ossification are invaded by blood vessels to form another focus of endochondral ossification which almost fills the epiphysis, cartilage only remaining over the articular ends of the bone and in the thin growth plate separating the epiphysis from the metaphysis.

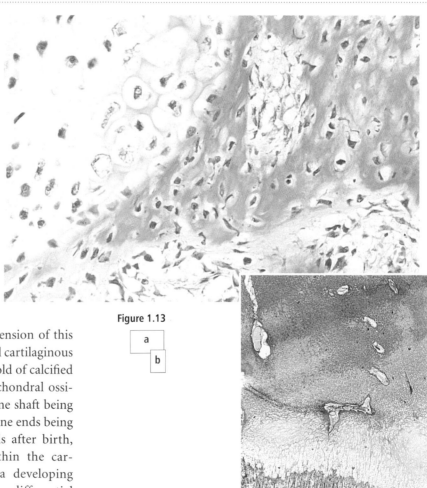

Figure 1.13

a

b

Figure 1.14 **Bone growth by endochondral ossification**
Longitudinal bone growth occurs by endochondral ossification at the growth plate which lies between the epiphysis and
the metaphysis (a). Cartilage cells in the growth plate exhibit
a columnar arrangement and are organized into various
zones (b). Beneath the epiphyseal bone, there is a zone of
reserve (or resting) cells with isolated chondrocytes surrounded by abundant cartilage matrix. Beneath this there is a
zone of cell proliferation in which the chondrocytes proliferate
and form closely packed columns. In the underlying zone of
maturation and zone of hypertrophy, chondrocytes accumulate glycogen and become swollen and vacuolated. Beneath
this there is a zone of provisional calcification in which the
cartilage matrix between hypertrophied chondrocytes undergoes calcification; the cell wall of the chondrocytes becomes
calcified, the cells die, and the empty lacunae are invaded by
capillaries from the underlying bone marrow. Osteoblasts lay
down osteoid on the spicules of calcified cartilage matrix (c).
This is then rapidly mineralized to form woven bone (primary
spongiosa) in the underlying metaphysis. This newly formed
bone is also resorbed by osteoclasts. Subsequently, this woven
bone is replaced by lamellar bone (secondary spongiosa). The
external surface of the growth plate is surrounded by a peri-
chondrial ring of Ranvier which consists of a collar of dense
fibrous tissue which forms within the perichondrium covering
the growth plate. This provides mechanical support for the
junction between the epiphysis and the diaphysis.

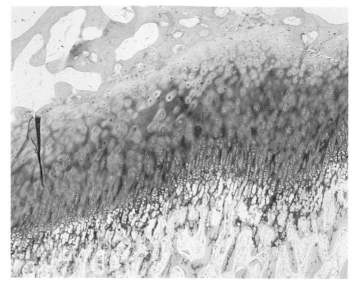

Figure 1.14

a

b

c

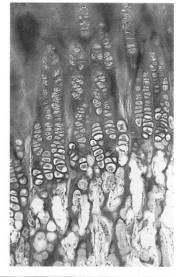

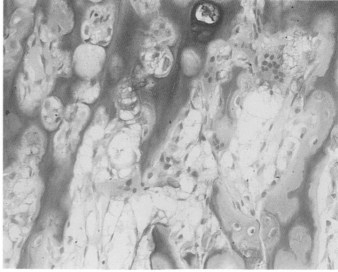

Figure 1.15 **Bone remodelling** Bone is in a dynamic state of formation and resorption in response to constantly changing mechanical stresses and the demands of mineral homeostasis. Bone remodelling occurs continuously throughout life and is carried out in microanatomical units which are termed bone multicellular units. In these units, a closely coupled sequence of bone resorption and bone formation takes place. The sequence is initiated by a phase of osteoclastic bone resorption, which is followed by a phase of reversal (marked by deposition of a cement line which indicates the extent of the resorption which has taken place). This is then followed by a phase of bone formation, which is carried out by osteoblasts. In cortical bone, remodelling takes place in a cutting cone with resorption by osteoclasts (arrowed) occurring at the tip of the cone, osteoblastic new bone formation following in its wake (a); this eventually results in refilling of the area resorbed and formation of a new osteon. A similar sequence of remodelling changes occurs in trabecular packets in cancellous bone. In normal bone, this cycle of trabecular bone remodelling takes approximately 5–6 months to complete. Remodelling of bone also occurs in response to physical forces, bone being deposited in sites subjected to stress and resorbed from sites where there is little stress, in accordance with Wolff's law. 1.15b shows an area of increased osteoblastic and osteoclastic activity associated with remodelling of subchondral bone in an osteoarthritic femoral head.

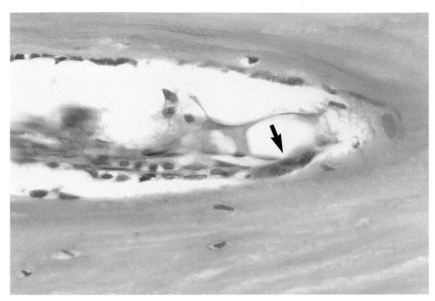

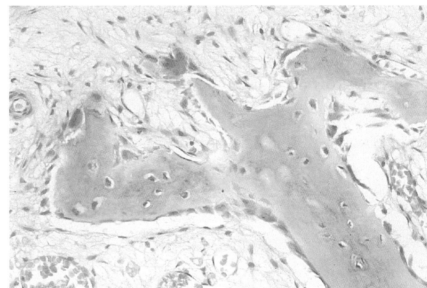

Figure 1.15

a

b

Joints and periarticular tissues

Figure 1.16 Joint structure
Joints are sites of articulation between opposing bone ends. These are covered by articular cartilage and held together by a sleeve of connective tissue, the joint capsule; the latter is covered by a synovial membrane. The joint capsule is composed of fibrous tissue and is continuous with the fibrous periosteum covering the opposing bones. Joints are classified as either diarthrodial (synovial), where there is a joint cavity containing synovial fluid and extensive movement of one bone upon another is possible, or non-diarthrodial, where limited movement of one bone upon another is permitted. In the latter, the joint cavity is filled with fibrocartilage (symphysis), hyaline cartilage (synchondrosis), or fibrous tissue (syndesmosis). The figures show: (a) an interphalangeal synovial joint of the toe; (b) the junction between the synovial membrane and articular cartilage; (c) a syndesmosis from the cranial suture of a child.

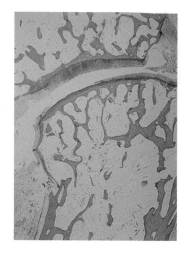
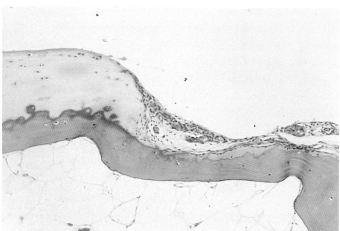
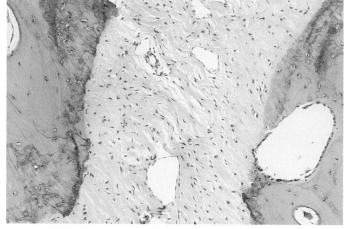

Figure 1.16

| a | b |
| c |

Figure 1.17 Articular cartilage The articular surface of bone in a synovial joint consists of smooth-surfaced hyaline articular cartilage which rests on a subchondral bone plate (a). The cartilage contains chondrocytes and an abundant extracellular matrix which is chiefly made up of type II collagen fibres, proteoglycans, and water. These proteoglycans consist mainly of glycosaminoglycans, chondroitin sulphate, and keratan sulphate; these are attached to a core protein and linked to hyaluronic acid to form large proteoglycan aggregates in cartilage. These in turn are bound to thin collagen fibrils and, being strongly negatively charged, hold large amounts of water.

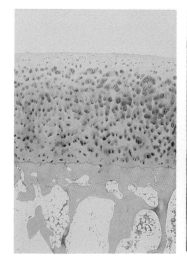
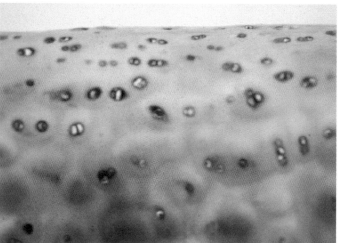

Figure 1.17

| a | b |

Cartilage cells are flattened in the superficial zone which is exposed to the maximal forces of articulation (b). Collagen fibres in this zone are also thinner and frequently arranged parallel to the articular surface. In the underlying mid-zone, cells are more rounded and surrounded by abundant matrix. In the deep zone, cells are few in number and frequently grouped in clusters (c). At the junction of articular cartilage with the subchondral bone plate, there is a basophilic tidemark (arrow) beneath which any cartilage is calcified. Blood vessels occasionally pass through the subchondral bone into calcified cartilage but in a normal junction do not usually extend into the overlying uncalcified cartilage. As articular cartilage is derived from epiphyseal cartilage (from which the growth plate or physis develops), it may exhibit physis-like changes, both during growth and in reaction to pathological conditions involving the articular surface.

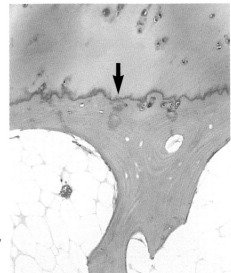

Figure 1.17

c

Figure 1.18 **Fibrocartilage** Fibrocartilage is a form of cartilage containing a high density of collagen fibres. It consists of alternating layers of hyaline cartilage and thick bundles of collagen fibres oriented in the direction of stress. 1.18a shows the fibrocartilage of the intervertebral disc; the abundant collagen fibres in this matrix are shown under polarized light in (b). Fibrocartilage is also found in the menisci of the knee, other intra-articular disc structures (e.g. in ribs, temporomandibular joint, and sternoclavicular joint), and at sites of tendinous or ligamentous insertion into bone.

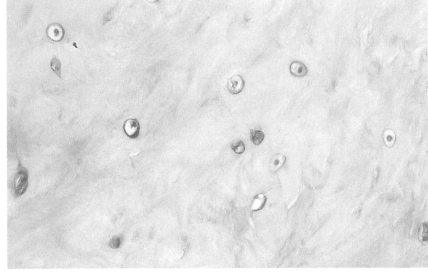

Figure 1.18

a

b

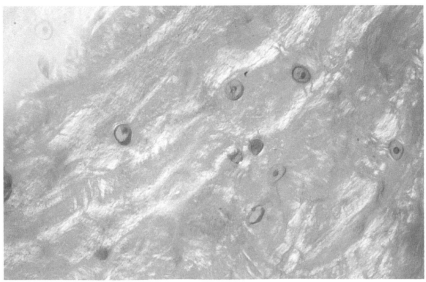

Figure 1.19 **Synovial membrane** The synovial membrane is found on the inner surface of the joint capsule which unites the articulating bone ends. It is covered by a synovial intima (arrow), a thin layer of synovial lining cells, one or two cells thick (a). A subintima of well-vascularized adipose tissue or fibrous tissue lies beneath the intima. The synovial membrane covers all surfaces within the joint cavity except articular cartilage and meniscal fibrocartilage. It is often folded to produce small villi which project into the joint cavity. Synovial lining cells are essentially of two types: A (macrophage-like) cells and B (fibroblast-like) cells. Type B cells, which secrete hyaluronic acid, are relatively more numerous in the normal synovium but type A cells, which are phagocytic, are much more prominent in the reactive synovium seen in most forms of joint pathology. This is readily shown by immunohistochemical staining of a normal synovial membrane (b) and inflamed synovial membrane (c) using the anti-macrophage monoclonal antibody, Mac 387 (b).

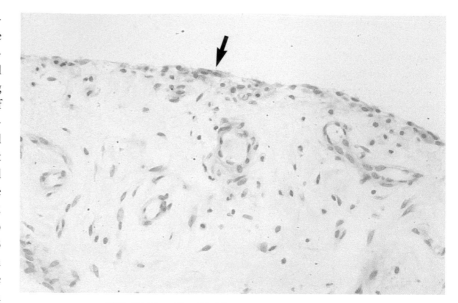

Figure 1.19

a

b

c

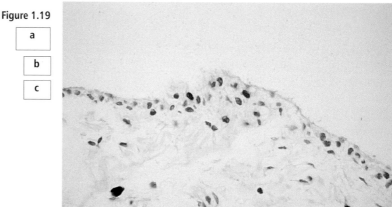

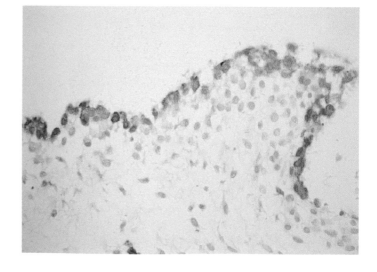

Figure 1.20 **Tendons and ligaments** Tendons are cord-like structures which join a muscle to bone; ligaments join one bone to another. Both tendons and ligaments are composed of dense connective tissue containing parallel bundles of collagen fibres. Rows of flattened fibroblasts, which are oriented in the direction of pull to which the tendon or ligament is subjected, lie between the collagen bundles. 1.20a shows part of a tendon sheath of one of the extensor muscles of the hand. At sites of friction, tendons are covered by a synovial tendon sheath. This sheath is composed of two layers of connective tissue, the outer being continuous with the surrounding fibrous tissue and the inner directly covering the collagen of the tendon sheath. Both surfaces are covered by synovial lining cells (arrow). At sites of attachment to bone, both tendons and ligaments undergo a transition into fibrocartilage and may exhibit a line of calcification (b). The collagen fibres of these structures penetrate deeply through the compact bone of the cortex.

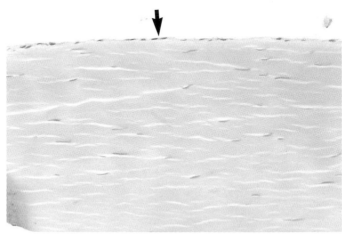

Figure 1.20

a

b

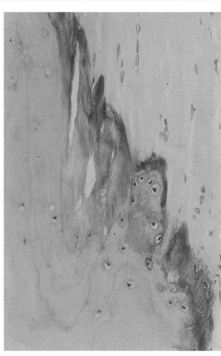

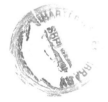

2

Repair, necrosis, and reactive changes in skeletal tissue

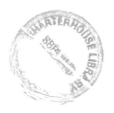

Fracture healing

A fracture is a break in the continuity of a bone caused by mechanical forces. It may be caused by a single violent force or by a bone being subjected to repeated injuries or large loads (fatigue/stress fracture). Fractures may be simple (closed), where there is no communication between the fractured bone ends and the body surface, or open (compound) when the fracture communicates with a wound on the body surface. Fractures are also described grossly on the basis of their shape or pattern, e.g. transverse, oblique, spiral, comminuted, crush, or greenstick. A pathological fracture occurs through an area of bone weakened by disease. A summary of the sequence of pathological changes seen in fracture healing is shown in Table 2.1.

Table 2.1 Morphological changes in fracture healing*

Time post-fracture (days)	Histological features
0–3	Haemorrhage; fibrin clot; early acute and late chronic inflammatory infiltrate; marrow necrosis; granulation tissue
3–7	Chronic inflammation (macrophages ++); granulation tissue; osteoclastic bone resorption; early osteoid/woven bone formation
7–35	Progressive increase in bone necrosis; chronic inflammation; reparative fibrous tissue; primary callus; woven bone and cartilage formation
35+	Secondary callus; replacement of woven by lamellar bone; osteoblastic and osteoclastic activity

* Exact timetable of histological changes depends on fracture stability, vascularization, degree of comminution, etc.

Figure 2.1 **Fracture repair: initial response** Immediately following a fracture, there is disruption of blood vessels in the medulla, cortex, periosteum, and surrounding soft tissues. This results in the formation of a haematoma which lies between the bone ends and extends beneath the periosteum and into soft tissues around the fracture site. Areas of haemorrhage are present in the bone marrow (a). Necrosis in fatty or haematopoietic marrow, evidenced by the indistinct outline and change in nuclear staining of marrow cells, first becomes evident several hours after the fracture has occurred (b). Disappearance of osteocyte nuclei from lacunae in bone is not generally seen until 7–14 days post-fracture.

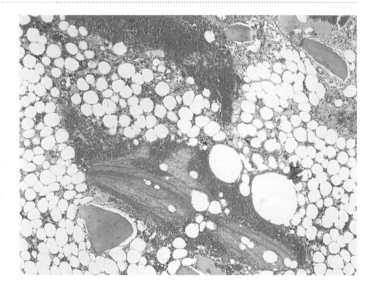

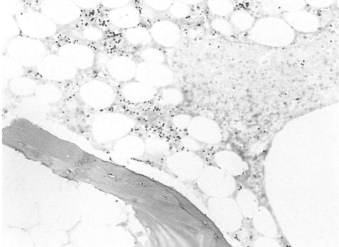

Figure 2.1

a

b

Figure 2.2 **Fracture healing: early reparative changes** In the first few days after a fracture has occurred, there is granulation tissue formation with ingrowth from the surrounding viable bone of fibroblasts and capillaries into the fibrin clot between the fractured bone ends (a). This is accompanied by an inflammatory infiltrate, initially containing neutrophil polymorphs, but later containing more chronic inflammatory cells amongst which macrophages are prominent. Macrophages remove red cells and necrotic fat and tissue debris and often have a foamy cytoplasm (b).

Figure 2.2

| a | b |

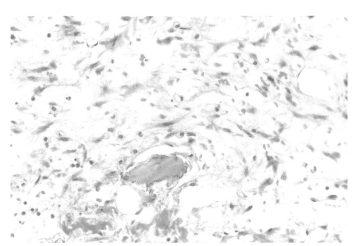
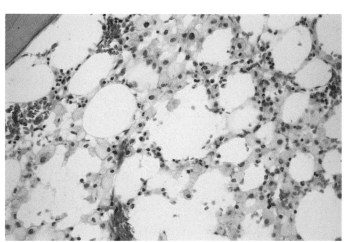

Figure 2.3 **Fracture healing: primary callus** Fracture healing is characterized by the formation of callus, a skeletal repair tissue which unites the fractured bone ends. Primary callus is formed initially and consists of newly formed bone and cartilage which is produced by proliferating osteoprogenitor cells derived from the periosteum, endosteum, and marrow stroma. Callus which lies within reparative tissue in the medulla is termed internal callus (a). External callus develops around the fractured bone ends and is in contact with surrounding soft tissues, including muscle (arrow) (b).

Figure 2.3

| a | b |

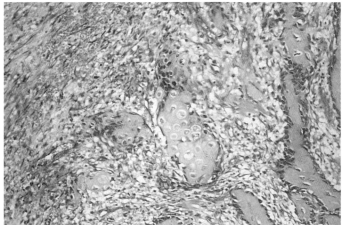
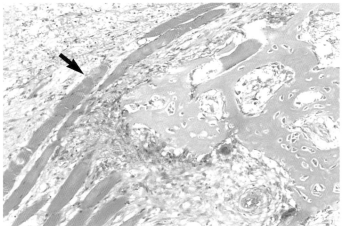

Figure 2.4 **Fracture healing: primary callus**

Osteoid and woven bone formation is seen by the end of the first week in most fractures. Osteoblasts lay down osteoid and woven bone partly on the surface of pre-existing necrotic bone trabeculae (a). Cartilage formation is seen within primary callus, particularly where it is formed rapidly in an area subjected to continued mechanical stress or where there is a poor blood supply; these conditions are found most commonly in external callus (b). Cartilage formed in fracture callus is usually surrounded by organized woven bone; it is often cellular and chondrocytes may show some pleomorphism (c). Internal callus, which is relatively well vascularized and mechanically more stable, less commonly contains cartilage and is composed mainly of a well-organized network of woven bone (d).

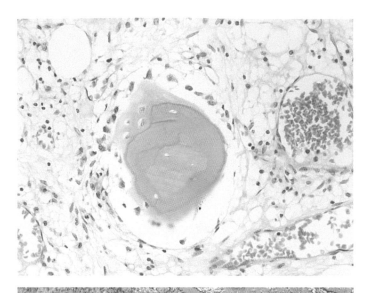

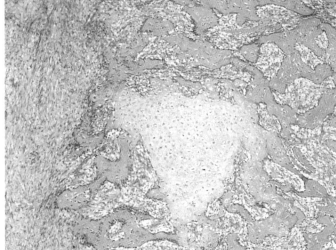

Figure 2.4

| a |
| b |
| c | d |

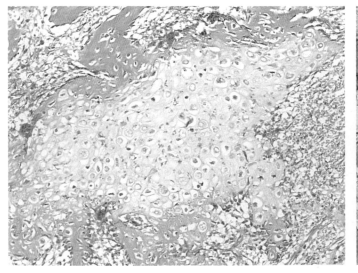

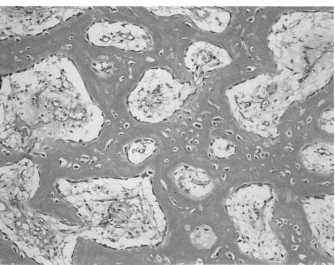

Figure 2.5 **Fracture healing: secondary callus** Secondary callus is the term used to describe the mature lamellar bone which gradually replaces the woven bone of primary callus. In this way, the normal cortical and cancellous bone architecture is restored following injury. 2.5a shows osteoblasts laying down new bone in apposition on the surface of woven bone in primary callus; the lamellar nature of the newly formed bone is shown by polarization microscopy (b). At the same time there is resorption of primary callus by osteoclasts. This process of gradual remodelling occurs over a period of several months and is more rapid in children.

Figure 2.5

| a | b |

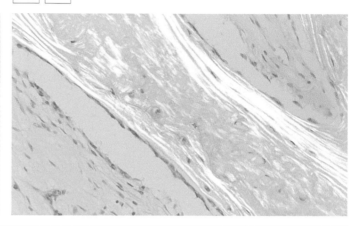

Figure 2.6 **Fracture non-union and pseudarthrosis** Union between the bone ends following a fracture may be delayed or fail to occur (non-union). This may be due to several factors such as interposition of soft tissue between the fractured bone ends, wide separation of the fractured ends, pathological fracture, or lack of immobilization. In a non-union (a), the bone ends are usually united by fibrous or fibrocartilaginous connective tissue containing necrotic bone trabeculae or areas of reactive new bone formation. Fibrocartilaginous tissue generally predominates if the fracture site is mobile or poorly vascularized; non-union tissue may also contain areas of fibro-osseous metaplasia. Clefts covered by fibrinous material may form within the non-union tissue of an unstable fracture (b). This effectively results in the formation of a pseudarthrosis with the bone ends covered by organized fibrous or fibrocartilaginous tissue (c); rarely, a true synovial lining develops over the pseudarthrosis. The bone beneath the fracture non-union or pseudarthrosis often shows evidence of remodelling changes with prominent cement lines and osteoblastic and osteoclastic activity.

Figure 2.6

| a |
| b | c |

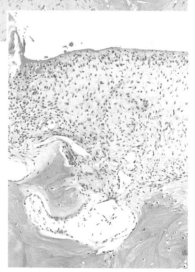

Figure 2.7 **Stress fracture** A stress fracture occurs in normal bone as a result of repeated injury or mechanical loading. This type of fracture occurs at a number of well-recognized sites and is often associated with particular occupations or activities (e.g. a march fracture of the second metatarsal bone occurring in military recruits). Fractures of the tibia and fibula (a) commonly occur in athletes or dancers. Clinically, these lesions present with pain and swelling and radiologically they show a pronounced periosteal reaction; these features may give the impression that the lesion is infective or neoplastic in nature. Histologically, features are essentially those of fracture callus which may be hypercellular but usually shows evidence of reactive osteoid or new bone formation (b).

Figure 2.7

a

b

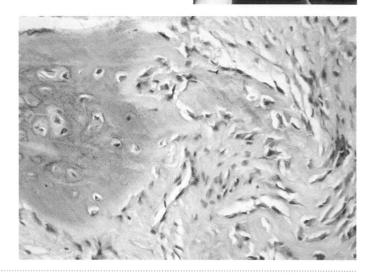

Figure 2.8 **Pathological fracture** A pathological fracture is one which occurs secondary to an underlying systemic or localized disease of the affected bone. Systemic causes include metabolic bone diseases such as osteoporosis, hyperparathyroidism, osteomalacia, and congenital conditions such as osteogenesis imperfecta. Localized lesions which weaken the bone include benign and malignant tumours and infection. The most common cause of a pathological fracture is a malignant tumour, usually metastatic carcinoma or myeloma. Pathological fractures are often of unusual morphology and occur in unusual locations within a particular bone. The figure shows a transverse pathological fracture of the femoral shaft occurring secondary to myeloma. There is usually little evidence of callus formation in pathological fractures due to a malignant lesion; this is seen more commonly in fractures associated with slow-growing benign lesions.

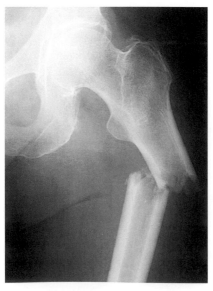

Figure 2.8

Figure 2.9 Encysted haematoma Rarely, haemorrhage in bone may result in the formation of a large haematoma which becomes encysted. This occurs most commonly in patients with blood dyscrasias (e.g. haemophilia) but may rarely occur idiopathically. 2.9a shows the radiological appearances of an idiopathic encysted haematoma of the left ilium; the lesion is osteolytic and well defined. Histologically, it consists of an area of haemorrhage and thrombus formation within bone (b).

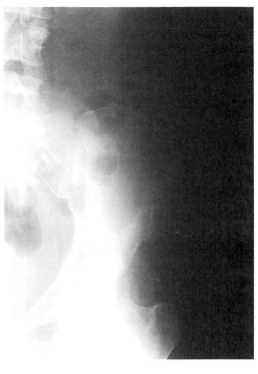

Figure 2.9

a

b

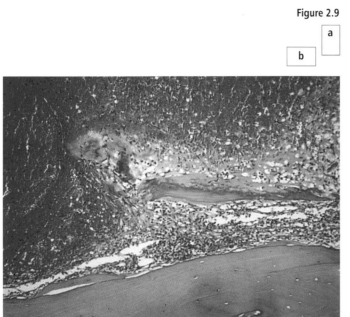

Bone necrosis (osteonecrosis)

Figure 2.10 Osteonecrosis Osteonecrosis is seen in relation to many diseases which affect bone (Table 2.2). When extensive it may result in bone infarction. This occurs most commonly in the epiphysis and involves subchondral bone. Medullary infarcts may also occur in the diaphysis or metaphysis. Histologically, osteonecrosis is most easily recognized by the absence of osteocyte nuclei from lacunae (arrow). This figure shows extensive loss of osteocyte nuclei in cortical bone. Note that osteocytes in lamellae lying nearest to vessels within Haversian canals are still viable and have retained their nuclei.

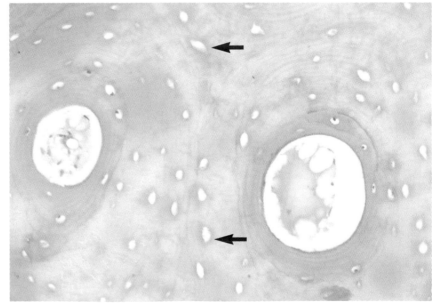

Figure 2.10

Table 2.2 Conditions associated with osteonecrosis

Trauma
Idiopathic
Corticosteroid treatment
Caisson disease
Sickle cell anaemia
Radiation treatment
Gaucher's disease
Alcoholism
Renal transplantation
Non-steroidal anti-inflammatory drugs
Immunosuppressive therapy
Hyperlipidaemia
Hyperuricaemia
Chronic pancreatitis
Pregnancy
Infection
Neoplasia in bone
Blood dyscrasias

Figure 2.11 Subchondral avascular bone necrosis and infarction Osteonecrosis and segmental infarction occur most frequently in the subchondral region of the epiphysis. The femoral head is most commonly affected. In most cases subchondral bone necrosis is associated with previous fracture but it may also occur without cause (idiopathic avascular necrosis). Subchondral bone necrosis is also a feature of other conditions such as Cushing's disease, corticosteroid treatment, Gaucher's disease, Caisson disease, alcoholism, or sickle cell anaemia. Clinically, subchondral infarcts cause chronic pain which is initially associated with activity, but later pain becomes progressively more constant until finally it is present at rest. Subchondral infarcts often result in collapse of the articular surface and predispose to the development of a severe secondary osteoarthritis. 2.11a shows bilateral subchondral avascular necrosis occurring in a case of Cushing's disease. This is initially seen as a subchondral crescent of radiolucency; irregular areas of radiolucency and radiodensity are later evident within the infarcted area which may have a sclerotic border. Grossly, following infarction, the bone initially appears normal but later the infarcted area becomes paler and well demarcated. A subchondral fracture may develop within the infarcted area, resulting in partial or complete separation of the articular cartilage and underlying subchondral bone from the remainder of the epiphysis (b). These subchondral fractures in avascular necrosis are often best appreciated in specimen radiographs (c).

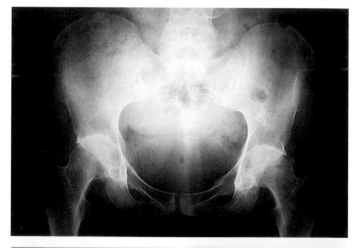

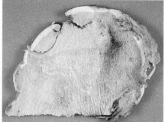 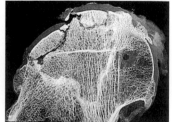

Figure 2.11

a

b c

Figure 2.12 **Subchondral avascular bone necrosis and infarction** Histologically, the earliest changes of bone necrosis are seen in the marrow where there is serous exudation, necrosis of fatty and haematopoietic marrow, fat cysts, and occasionally an inflammatory cell infiltrate (a). Loss of osteocyte nuclei from lacunae is not usually seen until the second week after the onset of ischaemia and may initially be patchy with marrow necrosis still prominent (b) There is extension of well-vascularized fibroblastic granulation tissue from surrounding viable bone into the fibrin present within the infarcted area. This granulation tissue contains stromal osteoprogenitor cells which differentiate into osteoblasts that lay down osteoid and new bone (c). In subchondral infarcts, the articular cartilage usually remains viable down to the calcified zone but the bony end plate and underlying bone trabeculae are necrotic (d).

Figure 2.12

| a |
| b |
| d |
| c |

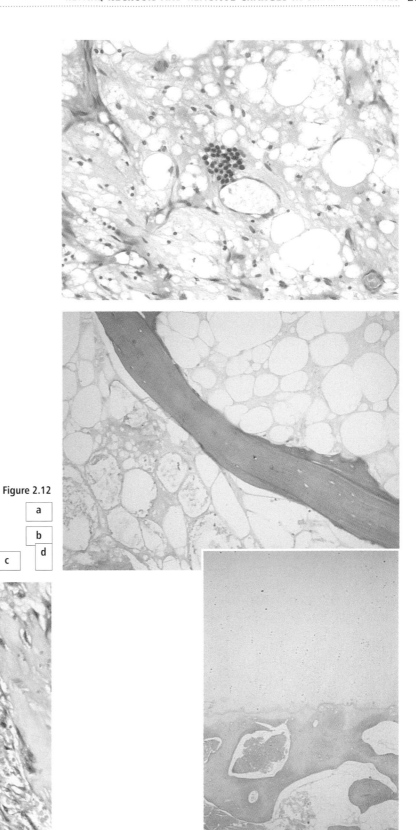

Figure 2.13 **Subchondral avascular bone necrosis and infarction** In the process of infarct healing, osteoblasts (arrow) lay down new bone on the surface of necrotic bone which at the same time is resorbed by osteoclasts (a); this process is termed 'creeping substitution'. In late stages of bone infarction there is often little evidence of active repair. Necrotic bone trabeculae are surrounded by bone marrow which is filled with necrotic acellular material or collagenous fibrous tissue in which there are focal areas of calcification (arrow) (b). The articular surface (arrow) becomes separated from the underlying bone (c); cellular fibrous tissue (arrow) is often seen on the surface of articular cartilage (d). Following collapse of the articular surface, changes of advanced secondary degenerative arthritis ensue and there is often extensive deposition of bone and cartilage fragments in the synovial membrane.

Figure 2.13

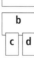

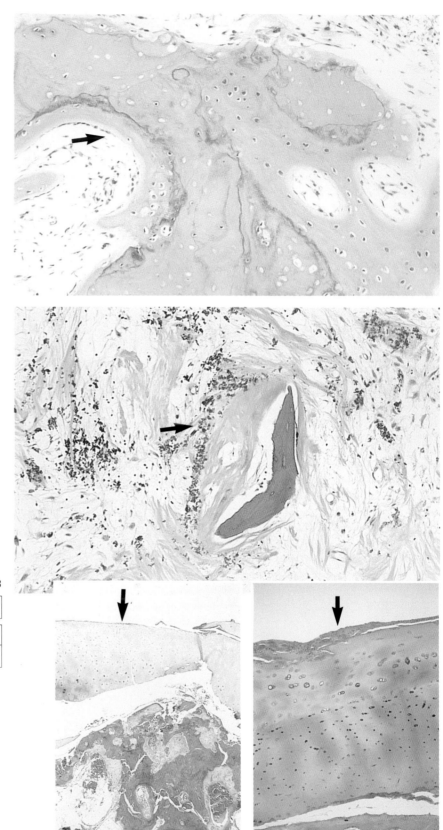

Figure 2.14 **Medullary bone necrosis and infarction**
Medullary infarcts may occur spontaneously but are also a recognized complication of conditions which cause subchondral bone necrosis such as sickle cell disease, Gaucher's disease, and Caisson disease. These infarcts are usually painful, but may be asymptomatic and discovered incidentally on radiographs. 2.14a shows two medullary infarcts in the shaft of the lower femur. The infarcted areas are well defined, have an irregular sclerotic border, and contain focal areas of calcification. 2.14b shows the gross appearances of an acute medullary infarct in a case of sickle cell anaemia. The infarct usually lies within the metaphysis or diaphysis, is relatively well defined, and paler than surrounding red marrow. Histologically, changes are similar to those seen in subchondral bone necrosis. As biopsied lesions are often old, there is usually little evidence of active repair; necrotic bone trabeculae show loss of osteocyte nuclei and surrounding fibrous tissue often contains areas of calcification (c). Rarely, medullary infarction may be complicated by the development of a primary malignant bone tumour, most often, but not always, a malignant fibrous histiocytoma.

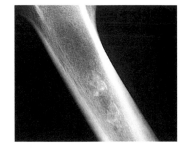
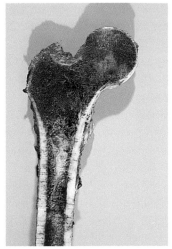
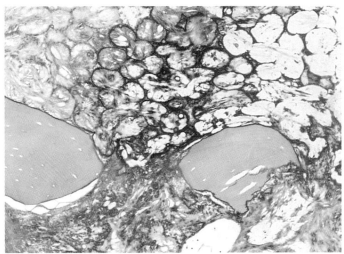

Figure 2.14

 a | b

c

Figure 2.15 **Osteochondritis dissecans** In this condition, part of the articular surface becomes separated totally or partially from the underlying bone. This occurs most commonly following infarction of the subarticular surface of the medial femoral condyle near the intercondylar notch (a). It may also occur in other joints such as the elbow (b). Radiologically, a well defined defect, extending up to the articular surface, is seen in the subchondral bone. Histologically, if the segment of the articular surface maintains an attachment to the underlying epiphysis, the subchondral bone remains viable, but if it loses this attachment the subchondral bone shows features of avascular necrosis. The surface of the detached necrotic bone and cartilage fragment is commonly covered by fibrous tissue and fibrocartilage (c).

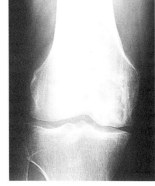
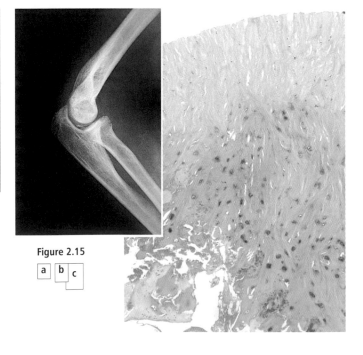

Figure 2.15

a | b | c

Figure 2.16 Osteochondritis juvenilis This term is used to describe a large number of eponymous conditions occurring in the epiphysis and apophysis of children and adolescents. Although primary avascular necrosis of epiphyseal bone prior to closure of the growth plate was thought to be the common pathology underlying these various conditions, other mechanisms are now known to be involved. True avascular necrosis is the cause of Perthes' disease, where there is necrosis of the femoral capital epiphysis (a). This occurs more commonly in male children and the age of onset is usually between 5 and 11 years. There is often a family history and the condition is bilateral in 10 per cent of cases. Other common sites at which osteochondritis due to true avascular necrosis occurs are the carpal lunate bone (Kienböck's disease), the tarsal navicular bone (Köhler's disease), and the head of the second metatarsal bone (Freiberg's disease). A partial or total avulsion of the tendon insertion that removes a flake of bone, which only then becomes necrotic, is thought to underlie the pathology of Osgood–Schlatter's disease of the tibial tubercle, Sever's disease of the calcaneal apophysis, and Sinding–Larsen disease of the lower pole of the patella. 2.16b shows magnetic resonance imaging changes of oedema and inflammation at the site of tendon insertion (arrow) in Osgood–Schlatter's disease.

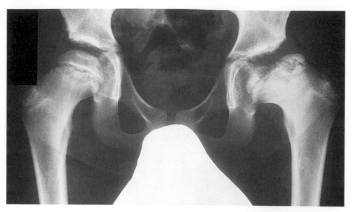

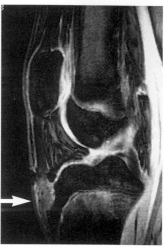

Figure 2.16

a

b

Figure 2.17 Subperiosteal new bone formation Periosteal new bone formation may occur in a wide variety of bone conditions which result in elevation of the periosteum from the cortex (e.g. trauma, infection, neoplasia); organized subperiosteal new bone formation may also occur in the context of a vasculitis such as polyarteritis nodosa or in association with varicose veins. Radiologically, the latter may be evident as roughening of the external surface of the tibia (a). Histologically, there is periosteal oedema, congestion, fibrosis, and new bone formation (b). A marked periosteal reaction with inflammation may also be seen in infantile cortical hyperostosis. Hypertrophic pulmonary osteoarthropathy is also characterized by periosteal new bone formation which is typically symmetrical and occurs in the diaphysis of long bones.

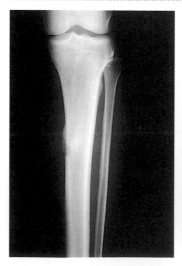

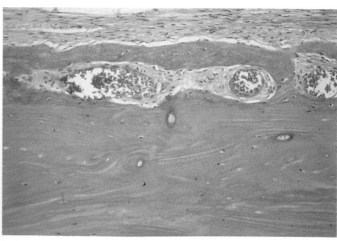

Figure 2.17

a b

Figure 2.18 **Bone grafting (transplantation)**
Bone grafts are commonly used to promote fracture healing or to fill a space within a bone which has been destroyed by disease or injury. Bone grafts may be composed of autologous compact or cancellous bone (autograft) or of homologous bone (homograft) derived from a bone bank. The transplanted bone is largely or entirely necrotic and effectively acts as scaffolding for the ingrowth of reparative granulation and fibrous tissue that contains osteoprogenitor cells; the latter differentiate into osteoblasts which form host bone. This figure shows osteoblasts (long arrow) laying down osteoid and woven bone on the surface of the necrotic bone graft which is also being resorbed by osteoclasts (short arrow); this process is similar to that of creeping substitution in avascular necrosis and results in removal and, where effective, replacement of necrotic graft bone by newly formed host bone.

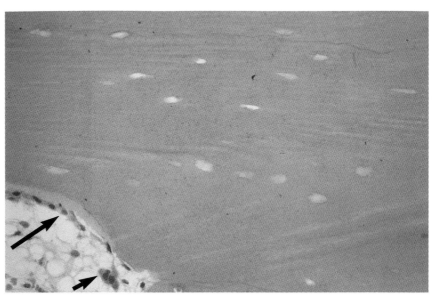

Figure 2.18

Figure 2.19 **Bone reaction to internal fixation devices**
Smooth or threaded pins, intramedullary rods, and screw and plate devices are used to fix fractures internally. The tissue surrounding these devices, when well fixed, is usually composed of a fibrous tissue membrane and underlying bone. 2.19a shows the bone and fibrous membrane around an intramedullary nail. Focal remodelling changes may be seen in the bone. Loosening of the fixation device results in thickening of the fibrous membrane. 2.19b shows the bone and membrane covering the track of a screw that has loosened. The membrane is thickened and composed largely of reparative fibrous and granulation tissue. Focal areas of fibrocartilaginous metaplasia and a bursa-like synovial lining may also be found in the membrane surrounding a loose fixation device. A macrophage and giant cell reaction to titanium and cobalt–chromium particles (c) may also be seen in the fibrous membrane surrounding a fixation device. Corrosion of implanted metallic fixation devices is characterized by the presence of black or brown particles within fibrous tissue and an associated chronic inflammatory cell infiltrate (d).

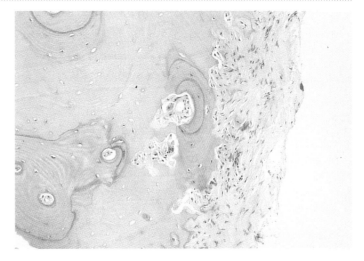

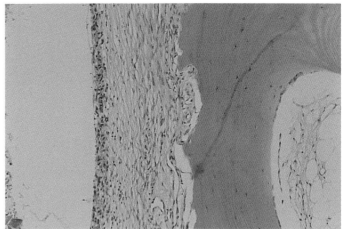

Figure 2.19

a

b

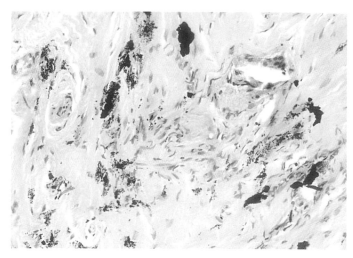

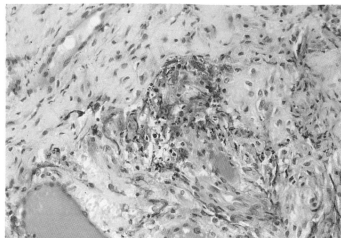

Figure 2.19 continued

c d

Figure 2.20 Subungual exostosis A subungual exostosis is a benign painful lesion which projects from the distal portion of a terminal phalanx, usually the great toe. It occurs over a wide age range and is thought to arise by osseous or cartilaginous metaplasia of periosteal cells following trauma or infection. The lesion arises from the dorsal aspect of the tip of the terminal phalanx and lies in the dermis and subcutaneous tissue beneath the nail (a). It is composed of fibrous tissue, cartilage, and bone in which there is evidence of fibrocartilaginous and occasionally fibro-osseous metaplasia (b). Complete excision is required for cure.

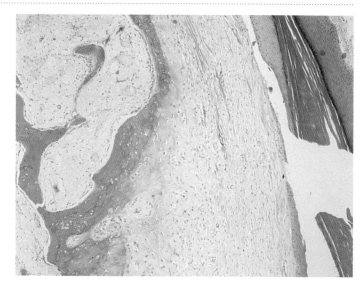

Figure 2.13

a

b

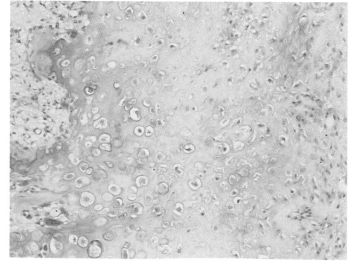

Figure 2.21 Avulsion/traction exostosis (bony spur) These outgrowths often occur at sites of ligamentous or tendinous attachment and are most likely induced by external traction. They are composed of collagenous fibrous tissue which usually undergoes direct fibro-osseous metaplasia; in some cases there is an intermediate zone of fibrocartilage which undergoes endochondral ossification. This figure shows a calcaneal spur in which there is fibro-osseous metaplasia with woven bone lying between collagenous fibrous tissue (left) and underlying lamellar bone (right). Woven bone exhibits remodelling changes.

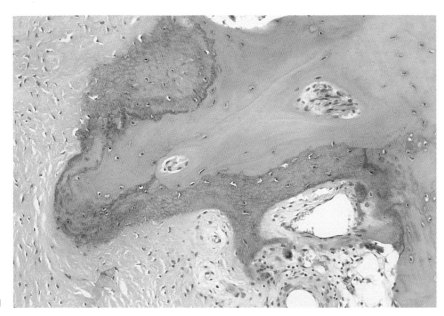

Figure 2.21

Figure 2.22 Myositis ossificans This is a benign, solitary, ossifying reactive condition which occurs chiefly in adolescents or young adults who present with a painful lump of several weeks duration, usually in the upper arm or thigh. A history of trauma is often, but not always, elicited. Radiographs (a) and computed tomography scans (b) show that the mass (arrowed) lies in soft tissue in close proximity to but separated from the external bone surface. Histologically, it essentially shows features of external callus with formation of a network of woven bone within reparative fibrous and granulation tissue. There is a characteristic zonal maturation pattern, central areas of the lesion being more cellular and immature (c) than peripheral areas (d) of lesion. The intermediate zone (c) is composed of poorly organized woven bone, areas of osteoid formation, and focally, areas of cartilage which undergo endochondral ossification. This lesion often needs to be distinguished from parosteal osteosarcoma and other surface tumours of bone. It is unrelated to fibrodysplasia (myositis) ossificans progressiva (see Chapter 4).

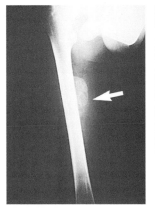
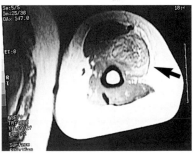

Figure 2.22

| a | b |
| c | d |

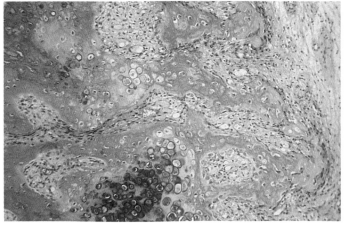
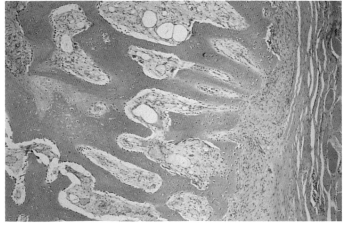

Figure 2.23 Heterotopic ossification Heterotopic ossification in soft tissue around bones and joints may be seen in a number of clinical settings. It may follow surgical procedures for joint disease, particularly surgery of the hip, or may develop after major trauma, often in association with neurological injuries. Bone generally forms by direct fibro-osseous metaplasia or fibrocartilaginous metaplasia with subsequent endochondral ossification. This figure shows largely mature (lamellar) heterotopic bone, which is covered by fibrous tissue apposed to muscle (right).

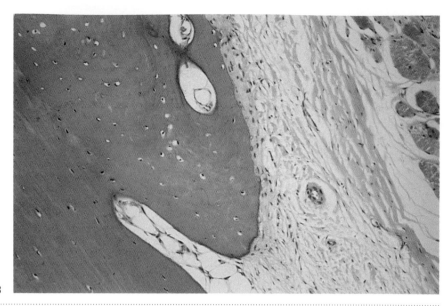

Figure 2.23

Figure 2.24 Radiation effects on bone Heavy doses of radiation, whether from external or internal sources, produce several pathological changes in bone. This includes thickening and obliteration of the lumen of small blood vessels, leading to bone necrosis (a). The bone marrow contains abnormally large stellate fibroblasts and there is extensive fibrosis with dense collagen formation. Weakening of the bone may result in pathological fracture. Osteomyelitis also occurs more commonly in necrotic irradiated bone, particularly in bones of the jaw. 2.24b shows osteomyelitis in irradiated bone with necrotic bone (right) and a partly necrotic inflammatory exudate (arrow). Damage to cartilage cells of the growth plate may lead to growth retardation. Sarcomas may also develop in irradiated bone after a latent interval of several years. 2.24c shows radiation-induced necrosis of bone associated with development of a fibrosarcoma.

Figure 2.24

a

b	c

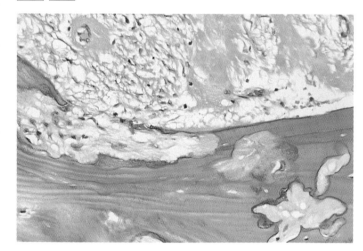

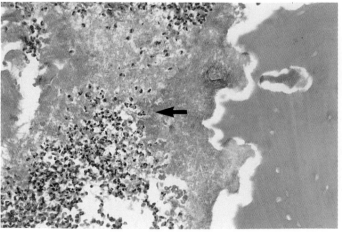

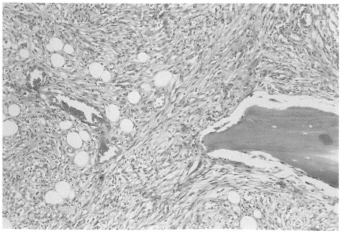

Figure 2.25 **Joint injury**

Traumatic injury to a joint may result in damage to articular cartilage, subchondral bone, the synovial membrane, and capsular tissues. Articular cartilage is an avascular tissue and has a limited ability to repair itself. Clusters of chondrocytes may be seen in the vicinity of defects in the cartilage matrix and reparative fibrous tissue may extend

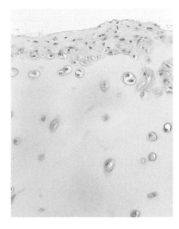 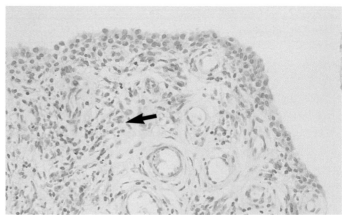

Figure 2.25

from the synovial membrane over the surface of the articular cartilage following injury (a). The underlying bone may show evidence of haemorrhage or fracture repair. Haemorrhage into the joint results in a siderotic synovitis (b). This is characterized by the presence of haemosiderin within synovial lining cells and subintimal macrophages (arrow). Scattered giant cells containing haemosiderin may also be noted.

Figure 2.26 **Meniscal injury and cystic degeneration**

Menisci are essentially avascular structures composed of dense fibrous tissue and fibrocartilage. Rotational injuries commonly result in meniscal tears which heal poorly; these tears occur most frequently in the posterior horn of the medial meniscus. There is fraying and separation of collagen fibres within the substance of the meniscus as well as on the surface (a). Fibroblasts and capillaries from surrounding tissues may be seen in the vicinity of the tear which may be covered by fibrin (arrow) (b). Meniscal cysts form as a result of mucinous or myxoid degeneration within meniscal connective tissue (c). The cysts are often multilocular and occur most frequently in the anteromedial part of the lateral meniscus.

Figure 2.26

a

b c

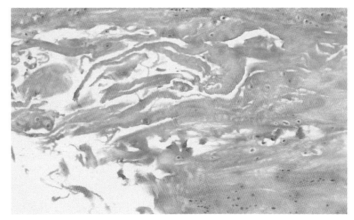

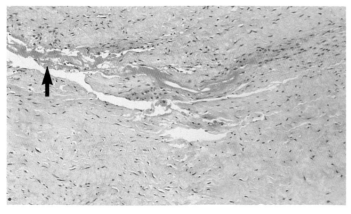 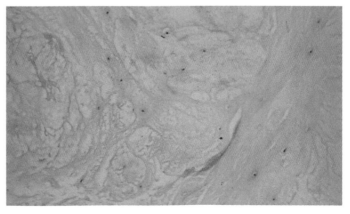

Figure 2.27 Ganglion A ganglion is a unilocular or multilocular cyst which contains mucinous material. It is usually located in connective tissue close to a joint capsule or tendon sheath but does not usually communicate with the joint cavity. It is found most commonly around the wrist, hands and feet, ankle or knee joint. It may arise from a detached fragment of synovial tissue or develop following myxoid degeneration within connective tissue. The cyst wall lacks a distinct lining and is composed of dense fibrous tissue which may contain focal areas of mucinous degeneration.

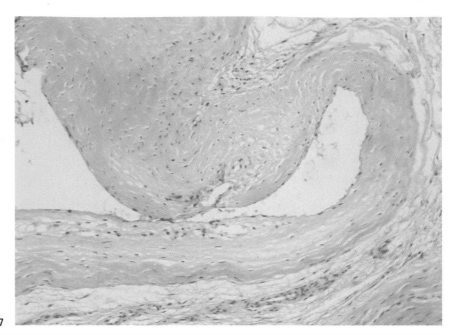

Figure 2.27

Figure 2.28 Bursa A bursa is a cavity or space which is lined by synovial tissue. It may communicate with a joint space or synovial cavity of a tendon sheath but may also form spontaneously in connective tissue which is subject to continuous movement or mechanical trauma, such as over a bony prominence; the latter may be occupation-related (e.g. a pre-patellar bursa in housemaid's knee). The wall of the bursa is of variable thickness and composed of cellular or collagenous connective tissue. It may be covered in part by a synovial lining but the surface is commonly ulcerated and covered by a fibrinous exudate (a). Fibrin may accumulate in the cyst cavity or wall and become organized, giving the bursa an appearance similar to that of a rheumatoid nodule (b). A variable inflammatory infiltrate may be present within the wall. Inflammation of bursae may occur in other conditions such as rheumatoid arthritis, gout, and tuberculosis.

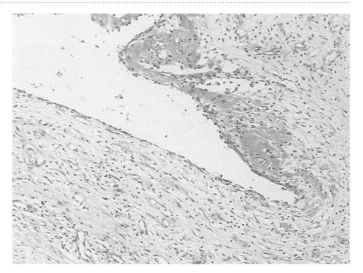

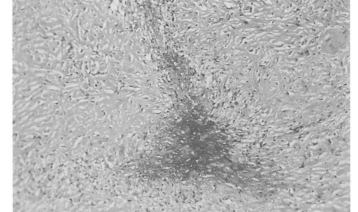

Figure 2.28

a

b

Figure 2.29 **Tendon/ligament injury and degenerative changes** Non-specific oedema, mucinous degenerative changes, or fibrocartilaginous metaplasia (a) may be seen in the dense connective tissue of ligaments and tendons in a variety of common orthopaedic conditions (e.g. trigger finger, golfer's/tennis elbow, DeQuervain's disease, and carpal tunnel syndrome). The symptoms are caused by swelling or fibrous thickening of the affected tissues. An inflammatory infiltrate is not usually prominent. The surface over a ruptured tendon is commonly ulcerated and covered by reparative fibrous or granulation tissue and fibrin (b). Calcific tendinitis may also be seen in collagenous connective tissue of a tendon, ligament, or joint capsule. It is characterized by the presence of amorphous calcium hydroxyapatite crystal deposits within the collagenous matrix of periarticular tissues (c). A macrophage and giant cell response to the calcified material is seen in some cases. It affects mostly the tendons about the shoulder but it has been described in many other locations. Calcific tendinitis was thought to be solely the result of trauma or degenerative changes within the collagenous matrix of tendons but genetic and metabolic factors are also thought to play a role.

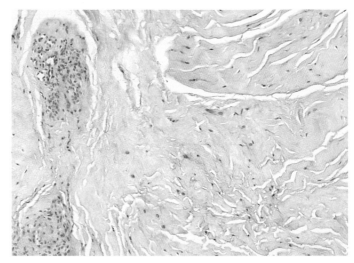

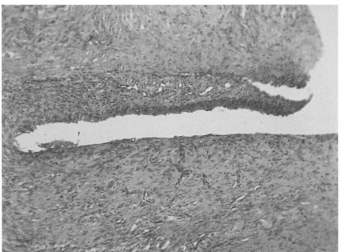

Figure 2.29

a

b

c

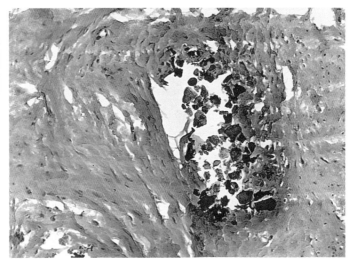

3

Infections of bone and joint

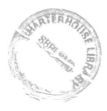

Introduction

Most infections of skeletal tissues are caused by bacterial organisms. Fungi, parasites, and other microbial organisms may also rarely be responsible. The nature of the infecting organism often determines the clinical course, distribution, and location of the infective lesion and the type of host inflammatory response seen in skeletal tissues. The infection may be centred in bone or joint tissues or both may be affected at the same time. In pathological terms, acute and chronic bone and joint infections are generally divided into those which are either pyogenic or non-pyogenic. Infective organisms may reach skeletal tissues by way of the bloodstream from a distant focus of infection or by direct spread either from a neighbouring focus of infection or a penetrating injury (e.g. compound fracture or surgical operation). Both the pathological changes and clinical course may be modified by antibiotic therapy.

Figure 3.1 **Acute pyogenic osteomyelitis** In the early stages of an acute osteomyelitis, radiological appearances are often normal or show only soft tissue swelling; as the infection develops, irregular areas of radiolucency are seen in the medulla, most often in the metaphyseal region. 3.1a shows a focus of early osteomyelitis of the proximal femur involving the apophyseal region of the greater trochanter. The MRI appearances of this lesion are shown in 3.1b. MRI and isotope scans are often useful for detecting early osteomyelitis.

Pyogenic infections of bone and joint

Pyogenic osteomyelitis occurs most commonly in young children; this infection most frequently results from haematogenous spread and is usually centred in the metaphysis of long bones. The organism responsible is usually *Staphylococcus aureus*. In neonates, osteomyelitis is often due to infection with group B streptococcus or Gram-negative organisms such as *Escherichia coli*; more than one bone is commonly affected. Patients with avascular necrosis associated with sickle cell disease or Gaucher's disease are prone to develop an osteomyelitis due to salmonellae. Elderly debilitated patients with genitourinary infection may develop a spinal osteomyelitis due to Gram-negative bacilli. Drug addicts are particularly prone to develop an osteomyelitis due to *Pseudomonas aeruginosa*, often in the spine or pelvis.

Subsequent radiological changes of osteomyelitis are essentially those of bone destruction, reactive bone sclerosis, and periosteal new bone formation. Focal areas of radio-opaque necrotic bone are seen within the infected region and more bone sclerosis is evident the longer the infection persists. 3.1c shows the radiographic appearances of a case of established pyogenic osteomyelitis of the lower femur. There is diffuse loss of bone from the medulla and cortex and new bone formation on the medial and posterior diaphysis.

Figure 3.1

a b c

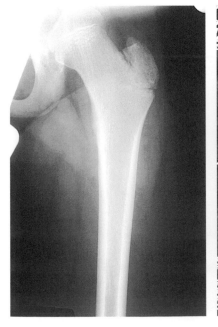
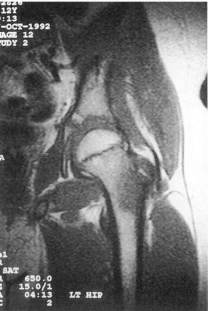
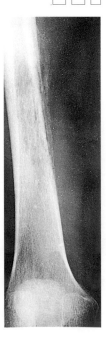

Figure 3.2 **Acute pyogenic osteomyelitis** In the early stages of an acute pyogenic osteomyelitis, there is medullary bone destruction associated with a heavy diffuse infiltrate of neutrophil polymorphs (a, b). This inflammatory infiltrate spreads rapidly through the marrow of the medulla and extends into vascular channels of the cortex (c); cortical bone contains empty osteocyte lacunae, indicating bone necrosis. Gram-positive cocci (arrow) within the inflammatory exudate are seen (d). Organisms, however, are not always present on Gram staining, and the nature and extent of the inflammatory infiltrate may be modified if there has been previous antibiotic treatment.

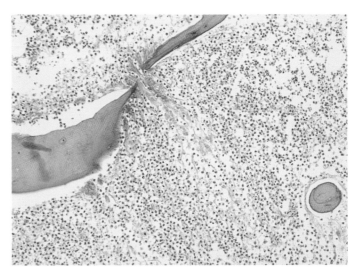

Figure 3.2

| a |
| b |
| c | d |

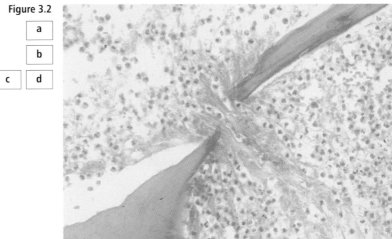

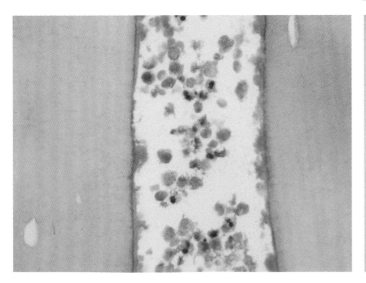

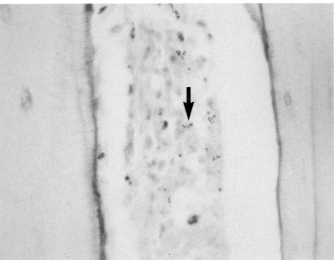

Figure 3.3 **Acute pyogenic osteomyelitis**
Continuing infection results in the formation of large abscesses within the medulla and beneath the periosteum which becomes elevated from the underlying cortex. Inflammatory swelling leads to the loss of both the endosteal and periosteal blood supply to the cortex, resulting in a large segment of the cortex becoming necrotic. This necrotic bone is termed a sequestrum. 3.3a shows part of a sequestrum with necrotic cortical bone and acute inflammatory cells lying within vascular channels. Elevation of the periosteum results in new bone formation. A sleeve of new bone (involucrum) develops around the necrotic cortex and medulla; this involucrum is initially composed of reactive woven bone trabeculae (b), but later may become organized into a neocortex of compact bone (c).

Figure 3.3

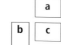

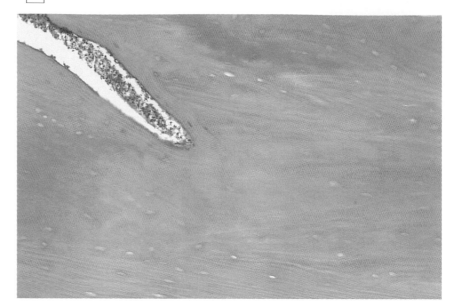

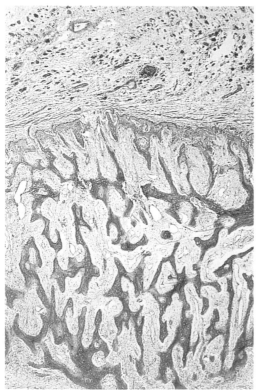

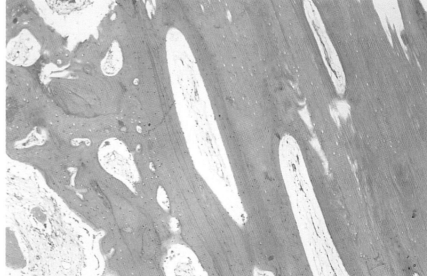

Figure 3.4 **Pyogenic osteomyelitis** Sinuses (cloacae) extend from the infected medullary cavity through the sequestrum and involucrum and open onto the skin surface; these tracks are usually lined by inflamed granulation tissue but may develop a lining of stratified squamous epithelium which grows down from the skin surface. 3.4a shows part of the squamous epithelial lining (arrow) of a chronic sinus which has extended into necrotic medullary bone. Particularly virulent pyogenic infections may extend directly into soft tissues, producing necrosis of muscle fibres and an associated heavy neutrophil polymorph infiltrate (b). Chronic inflammatory cells, mainly lymphocytes, plasma cells, and macrophages, may be present in addition to neutrophil polymorphs later in the course of a pyogenic osteomyelitis (c); this infiltrate may be present from the beginning if there has been antibiotic treatment.

Figure 3.4

a

b c

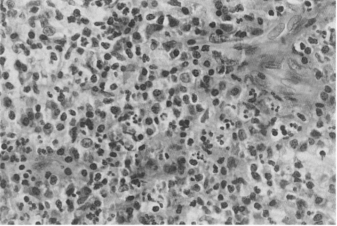

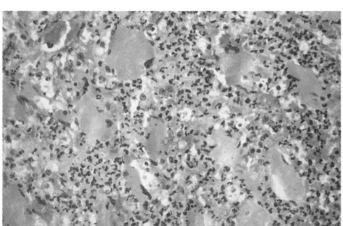

Figure 3.5 **Chronic osteomyelitis** Chronic osteomyelitis may follow acute osteomyelitis or arise *de novo* following infection with organisms of low virulence. There is bone swelling and pain. Chronic osteomyelitis following acute osteomyelitis typically shows radiological features of extensive irregular bone sclerosis and lysis with formation of abundant periosteal new bone. 3.5a shows a case of chronic osteomyelitis of the femur; in addition to marked bone destruction, there is involvement of the hip joint and extension of infection into the pelvis. 3.5b shows a case of chronic osteomyelitis of the lower femur developing *de novo* in which the radiological features of ill-defined medullary and cortical bone destruction, irregular sclerosis, and a periosteal reaction are difficult to distinguish from those of a primary malignant bone tumour.

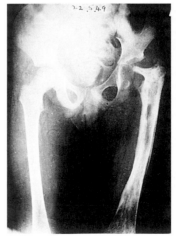
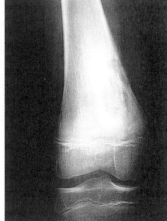

Figure 3.5

a b

Figure 3.6 **Chronic osteomyelitis** Bone changes in chronic osteomyelitis include marrow fibrosis and evidence of increased bone remodelling with prominent osteoblastic and osteoclastic activity and irregular cement lines in bone trabeculae (a). A diffuse, focally heavy inflammatory infiltrate, composed predominantly of lymphocytes, plasma cells, and macrophages with occasional scattered neutrophil polymorphs, is usually seen in the fibrous tissue filling marrow spaces (b). In long-standing chronic osteomyelitis, inflammation may not be pronounced and abundant marrow fibrous tissue surrounds necrotic bone trabeculae (c).

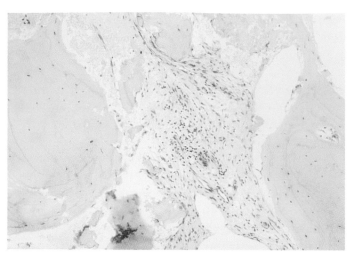

Figure 3.6

| a |
| b | c |

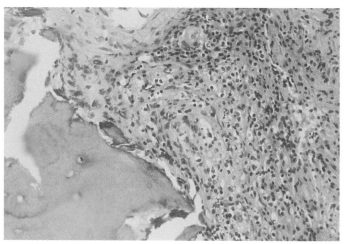

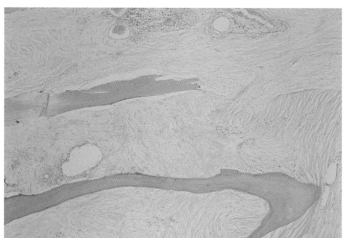

Figure 3.7 **Brodie's abscess** A Brodie's abscess is a localized area of infection within the bone. A central area of osteolysis is surrounded by dense sclerotic bone. 3.7a shows the radiological appearance of a Brodie's abscess of the upper tibia. The lesion usually lies in the metaphysis and often produces expansion of the affected bone. Histologically, it essentially shows the appearances

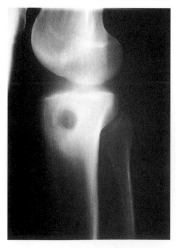

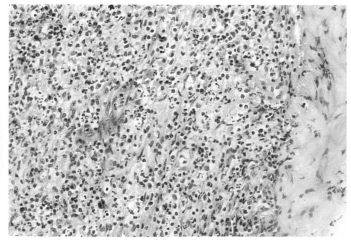

of an abscess cavity with granulation and fibrous tissue containing a variable mixture of acute and chronic inflammatory cells (b). The bone surrounding this area of inflammation is often thickened and sclerotic; there may also be subperiosteal new bone formation in the overlying cortex. Evacuation of the inflammatory tissue is usually required for healing.

Figure 3.7

| a | b |

Figure 3.8 **Complications of osteomyelitis: Marjolin's ulcer** Haematogenous spread of acute osteomyelitis may result in a septicaemia. Spread of infection locally may lead to an infective arthritis; the latter is particularly common in neonatal osteomyelitis where the metaphysis lies within the joint capsule. Other local complications include pathological fracture and growth disturbance due to growth plate damage. Long-standing chronic osteomyelitis may be complicated by secondary amyloidosis. Malignant change may also rarely develop in the squamous epithelial lining of a persistent sinus in chronic osteomyelitis. This is termed a Marjolin's ulcer. Carcinoma development is usually signalled by the onset of severe persistent pain or excessive discharge from a previously quiescent sinus in chronic osteomyelitis. 3.8a shows the gross features of a Marjolin's ulcer of the leg. The tumour usually extends into bone and is most commonly a well-differentiated keratinizing squamous cell carcinoma (b).

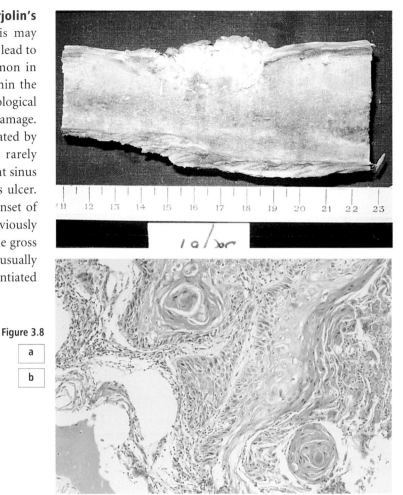

Figure 3.8

a

b

Figure 3.9 **Vertebral pyogenic osteomyelitis** Vertebral pyogenic osteomyelitis most commonly arises in the lumbar spine but less frequently may involve the thoracic or cervical spine. Infection usually begins within the vertebral body as a subacute osteomyelitis then spreads through the vertebral end plate to involve the disc (discitis). Radiologically, there is focal or diffuse destruction of the vertebral body with irregular lysis and sclerosis (a). The bone usually contains a mixed acute and chronic inflammatory infiltrate with lymphocytes, plasma cells, macrophages, and scattered neutrophil polymorphs (b). Marrow fibrosis is present and there is often bone necrosis and remodelling. Inflammatory cells (arrow) are seen within necrotic and degenerate fibrocartilage when there is disc involvement (c). Disc destruction is more common in pyogenic than non-pyogenic infections of the spine. More than one vertebral segment may be involved. Vertebral osteomyelitis is more common in diabetic patients and in elderly individuals with urinary tract infection due to Gram-negative bacilli. Drug addicts are also particularly prone to develop vertebral osteomyelitis due to infection with *Pseudomonas aeruginosa*.

Figure 3.9

a

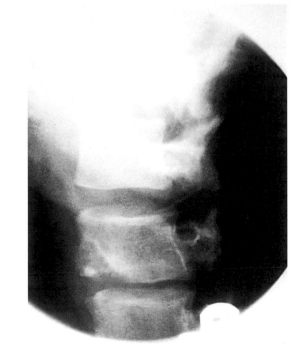

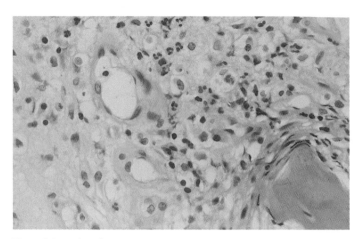

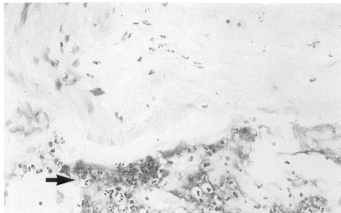

Figure 3.9 continued

b   c

Figure 3.10 Chronic recurrent multifocal osteomyelitis This form of osteomyelitis occurs predominantly in children and young adults. The onset is insidious with low-grade fever and swelling; there is pain and tenderness of the affected bones which radiologically show changes of osteomyelitis. Isotope bone scans reveal multiple sites of involvement. In most cases there is a subacute or chronic osteomyelitis with marrow fibrosis and scattered lymphocytes, plasma cells, and macrophages (as shown here). There may also be sclerotic thickening of cortical and cancellous bone. Organisms are usually isolated with difficulty. The clinical course is protracted and characterized by remissions and exacerbations.

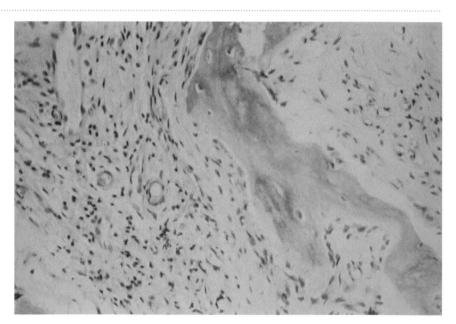

Figure 3.10

Figure 3.11 Pyogenic arthritis As for osteomyelitis, pyogenic arthritis may occur as a result of blood-borne infection or by direct spread from a focus of infection in neighbouring bones or from an open wound. It is most commonly due to *Staphylococcus aureus* but streptococci, *Haemophilus influenzae* (especially in children), and Gram-negative bacilli (especially in infants) may also be responsible. Haematogenous spread of a gonococcal infection may also cause a pyogenic arthritis. Predisposing factors include rheumatoid arthritis, diabetes, and steroid treatment. Grossly, the synovial

Figure 3.11

a

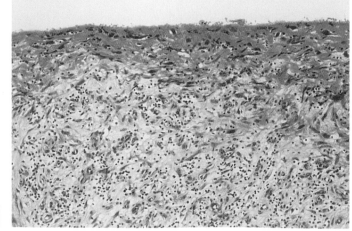

membrane is thickened, congested, and inflamed. The synovial lining is usually ulcerated and covered by an acute inflammatory fibrinous exudate containing numerous neutrophil polymorphs (a). The underlying subintima is composed of granulation tissue containing a heavy inflammatory infiltrate. Organisms may be identified in the inflamed synovium in the acute stage. The presence of Gram-positive cocci (arrow) is shown in 3.11b. The articular cartilage shows loss of matrix staining and necrosis of cartilage cells in the superficial zone; a pannus of inflamed fibrous tissue extends over the articular surface from the inflamed synovium (c). This tissue may become organized and lead to fibrous ankylosis of the joint.

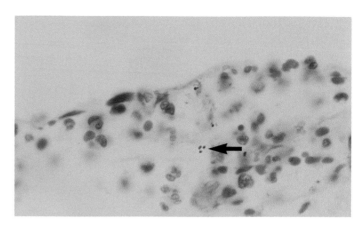

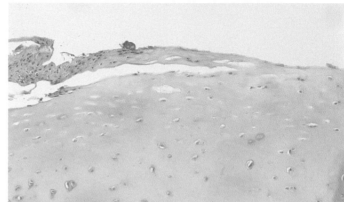

Figure 3.11

b

c

Non-pyogenic infections of bone and joint

Figure 3.12 **Tuberculosis of bone and joint** Infection with *Mycobacterium tuberculosis* usually involves both bone and joint tissues at the same time. It follows haematogenous spread from a primary focus of infection which is usually located in the lungs. Any bone or joint may be affected but lesions occur most frequently in the spine, long bones, and small tubular bones of the hands and feet. There may be multifocal involvement. In the spine, tuberculosis usually arises in the vertebral bodies and extends to involve the inter-vertebral disc and the bodies of adjacent vertebrae. Often more than one vertebra is involved (a). Bone destruction results in anterior angulation of the spine (kyphosis). 3.12b shows the radiological features of tuberculosis involving mainly L5. There is bone destruction, narrowing of the disc space, and swelling of surrounding soft tissues. Tuberculous infection within long bones usually begins in the metaphyseal or epiphyseal region, producing one or more areas of osteolytic bone destruction with little or no surrounding sclerosis or periosteal reaction. 3.12c shows a tuberculous lesion of the upper tibia.

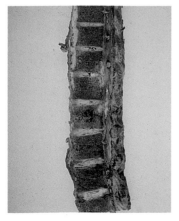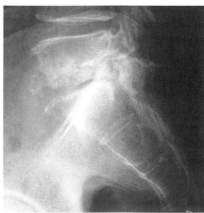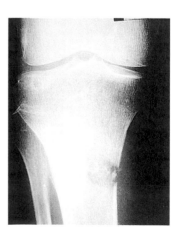

Figure 3.12

 c

Figure 3.13 Tuberculous osteomyelitis Tuberculous infection of bone is characterized by the presence of granulomas exhibiting central caseous necrosis (top left) with surrounding plump epithelioid macrophages and giant cells (arrow) (a, b). Lymphocytes and other chronic inflammatory cells are often seen at the edge of the granuloma. In some cases of tuberculous osteomyelitis, little or no cellular infiltrate is seen in marrow spaces which are filled with abundant caseous necrotic material (c). In other cases, tuberculoid granulomas are composed entirely of plump macrophages and a few giant cells and show little evidence of central necrosis. Acid-fast bacilli (arrow) may be identified by Ziehl–Neelsen staining (d).

Figure 3.13

| a | b | c | d |

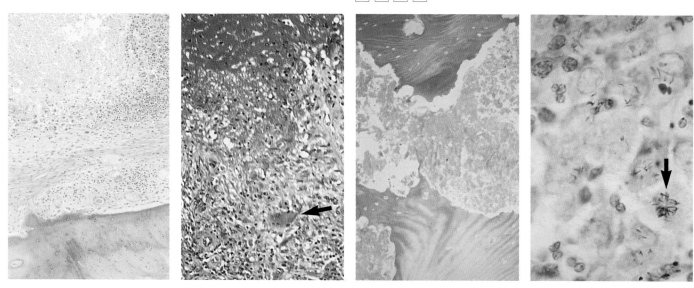

Figure 3.14 Tuberculous arthritis Granuloma formation and caseous necrosis are also seen in the synovial membrane of joints affected by tuberculosis (a, b). Inflamed synovial tissue extends pannus-like over the surface of articular cartilage as well as into subchondral bone, causing cartilage and bone destruction. Small melon-seed bodies composed of fibrin and necrotic material may be found in the joint or attached to the synovial membrane.

Figure 3.14

| a | b |

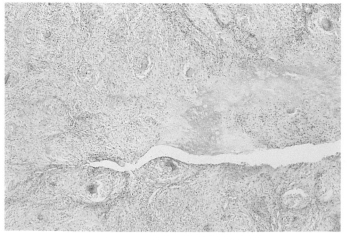
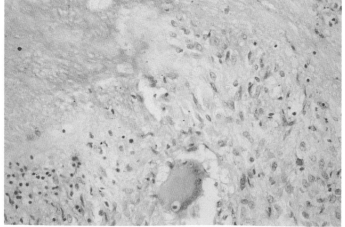

Figure 3.15 Leprosy Destructive cystic lesions of bone may be found in lepromatous leprosy. These show bone destruction with cellular and collagenous fibrous tissue containing numerous plump macrophages and occasional scattered giant cells (a, b). Inflammatory cells contain numerous acid-fast bacilli (*Mycobacterium leprae*). The bones of the hands and feet are most commonly affected. A severe neuropathic degenerative arthritis may also occur in tuberculoid leprosy as a consequence of loss of sensory innervation.

Figure 3.15

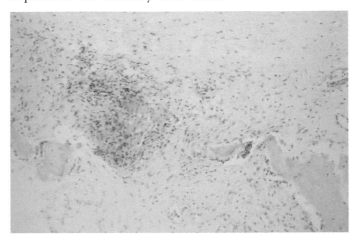
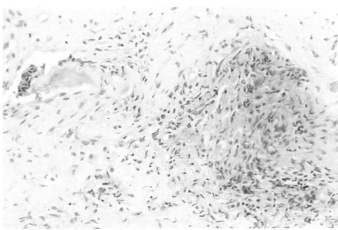

Figure 3.16 Infection with atypical mycobacterial organisms Infection with *M. avium*, *M. marinum*, and *M. kansasii* may produce a chronic swelling in a synovial joint or tendon sheath, particularly in the extremities. Infection may occur either by direct implantation or via the bloodstream. It results in a granulomatous synovitis. Granulomas (arrow) show little or no evidence of caseation necrosis and are composed of numerous epithelioid macrophages and giant cells (a, b). Acid-fast bacilli are not usually identified in tissue sections and microbiological diagnosis is required to distinguish this condition from tuberculosis and other causes of granulomatous synovitis such as sarcoidosis and brucellosis; the latter commonly involves the thoracolumbar and lumbar spine.

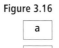

Figure 3.16

a

b

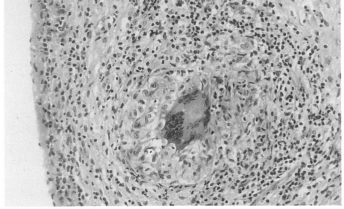

Figure 3.17 **Sarcoidosis** Sarcoidosis is a chronic (non-infective) granulomatous inflammatory disease which needs to be distinguished from mycobacterial and other infective causes of granulomatous osteomyelitis and arthritis. In sarcoidosis there is formation of non-caseating granulomas composed of epithelioid histiocytes and giant cells. The lungs are commonly affected but there may also be bone and joint involvement, particularly of small tubular bones of the hands and feet. Cystic erosions and punched out lesions (arrow) are seen radiologically in the bone (a). The bone lesions consist of non-caseating granulomas which are separated by a lymphocytic infiltrate (b). Similar discrete cellular granulomas are commonly seen in the synovial membrane (c).

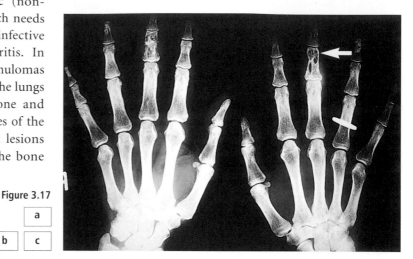

Figure 3.17

a

b	c

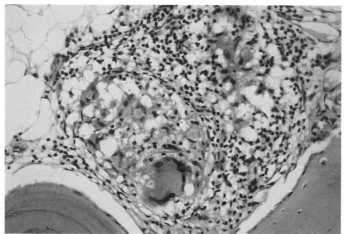

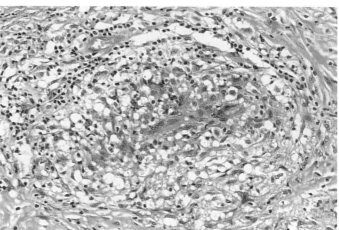

Figure 3.18 **Actinomycosis** Actinomycosis is a chronic, slowly progressive infectious disease caused by the aerobic Gram-positive organism *Actinomyces israelii*, a commensal organism found in the mouth and pharynx. Bone involvement occurs following spread from an adjacent focus of infection. Organisms usually spread from the oral mucosa, leading to an osteomyelitis of the jaw; pulmonary and abdominal actinomycosis may lead to vertebral osteomyelitis. Haematogenous spread may rarely occur. As shown here the lesion is composed of multiple, small, communicating abscesses containing clumps of organisms (sulphur granules); these are surrounded by inflamed granulation tissue in which there are numerous neutrophil polymorphs and macrophages. The organisms are positive on periodic acid–Schiff (PAS) staining.

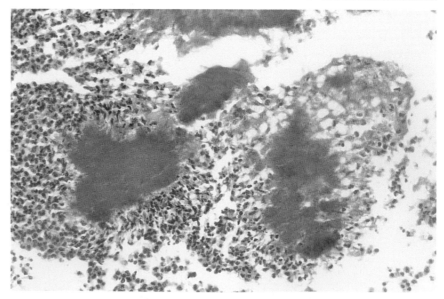

Figure 3.18

Figure 3.19 **Maduromycosis (mycetoma)** This condition is due to infection with various fungi or actinomycetes which are soil saprophytes or plant pathogens. Infection usually follows skin trauma and most commonly occurs in the feet. Lesions enlarge slowly and are associated with extensive tissue destruction; bone involvement is common. Mycetomas contain clusters of actinomycotic bacteria (see 3.18) or fungal hyphae. These grains or granules consist of colonies of organisms which are surrounded by numerous acute inflammatory cells (a). Fungal elements can be identified by Grocott staining (b).

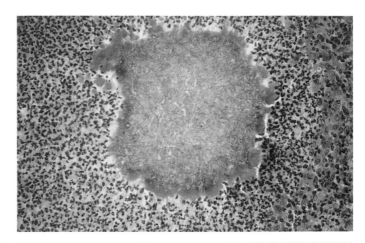

Figure 3.19

a

b

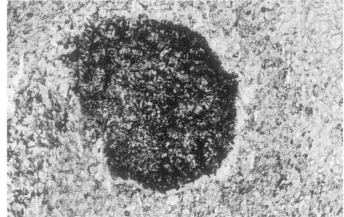

Figure 3.20 **Syphilis** In both congenital and acquired syphilis (due to infection with the spirochaete *Treponema pallidum*), pathological changes are seen in bone and joint with bone changes predominating. In congenital syphilis, growth abnormalities are common due to the presence of a heavy chronic inflammatory infiltrate in the metaphysis. The growth plate is weakened and may fracture. 3.20a shows the radiological appearances of a case of congenital syphilis. There is asymmetry of the lower femoral growth plate and extensive periosteal new bone formation. 3.20b shows gumma formation in the skull in acquired tertiary syphilis. There is irregular bone destruction and a sclerotic reaction. Histologically, syphilitic lesions contain numerous lymphocytes, plasma cells, and histiocytes (c); there may also be tissue necrosis.

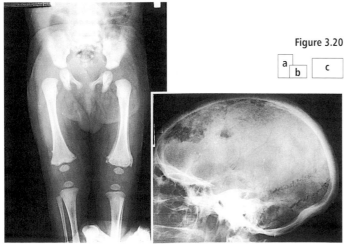

Figure 3.20

a
b   c

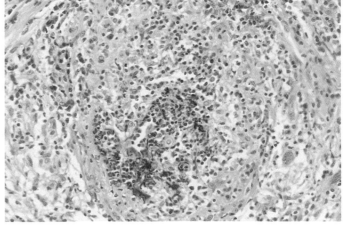

Figure 3.21 Yaws Yaws is due to infection with *Treponema pertenue*. It produces similar radiological and pathological changes to syphilis. There is irregular bone destruction and extensive subperiosteal new bone formation, resulting in irregular thickening of the shaft of long bones. Fusiform thickening of the central portion of the diaphysis of the tibia in a case of yaws is shown here. Pathological changes are similar to those of syphilis.

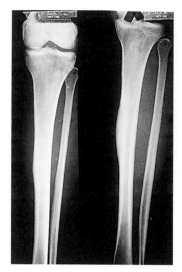

Figure 3.21

Figure 3.22 Lyme disease Lyme disease is caused by a spirochaete (*Borrelia burgdorferi*), which is transmitted to humans by ticks of the *Ixodes ricinus* complex. The disease is most commonly found in North America but has been reported in other countries. Infection results in the formation of characteristic skin lesions (erythema chronicum migrans) at the site of the tick bite and an arthritis involving one or more joints. Cardiovascular and neurological complications may also follow infection. In joints, there is thickening of the synovial lining and a moderate or heavy subintimal lymphocyte or plasma cell (arrow) infiltrate amongst which are scattered occasional lymphoid follicles and neutrophil polymorphs. Histological features may closely resemble those of rheumatoid arthritis. The spirochaete may rarely be isolated from the skin and synovium and serological tests are usually required for confirmation of the diagnosis.

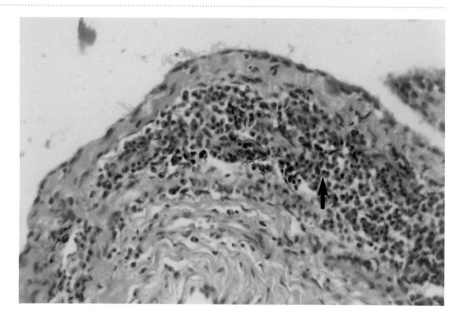

Figure 3.22

Figure 3.23 Hydatid cyst Infection with *Echinococcus granulosus* in humans results in the formation of hydatid cysts. These cysts are found most commonly in the liver and lung but may rarely occur in bone. Any bone may be affected but lesions are seen most commonly in the spine. 3.23a shows the radiological features of a hydatid disease of the tibia. The cysts are large and multiloculated; areas of radiolucency are separated by bony septa. The cyst wall is usually composed of granulation tissue containing a chronic inflammatory infiltrate and focal areas of giant cell response to chitinous material derived from the cyst wall (b, c). Scolices are rarely identified within the cyst.

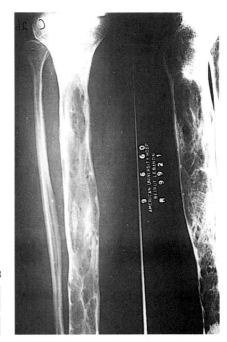

Figure 3.23

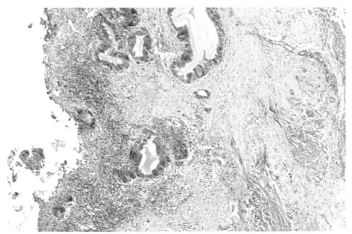

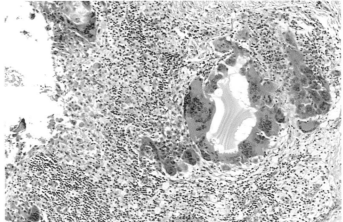

4

Disorders of skeletal development

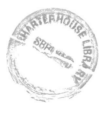

Introduction

Numerous disorders of skeletal development (skeletal dysplasias) have been described. These may affect the entire skeleton or only a part of the skeleton. In general, these conditions are characterized and diagnosed on the basis of their clinical and radiological features; molecular biology, however, is being increasingly used to identify and categorize disorders of skeletal development on the basis of the gene abnormality associated with each condition. Histology plays a role in indicating the nature of the tissue changes that cause abnormal skeletal development. Pathological changes may show evidence of disturbances predominantly affecting cartilage or bone formation, bone resorption, or exhibit accumulation of a metabolic product in skeletal tissues. In this chapter, a number of common or representative dysplastic conditions, which illustrate these pathological changes, are presented; other disorders of skeletal development which present primarily as arthritis, metabolic bone disorders, or bone tumours are more appropriately discussed in the chapters dealing with these conditions.

Skeletal dysplasias in which there is abnormal cartilage development

Figure 4.1 Achondroplasia This condition is due to expression of an abnormal dominant gene which has a relatively high mutation rate (1:10 000 births). It is associated with an abnormality in the fibroblast growth factor receptor 3 (FGFR3) gene present on the short arm of chromosome 4. Most cases are sporadic. Heterozygous achondroplasia is relatively common but homozygous achondroplasia is extremely rare. Skeletal radiographs show short tubular bones with small epiphyseal centres (a). There is sharp flaring of the metaphysis. Long bones are normal in diameter but commonly bowed. There may be cortical thickening at sites of muscle attachment. Vertebrae are relatively small and have square rather than rectangular outlines (b). Skull bones of the cranial vault and mandible, which are formed by intramembranous ossification, appear disproportionately large relative to hypoplastic facial bones and the bones of the base of the skull which are formed by endochondral ossification (c).

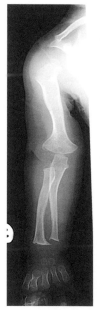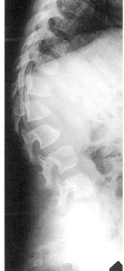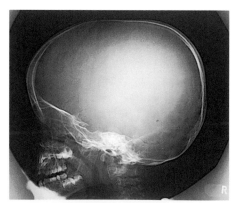

Figure 4.1

a b c

Figure 4.2 Achondroplasia Endochondral ossification may be little altered in heterozygous achondroplasia but cartilage columns in general are smaller than normal (a) and show a disturbance of endochondral ossification (b). The height of each chondrocyte zone in the growth plate is reduced and an ordered columnar arrangement of chondrocytes may be lacking. 4.2c (von Kossa stain) shows poorly organized columns of cartilage cells, a paucity of hypertrophic cells, and abnormal arrangement of metaphyseal bone. These changes are generally more pronounced in homozygous achondroplasia which is a lethal condition. Heterozygous achondroplasia is compatible with survival into adult life. Death may occur in infancy due to neurological complications (hydrocephalus). Spinal problems (disc prolapse and cord compression), respiratory problems, and premature degenerative arthritis may also complicate heterozygous achondroplasia.

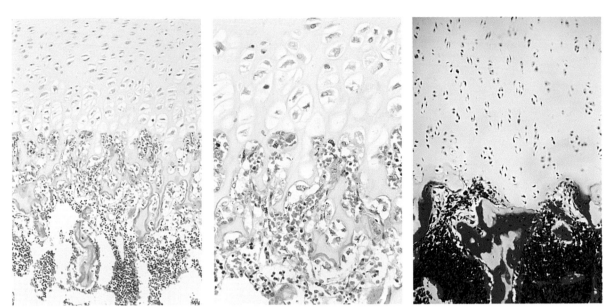

Figure 4.2

Figure 4.3 **Thanatophoric dysplasia** This was formerly regarded as a lethal form of achondroplasia but is now known to be a separate condition. It is the commonest form of lethal skeletal dysplasia. Most cases occur sporadically, but some are probably due to an autosomal dominant mutation. In this condition there is also an abnormality in the FGFR3 gene. Affected infants usually die of respiratory distress shortly after birth. Radiographs show a large head, prominent forehead, and craniofacial disproportion (a). The chest is narrow and the ribs are short and hypoplastic. The long bones are all short and curved; there is cupping of the epiphysis, and bony spikes are seen at the edge of the growth plate. The lumbar vertebral bodies are flattened and have an inverted 'U' appearance. Histological changes in the growth plate are variable but include disorganization of chondrocyte maturation with lack of column formation and a reduction in the zones of chondrocyte proliferation and hypertrophy (b). Other areas of the growth plate may appear relatively normal or show reduced endochondral ossification with the cartilage of the growth plate appearing to sit directly on the underlying bone (c).

Figure 4.3

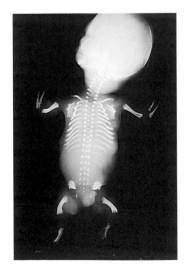

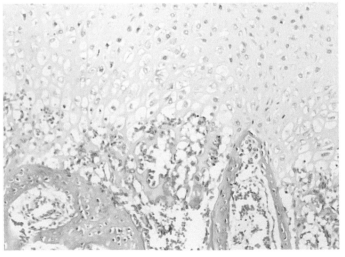

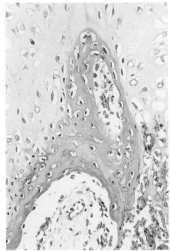

Figure 4.4 Pseudoachondroplasia This relatively common osteochondrodystrophy exists in several forms and may be inherited autosomal dominant or recessive; most cases, however, occur sporadically. There is an abnormality in the gene which encodes the cartilage oligomeric matrix protein (COMP) which is present on the short arm of chromosome 19. There is growth retardation with extreme shortening and deformity of the limbs similar to that seen in achondroplasia; craniofacial changes are not seen. Radiologically, in long bones, the metaphysis is widened and cup-shaped and the epiphysis irregular in outline (a). Early secondary osteoarthritis commonly develops in the knee (b) and other large weight-bearing joints. The vertebrae are biconvex and have central projections (c). Tubular bones of the hands and feet are shortened and the phalanges have a broad base. Intracellular inclusion bodies have been noted in cartilage cells.

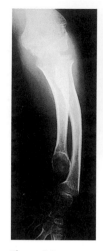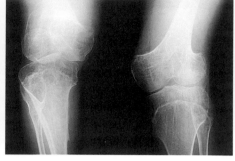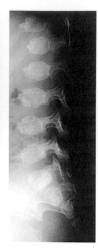

Figure 4.4

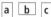

Figure 4.5 Achondrogenesis This very rare lethal condition exists in two forms: type I (inherited autosomal recessive) and type II (inherited autosomal dominant). 4.5 shows a case of achondrogenesis type II in which there is an abnormality in the type II collagen gene (*COL2A1*). Radiologically, bones are tiny, short, and square and there is little evidence of ossification in the skull or vertebral bodies. The ribs are short and often fractured. There is prominent metaphyseal flaring. Histologically, the growth plate cartilage appears hypocellular and chondrocyte lacunae appear large and may contain PAS-positive (diastase-resistant) inclusion bodies. Infants are usually stillborn and show marked micromelia, short trunk, prominent abdomen, and a disproportionately large head.

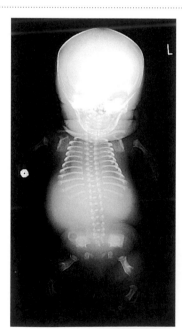

Figure 4.5

Figure 4.6 **Spondyloepiphyseal dysplasia congenita (SEDC)** This condition is usually compatible with life and presents as short-limbed dwarfism often associated with other abnormalities such as cleft palate and talipes equinovarus. There is severe kyphoscoliosis and thoracic deformity in childhood (a). This is associated with platyspondyly and hypoplasia of the odontoid process. There is also severe shortening of tubular bones and marked epiphyseal dysplasia (b). An abnormality in the *COL2A1* gene located on chromosome 12 has been reported.

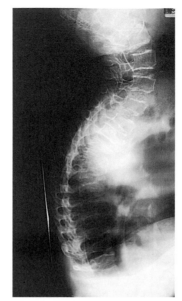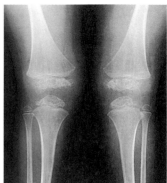

Figure 4.6

a b

Figure 4.7 **Multiple epiphyseal dysplasia** This relatively common group of chondrodysplasias shows variable features including slight shortness of stature, abnormal gait, and early onset degenerative arthritis. Abnormalities in the genes encoding COMP and type IX collagen have been reported. Radiologically, the epiphysis of long bones may show stippled opacities; later, in childhood and adolescence, it appears irregular and fragmented. Changes in the hip (shown here) may be confused with Perthes' disease. Histologically, the growth plate appearance and endochondral ossification are within normal limits. There is no consistent inheritance pattern.

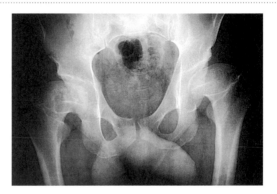

Figure 4.7

Figure 4.8 **Metaphyseal chondrodysplasia (metaphyseal dysostosis)** This heterogeneous group of conditions is characterized chiefly by metaphyseal abnormalities with essentially normal development of the epiphyses and axial skeleton. The Schmidt type is the most common and is inherited autosomal dominant. The abnormal gene encodes for type X collagen and is present on the long arm of chromosome 6. The dysplasia is characterized by bowing of the legs and moderately short stature, normal head and trunk, relatively short limbs, and enlarged metaphyses in growing bones. Skeletal radiographs show rickets-like changes in the growth plates which are expanded and irregular. This is shown here in joints of the wrist and hand. The growth plate is disorganized with loss of the normal columnar arrangement and clusters of abnormally large chondrocytes which are surrounded by dense fibrous tissue. Blood vessels may be seen amongst the cell clusters.

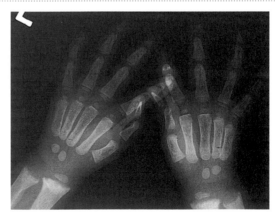

Figure 4.8

Figure 4.9 **Asphyxiating thoracic dwarfism** This condition is characterized by severe narrowing of the thorax and may lead to death from respiratory distress. Radiologically, ribs are short, horizontal, and have flared anterior ends (as shown here). Sternal ossification may be retarded in neonates. Tubular bones are often short. The pelvis is widened. Milder forms are compatible with life, the shape of the thorax tending to revert to normal during development.

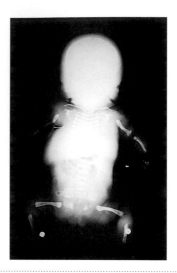

Figure 4.9

Figure 4.10 **Enchondromatosis (Ollier's disease; dyschondroplasia)** This is a non-hereditary disorder of bone characterized by the presence of multiple cartilaginous tumours in several bones. Lesions may be found in bones of all four limbs but most are confined to a single limb. They are commonly found in the small bones of the hands and feet and long tubular bones. The original case, as described by Ollier, showed a predominantly unilateral distribution. The lesions may lie centrally or peripherally within the bone. Patients present in childhood with either deformity or growth abnormality. 4.10a shows enchondromas within the proximal and middle phalanx in a case of Ollier's disease. The lesions are radiolucent and often larger and more confluent than solitary enchondromas; they show stippled calcification which becomes more pronounced with age. Histologically, the lesions are generally more cellular than solitary enchondromas (b). There are frequent binucleated cartilage cells (arrow) (c). The exact incidence of malignant change in enchondromatosis is unknown but estimates of 25 and 30 per cent have been reported. The association of multiple enchondromas and soft tissue haemangiomas is termed Mafucci's syndrome.

Figure 4.10

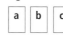

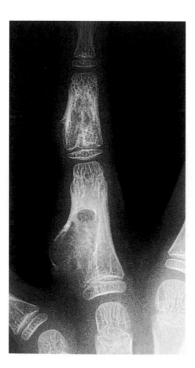
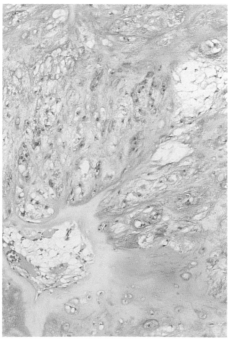
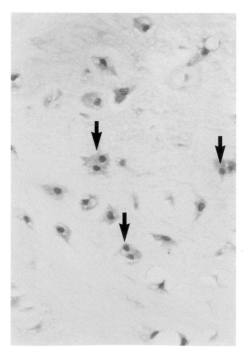

Figure 4.11 Hereditary multiple exostoses (diaphyseal aclasis) This condition is inherited autosomal dominant and is characterized by the presence of multiple osteochondromas in several bones. The specific genes for this disorder have not been identified and karyotypic abnormalities have been found on three different chromosomes (i.e. chromosomes 8, 11, and 19). The lesions enlarge during childhood, causing deformity and growth abnormalities. They are found most commonly in the metaphyseal region of long tubular bones. Radiologically, multiple asymmetric, sessile or pedunculated osteochondromas, which may be quite large, are seen in the vicinity of the metaphysis. 4.11a shows multiple osteochondromas in the femur and tibia. Grossly, confluent multiple lesions may give the impression of a single large mass and the cartilage cap may be thickened (b). Histologically, lesions resemble solitary osteochondromas. A fibrous perichondrium covers a cartilage cap of variable cellularity. During growth, endochondral ossification is evident at the base of the enlarging cartilage cap which may contain binucleated cells (c). The lesion ceases to grow once adulthood is reached. Enlargement of a lesion in an adult may indicate malignant transformation. The reported incidence of malignant change in these lesions varies widely (1–25 per cent), but it is generally thought to occur rarely.

Figure 4.11

a   b   c

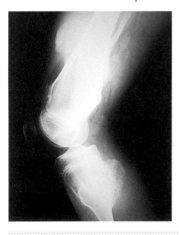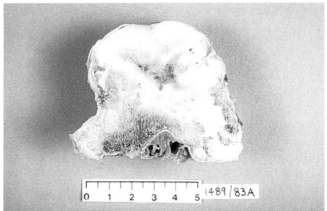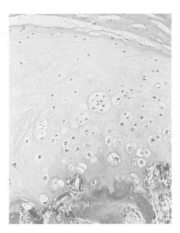

Figure 4.12 Dysplasia epiphysialis hemimelica (Trevor's disease) This is an uncommon familial disease in which an osteochondroma-like cartilaginous lesion develops in the epiphysis. Isolated, irregular centres of ossification in the epiphysis enlarge and fuse to form a cartilage-capped bony protuberance. 4.12a shows radiological findings of a lesion in the medial femoral condyle. The condition is usually diagnosed in early childhood when the patient presents with a painless mass or deformity. Lesions are most commonly seen around the ankle or knee but may occur elsewhere. They may result in a varus or valgus deformity or cause growth arrest or leg length discrepancy. Males are affected more commonly than females. Histological features resemble those of an osteochondroma with a broad cartilage cap covered by a fibrous perichondrium and endochondral ossification occurring at the base of the cap during growth (b). The lesion is benign and treated surgically by excision.

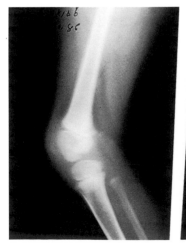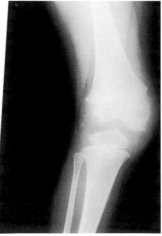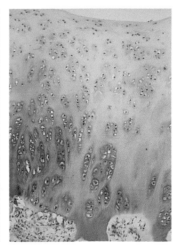

Figure 4.12

a   b

Skeletal dysplasias associated with abnormal bone formation

Osteogenesis imperfecta

Osteogenesis imperfecta (OI) is a group of hereditary bone diseases characterized by defective synthesis of the type I collagen molecule, a major matrix component of bone and other connective tissues. In bone, this abnormality results in osteopenia and a varying tendency to undergo pathological fracture.

With rare exceptions, OI is always the result of mutations in the genes *COL1A1* (located on the long arm of chromosome 17) and *COL1A2* (located on the long arm of chromosome 7) which code respectively for the α_1 and α_2 chains from which the collagen type I triple helix is formed. OI is divided into four main types on the basis of clinical expression and apparent mode of inheritance. Recent biochemical and molecular findings have shown that the four types are not strictly absolute as different mutations may lead to similar patterns of clinical expression.

Figure 4.13 **Osteogenesis imperfecta type I** This mild form of OI is inherited autosomal dominant; about one third of cases, however, are new mutations. Patients typically have blue sclerae and exhibit mild or moderate osteopenia. Fractures rarely occur in infancy but may begin when the child begins to walk; they are generally few in number and heal normally. Deformity is uncommon or mild. There may be early-onset adult hearing loss. The absence or (rare) presence of dentinogenesis imperfecta determines whether the OI is typed as IA or IB respectively. Radiologically, the skeleton usually shows generalized osteopenia and there may be evidence of previous fracture and associated deformity. Spinal changes and wormian bones are not seen. In type I OI, osseous tissue is formed and organized normally into compact and cancellous lamellar bone but there is an increase in the number of osteocytes per unit area of bone tissue; this is often best appreciated in cortical bone examined under polarized light (a). The bone is normally mineralized but less bone than normal is present. 4.13b shows isolated, small, relatively thin bone trabeculae from a case of type I OI.

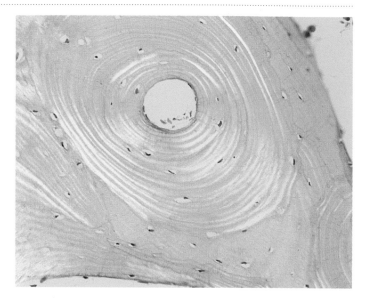

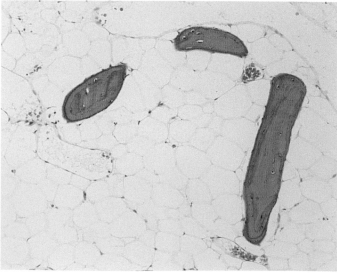

Figure 4.13

a

b

Figure 4.14 Osteogenesis imperfecta type II This is a severe (lethal) form of OI. Affected neonates are usually stillborn or die in the early neonatal period. They have numerous fractures and exhibit severe limb deformities. Radiologically, there is beading of the ribs and concertina deformity of the limb bones (a). There is poor ossification of the cranial vault and platyspondyly. Histologically, little lamellar bone is seen and woven bone is chiefly formed (b, c). In the growth plate, there is markedly reduced endochondral ossification and woven bone trabeculae that are formed often retain a central core of cartilage (d). This type of OI is usually due to a new dominant mutation; it was originally thought to be inherited autosomal recessive but this is now thought to occur rarely.

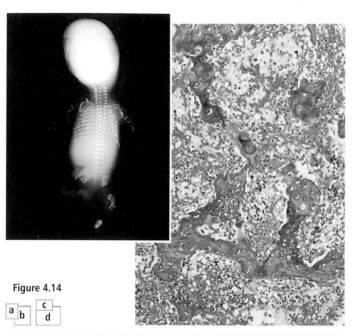
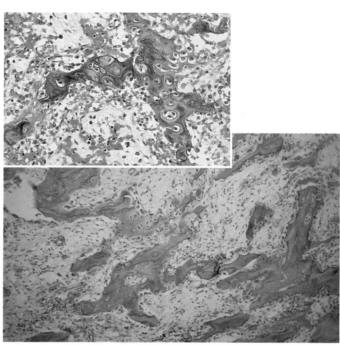

Figure 4.14

a		c
	b	d

Figure 4.15 Osteogenesis imperfecta type III This is a rare, progressive, deforming form of OI which is inherited autosomal recessive. Fractures are often present at birth and appear during infancy and throughout childhood. This results in progressive severe deformity, growth retardation, and scoliosis. Sclerae are usually white. Hearing loss and dentinogenesis imperfecta may be present. Radiologically, there is marked osteopenia with numerous fractures and severe limb deformity. 4.5a shows marked bowing deformity and osteopenia in bones of the upper limb in a case of type III OI. In the metaphysis and epiphysis of long bones, there is 'popcorn' calcification with numerous round cartilage nodules having a sclerotic margin and a central area of radiolucency. These are shown (b) grossly in a bisected knee joint and (c) radiologically. They are thought to result from a growth plate abnormality. Hyperplastic fracture callus may be noted in limb bones. Centres of intramembranous ossification in the cranial vault fail to unite with each other, producing the radiological appearance of wormian bone (d).

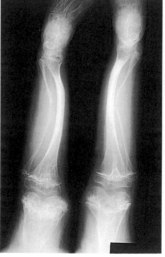
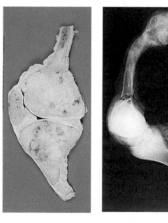
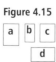
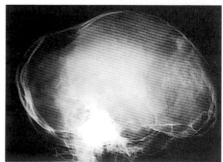

Figure 4.15

a	b	c
	d	

Figure 4.16 Osteogenesis imperfecta type III In type III OI, a variable but usually prominent amount of woven bone is seen in both the cortex and medulla. The bone trabeculae are usually thin and show prominent osteoblastic rimming (a, b); there is also usually increased osteoclastic activity. In older patients, bone is partly lamellar in type but areas of woven bone remain prominent. There are prominent cement lines in the bone which usually shows an increase in the number of osteocytes.

Figure 4.16

| a | b |

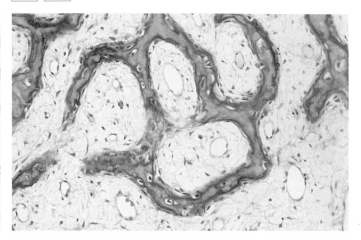

Figure 4.17 Osteogenesis imperfecta type IV In this mild/moderate form of OI, which is inherited autosomal dominant, fractures may occur at a young age but tend to decrease in frequency as the patient grows older. There may be short stature and the degree of severity and deformity is variable. The sclerae may be light blue at birth but this colour fades with increasing age. Dentinogenesis imperfecta is relatively common but may be absent. Radiologically, there is osteopenia which may lead to vertebral fracture and collapse (a). Histologically, bone is almost entirely lamellar in type but appears disorganized with increased prominence of irregularly arranged cement lines; there is also an increase in the number of osteocytes. These features are seen in cortical bone in 4.17b. Examination under polarized light shows that, unlike normal lamellar bone, numerous small segments of lamellar bone rather than long uninterrupted lamellae are present in OI type IV (c). Other conditions in which there is a disturbance of type I collagen formation, such as Marfan's syndrome, may also be complicated by osteopenia.

Figure 4.17

| a | b |
| | c |

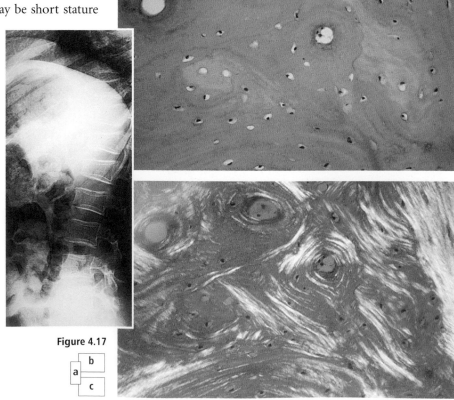

Sclerosing bone dysplasias

Figure 4.18 Osteopetrosis This rare inherited skeletal disorder is characterized by generalized osteosclerosis which results in thickening of cortical bone and narrowing of the medullary cavity. This condition results from impaired bone resorption that may be due to one of several abnormalities of osteoclast formation or function. Some forms of animal and human osteopetrosis may be cured by bone marrow transplantation. A gene abnormality affecting production of macrophage colony-stimulating factor, which is required for osteoclast formation, has been localized to the short arm of chromosome 1. Malignant osteopetrosis, which is inherited autosomal recessive, produces extensive bony overgrowth. This results in a severe leucoerythroblastic anaemia, granulocytopenia, and bleeding as well as pathological fractures and neurological complications. It usually results in death *in utero* or in early infancy. Benign osteopetrosis is inherited autosomal dominant. It is usually asymptomatic but may present with pathological fractures or neurological problems associated with stenosis of the neural foramina. There may also be problems with dental extractions, bone infections, and early onset degenerative arthritis. Radiologically, generalized osteosclerosis is evident with loss of distinct separation between the cortex and medulla (a). The spine shows a pronounced 'rugger jersey' appearance due to sclerosis of the vertebral end plates (b).

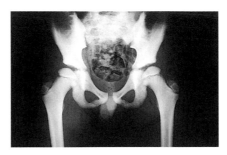

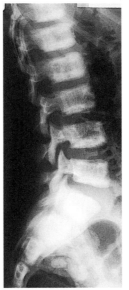

Figure 4.18

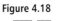

Figure 4.19 Osteopetrosis Histologically, in benign osteopetrosis, bone trabeculae contain residual cartilage which is surrounded by lamellar bone (a). Osteoclasts are usually few in number. Sclerotic bone may show evidence of osteonecrosis (b). Osteomyelitis, particularly of the jaw bones, is a complication of this condition. In malignant osteopetrosis, sclerosis and thickening of bone trabeculae, which may contain a central core of cartilage, is also seen. Osteoclasts may be absent or reduced in number but, in some forms of osteopetrosis, may be quite numerous. Osteopetrosis needs to be distinguished from other sclerosing bone dysplasias and other bone conditions where osteosclerosis may be a feature, such as fluorosis, heavy metal poisoning, excessive vitamin A or vitamin D intake, Paget's disease, osteonecrosis, osteomyelitis, bone metastases, and osteosarcoma.

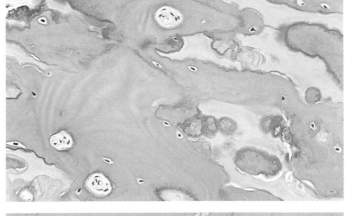

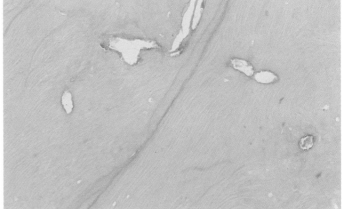

Figure 4.19

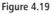

a

b

Figure 4.20 **Progressive diaphyseal dysplasia (Camurati– Engelmann disease)** This rare bone disease is inherited autosomal dominant with variable penetrance. It is characterized by new bone formation which occurs progressively on both the periosteal and endosteal surfaces of long bones. Any bone may be affected. The tibia and femur are most frequently involved. Most cases present in childhood. Radiologically, the diaphysis of the long bones shows variable amounts of periosteal and endosteal cortical thickening. These changes are shown in both femora in (a). Histologically, in the early stages, there is increased endosteal and periosteal new bone formation with bone surfaces covered by plump osteoblasts and osteoid (b). Bone formed is originally woven in type but later remodelled to lamellar bone. Clinical progression is variable.

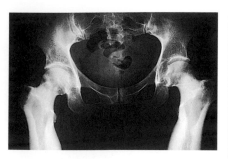
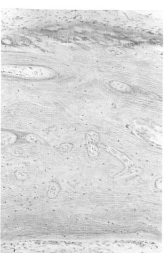

Figure 4.20

Figure 4.21 **Melorheostosis** In this rare condition, several areas of bone sclerosis are seen in the shaft of long bones, both on the external surface, beneath the periosteum, and on the internal surface of the cortex, extending into the medullary cavity. Bone sclerosis often appears to start proximally and progress distally. The disease may be confined to one limb but may be more extensive and bilateral. Patients complain of limb pain and joint stiffness. The condition may cause growth abnormalities in childhood. Radiologically, there is irregular patchy osteosclerotic thickening of the endosteal and periosteal surfaces of the long bones; this often gives the appearance of dripping candle wax covering the shaft. These features are shown in the radius in (a). Periosteal and endosteal thickening of cortical bone is seen histologically (b, Goldner stain). Endosteal thickening predominates during infancy and childhood and periosteal new bone formation is more evident in adulthood. Bone formed is largely lamellar in type.

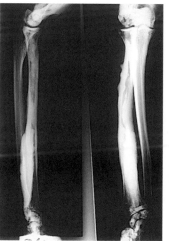
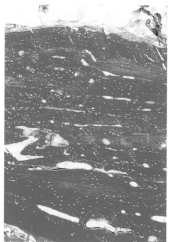

Figure 4.21

Figure 4.22 **Osteopoikilosis** In this rare condition, which is inherited autosomal dominant, numerous discrete islands of bone are found in the medulla. Involved bones are normal in outline. Lesions may be distributed symmetrically and are found most commonly in large tubular bones and small bones of the hands and feet. They are usually asymptomatic. Radiologically, multiple discrete radio-opaque lesions are seen in the medulla, most commonly in the epiphysis and metaphysis. 4.22a shows the radiological appearances of osteopoikilosis of the tibia. Histologically, each lesion is a discrete enostosis or bone island composed of sclerotic compact lamellar bone; the edges of the lesion merge with surrounding cancellous bone trabeculae (b).

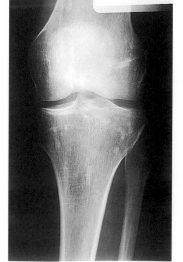

Figure 4.22

a

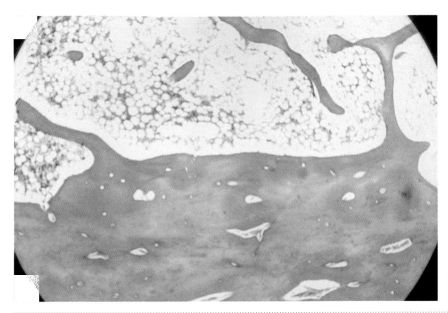

Figure 4.22 continued

b

Abnormal bone growth and remodelling due to inherited disorders of metabolism

Figure 4.23 **Mucopolysaccharidoses (MPS)** In this group of inherited lysosomal diseases, there is deficiency of specific enzymes involved in the degradation of glycosaminoglycans. As a consequence, large fragments of glycosaminoglycans are stored in many cells of the body including connective tissue cells of the skeleton. This results in growth retardation, abnormal facies (gargoylism), bowing deformity of the limbs, thoracolumbar kyphosis, and joint stiffness. Radiological changes in a case of MPS type II are shown. There is generalized rarefaction of tubular bones in the forearm and the epiphyses and metaphyses are irregular in outline (a); there is delay in the appearance of epiphyseal ossification centres. In the spine, vertebral bodies are hypoplastic and have a beak-like anterior projection (b). MPS II is due to accumulation of dermatan sulphate and heparan sulphate and is inherited X-linked recessive. Other mucopolysaccharidoses are inherited autosomal recessive; gene abnormalities have been localized to different chromosomes coding for the specific enzyme involved. Accumulated mucopolysaccharides are present in the cells of many tissues throughout the body, especially in fibroblasts and other connective tissue cells as well as mononuclear phagocytes in reticuloendothelial tissues.

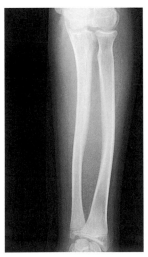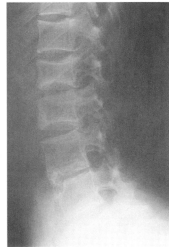

Figure 4.23

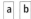

Figure 4.24 Morquio's syndrome (MPS IV) This form of MPS is due to accumulation of keratan sulphate and is characterized by the development of several skeletal deformities. Abnormalities in genes located on the short arm of chromosome 3 and on the long arm of chromosome 7 have been found. Children appear normal at birth but later show marked dwarfism, kyphoscoliosis, genu valgum, and flexion contractures. Radiological features are shown in long bones around the knee joint (a) and spine (b). Developing bones have small secondary centres of ossification which appear to ossify irregularly or not at all. Vertebral bodies are hypoplastic and flattened; there is 'beaking' of lumbar vertebrae. Endochondral ossification at the growth plate is depressed and collections of foam cells may be seen (c). Glycosaminoglycan-containing macrophages also fill the marrow spaces and may produce cortical defects.

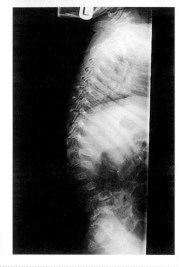
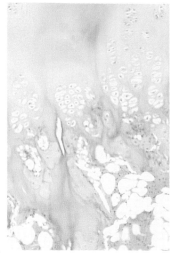
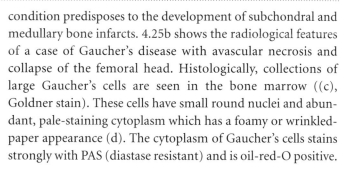

Figure 4.24

a

b c

Figure 4.25 Gaucher's disease Gaucher's disease is an inherited disorder characterized by the absence or deficiency of the enzyme glucocerebrosidase. The gene abnormality has been localized to the long arm of chromosome 1. This results in the accumulation of glucocerebroside in mononuclear phagocytes of the bone marrow and lymphoreticular system. It is encountered most frequently amongst Ashkenazi Jews. Early onset of this disease is associated with the development of a neuropathy and has a poor prognosis. The adult chronic non-neuropathic form of Gaucher's disease, inherited autosomal recessive, may cause bone pain and pathological fracture. It is associated with early onset degenerative joint disease, medullary and subchondral bone infarction, osteomyelitis, and development of spinal deformities. 4.25a shows the radiological features of Gaucher's disease in the humerus. Accumulation of Gaucher's cells results in the formation of multiple areas of radiolucency, widening of the medulla, and thinning of the cortex. This condition predisposes to the development of subchondral and medullary bone infarcts. 4.25b shows the radiological features of a case of Gaucher's disease with avascular necrosis and collapse of the femoral head. Histologically, collections of large Gaucher's cells are seen in the bone marrow ((c), Goldner stain). These cells have small round nuclei and abundant, pale-staining cytoplasm which has a foamy or wrinkled-paper appearance (d). The cytoplasm of Gaucher's cells stains strongly with PAS (diastase resistant) and is oil-red-O positive.

Figure 4.25

a b

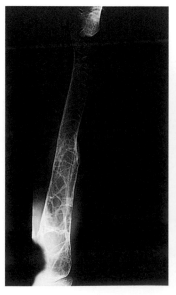
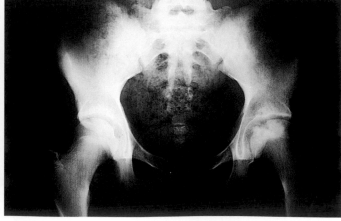

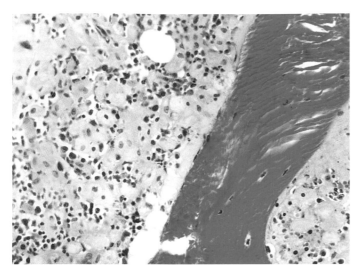

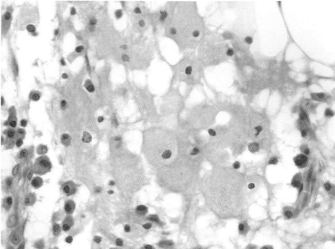

Figure 4.25 continued

| c | d |

Developmental conditions exhibiting heterotopic ossification

Figure 4.26 Fibrodysplasia (myositis) ossificans progressiva (FOP) This rare condition is characterized by progressive heterotopic ossification within soft tissues of the trunk and extremities. Most cases are sporadic but the condition is thought to be transmitted autosomal dominant with variable expression. Associated skeletal abnormalities include abnormal short big toes or thumbs and variable fusion of the cervical spine. Clinically, a painful, firm soft-tissue swelling develops in the muscles of the neck, paraspinal muscles, or upper and lower limb girdles; both clinically and pathologically this may be misdiagnosed as a sarcoma. The soft tissue mass undergoes progressive ossification, leading to development of muscle and joint contractures with resultant kyphoscoliosis and limitation of thoracic movement. Patients often survive into early adulthood but usually die of respiratory complications. 4.26a shows ossification of the left chest wall in a case of FOP. Radiological confirmation of abnormalities of the great toe and hands and feet should also be sought in this condition. Histologically, early lesions consist of cellular connective tissue which is oedematous and shows active fibroblast proliferation (b); focal areas of fibro-osseous and fibrocartilaginous metaplasia later develop in this tissue (c, d). Ossification is progressive and results in the formation of a confluent bony mass. There is associated muscle atrophy and fibrosis.

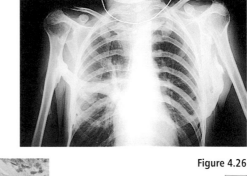

Figure 4.26

| a |

| b |
| d | c |

Figure 4.27 **Progressive osseous heteroplasia (POH)** This condition has only recently been separated from FOP. It is characterized by the formation of heterotopic bone in the dermis and subcutaneous tissues as well as in deeper soft tissues. Bone formation is usually first noted in childhood and may be confined to a specific body region or part of a limb. The trunk is not commonly involved. 4.27a shows the radiographic appearances of ossification of superficial and deep soft tissues of the left thigh in a case of POH. Numerous bone trabeculae are seen in subcutaneous fat and muscle (b). Bone formed is initially woven in type but later remodelled to well organized, mature, compact, and cancellous bone (c). Bone is formed almost entirely by fibro-osseous metaplasia and little or no cartilage is seen.

Figure 4.27

a

b c

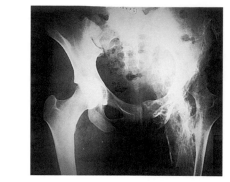

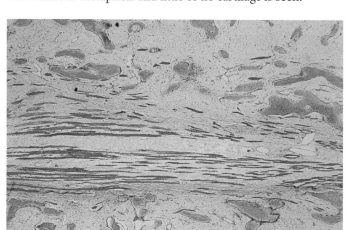

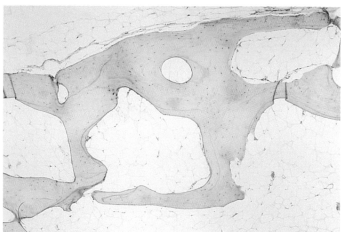

Other abnormalities of skeletal development and growth

Figure 4.28 **Polyostotic fibrous dysplasia** Fibrous dysplasia is a relatively common abnormality of skeletal development which is characterized by the formation of single or multiple fibro-osseous lesions in bone. The disease is more commonly monostotic than polyostotic. Some patients with polyostotic fibrous dysplasia may also exhibit precocious puberty and cutaneous pigmentation (Albright's syndrome). An abnormal gene has been localized to the long arm of chromosome 20; this affects the structure and function of a G-protein-coupled receptor. Small lesions are often asymptomatic but large lesions may cause swelling, deformity, bone pain, and pathological fracture. Lesions may present at any age but are usually noted in childhood or adolescence. They occur most commonly in the ribs, large tubular bones, skull, and facial bones but any bone may be affected. Polyostotic disease may exhibit involvement of only one side of the body or produce lesions in only one limb. Radiologically, lesions are well defined and have

Figure 4.28

a
b

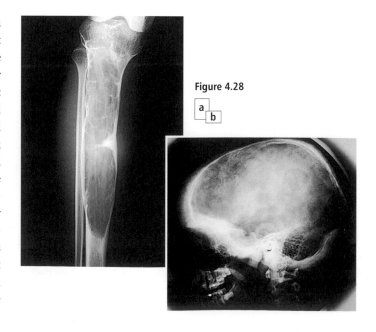

a somewhat radio-opaque ground-glass appearance; they often expand the bone and may be lobulated or predominantly lytic. (a) A large lesion in the tibia; (b) a large lesion in the skull from two cases of polyostotic fibrous dysplasia. Histological features of polyostotic fibrous dysplasia are similar to those of the monostotic condition (see Chapter 7). This is characterized by the presence of abundant cellular fibrous tissue containing irregular spicules of woven bone which typically are not covered by prominent osteoblasts (c); osteoclastic remodelling of woven bone trabeculae is seen.

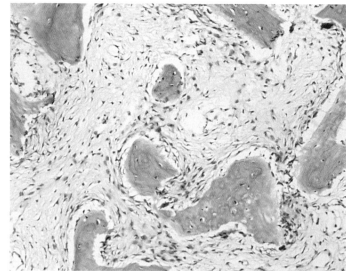

Figure 4.28

c

Figure 4.29 **Congenital pseudarthrosis** This congenital abnormality may be noted at birth or during early childhood. Neurofibromatosis is present in a high percentage of children with this condition. It consists of a fibrous defect in the diaphysis of the affected bone, usually the distal tibia. Radiologically, a lytic defect is present in the lower tibia and there is a bowing deformity of the tibia and fibula (a). The bone ends are covered by cellular and collagenous connective tissue which also fills the defect (b, c). A synovial lining may rarely form over parts of the fibrous tissue.

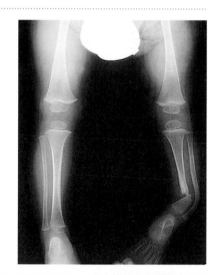

Figure 4.29

a

b c

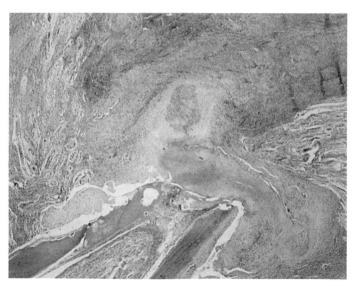

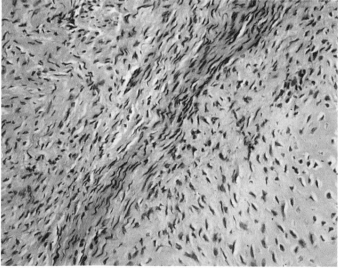

Figure 4.30 **Slipped capital femoral epiphysis (adolescent coxa vara)** This condition occurs predominantly in early adolescence, more commonly in males than females. It is due to spontaneous separation of the epiphysis from the metaphysis along the growth plate, resulting in a displacement, usually posterior, of the epiphysis from the diaphysis. Malalignment of the femoral head and neck results. Complications include avascular necrosis and secondary osteoarthritis. An increased incidence of chondrolysis has been noted in association with a slipped epiphysis in some patients. Specimens taken just after the displacement has occurred are rarely seen, but following healing, the growth plate is irregular, fragmented, and folded (as shown here).

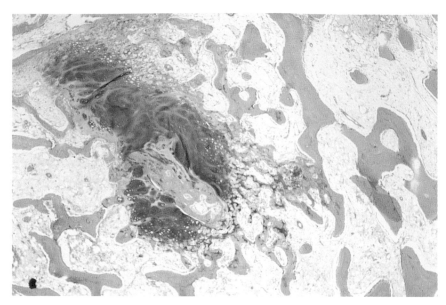

Figure 4.30

Figure 4.31 **Congenital dislocation of hip (CDH)** This common abnormality is not truly congenital but develops after birth. A familial predisposition has been noted. The left hip is more commonly affected but the condition may also affect both hips. The roof of the acetabulum is poorly formed and shallow, leading to instability of the hip and subluxation. The femoral head becomes flattened and comes to lie over the edge of the acetabulum. Both the acetabulum and femoral head develop abnormally. As a result there is early development of secondary osteoarthritis of the hip. Shown is a specimen radiograph of a femoral head showing osteoarthritic changes secondary to CDH. There is erosion and flattening of the articular surface, which is dome- or mushroom-shaped, and hypoplasia of the capital epiphysis.

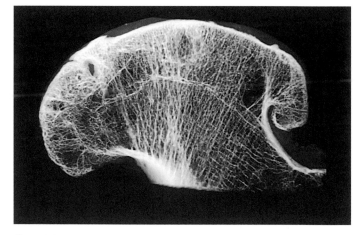

Figure 4.31

5

Metabolic and endocrine disorders of the skeleton

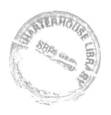

Introduction

Histopathology plays an important role in the evaluation of metabolic bone disorders. Pathological findings should always be interpreted in the light of the clinical and radiological findings and the results of biochemical and other investigations. The histopathological diagnosis of metabolic bone disorders requires an assessment of the relative amounts of mineral and organic matrix in bone. For this purpose undecalcified specimens need to be examined. This assessment is aided by histomorphometric analysis of matrix components and the number and activity of different cells in bone. Useful information on the status of bone mineralization is also provided by dynamic studies of the bone remodelling system; this follows the administration of fluorochromes such as tetracycline which are deposited at sites of bone mineralization. Changes in the range of normal histomorphometric values vary depending on the age and sex of the patient, the patient population, the bone which is sampled, as well as the technique of histological preparation. A general guide to the changes in bone histomorphometry occurring in a number of common metabolic bone disorders is shown in Table 5.1.

Table 5.1 Changes in bone histomorphometric values in selected metabolic bone disorders

	Trabecular bone volume	Osteoid volume	Active osteoblastic surface	Resorption surface	Number of birefringent lamellae	Mineral apposition rate	Osteoid maturation time
Primary hyperparathyroidism	↓/Normal	↑	↑	↑	<4	↑	Normal
Osteomalacia (vitamin D deficiency)	↑/Normal	↑	↑	Normal/↑	>4	↓	↑
Osteoporosis (inactive)	↓	Normal	↓	Normal	<4	↓/Normal	↑/Normal
Osteoporosis (active)	↓	↑	↑/Normal	↑	<4	↑/Normal	↑/Normal
Paget's disease (active)	↑	↑	↑	↑	<4	↑/Normal	Normal

Figure 5.1 **Primary hyperparathyroidism** Primary hyperparathyroidism is most commonly due to a single parathyroid adenoma; multiple adenomas are usually seen in association with multiple endocrine neoplasia, particularly type I. It may also rarely result from primary parathyroid hyperplasia, parathyroid carcinoma, or ectopic parathyroid hormone (PTH) production by tumours. Primary hyperparathyroidism occurs mainly in middle-aged adults and is more common in females than males. Patients may present with renal stones or vague non-specific complaints due to hypercalcaemia but most are asymptomatic. Clinical bone disease is seen in less than 10 per cent of patients. Laboratory investigations reveal hypercalcaemia, hypophosphataemia, and raised serum alkaline phosphatase. Diagnosis is confirmed by finding an elevated PTH level. Radiologically, there is thinning of the cortex, medullary osteopenia, and subperiosteal bone resorption. These changes are often best seen in the hand, particularly on the radial side of the middle phalanges (as shown here); there may also be discrete cystic lesions and erosion of the tufts of the distal phalanges.

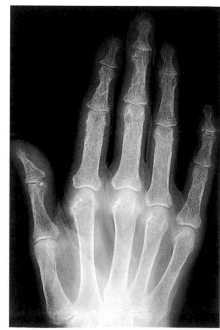

Figure 5.1

Figure 5.2 **Primary hyperparathyroidism** A marked increase in osteoclast numbers and resorptive activity is seen in the bone of patients with hyperparathyroidism (a). There is dissecting resorption of bone trabeculae and paratrabecular fibrosis (b, c). Bone trabeculae are thin; they contain an increased number of cement lines and a variable amount of woven bone (c). The bone cortex shows subperiosteal resorption and widening of Haversian canals by osteoclastic resorption. Bone trabeculae are also covered by a prominent osteoid seam (arrow) which measures less than four birefringent lamellae in thickness (d, von Kossa stain). Correspondingly, there is an increase in the fraction of the trabecular bone surface exhibiting tetracycline uptake (e).

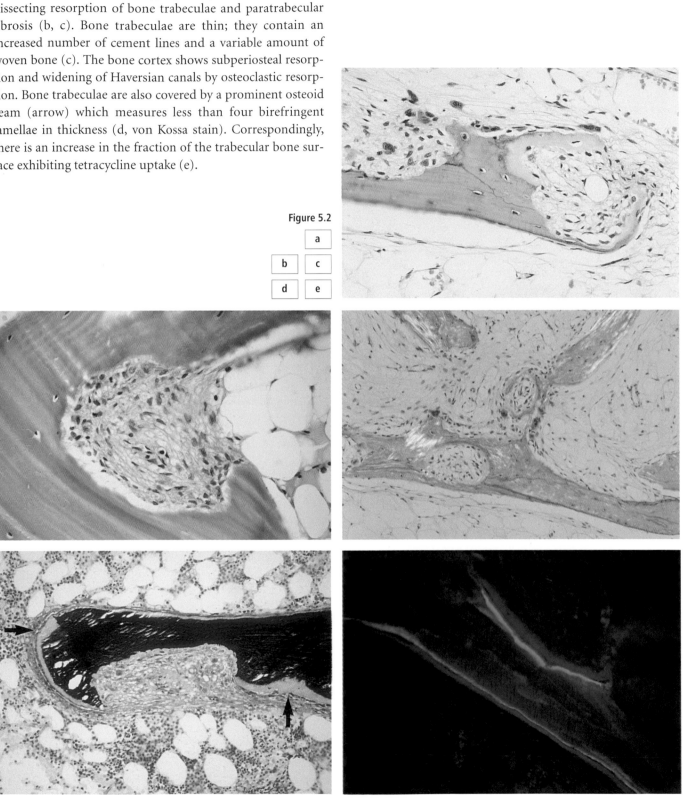

Figure 5.2

	a
b	c
d	e

Figure 5.3 **Brown tumour** This is a large, discrete tumour-like area of osteolysis that arises as a result of hyperparathyroidism. It may be found in any bone but most commonly occurs in the jaw or long tubular bones. 5.3a shows the radiological appearances of a brown tumour of the tibia. The lesion is composed of abundant cellular fibrous tissue containing numerous scattered osteoclast-like giant cells (b, c). Histological appearances are virtually identical to those of giant cell tumour of bone. Unlike brown tumour, the latter usually arises in the epiphysis of a long bone. Histological evidence of hyperparathyroidism may be seen in the bone surrounding a brown tumour. Estimation of serum calcium and phosphate may be necessary to exclude the possibility of a brown tumour when evaluating a giant cell-rich lesion of bone.

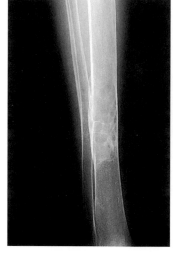

Figure 5.3

a

b c

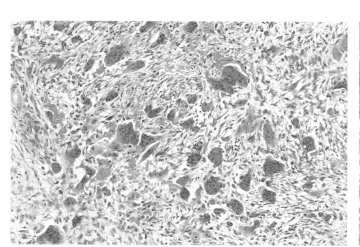

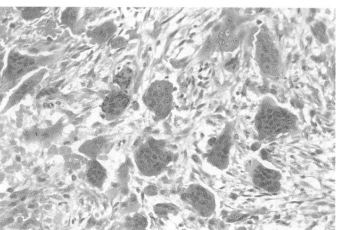

Figure 5.4 **Secondary hyperparathyroidism** Increased secretion of PTH, resulting from hyperplasia of all four parathyroid glands in response to a chronically low serum calcium (secondary hyperparathyroidism), is usually due to renal failure or osteomalacia. Changes in bone are similar to those seen in primary hyperparathyroidism (a, b). Primary and secondary hyperparathyroidism can usually be distinguished by the fact that, although osteoid is present in increased amounts in primary hyperparathyroidism, osteoid seams do not contain more than four birefringent lamellae. 5.4c shows a bone biopsy (stained with toluidine blue) from a case of chronic renal failure with secondary hyperparathyroid bone disease. Under polarized light it can be seen that thickened osteoid seams contain more than four birefringent lamellae. Results of tetracycline labelling are also useful in making this distinction (see below).

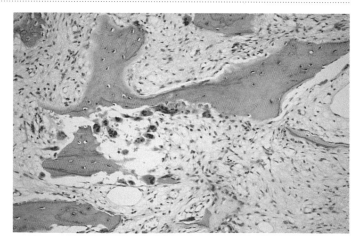

Figure 5.4

a

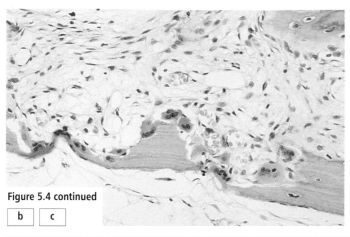
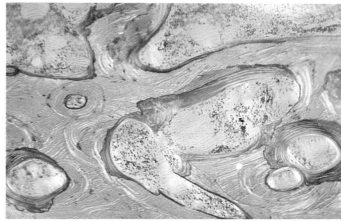

Figure 5.4 continued

b c

Osteomalacia and rickets

A number of conditions which are characterized by failure of normal mineralization of the bone matrix result in the skeletal changes of osteomalacia in adults and rickets in children. These conditions are usually caused by a lack of vitamin D or diseases affecting organs which are involved in vitamin D metabolism (e.g. malabsorptive disorders, renal failure).

Essentially, in both rickets and osteomalacia there is delayed or inadequate mineralization of the osteoid formed by osteoblasts. This undermineralized bone is weaker and more prone to fracture and deformity. Laboratory investigations in patients with vitamin D deficiency rickets/osteomalacia characteristically show low serum calcium, phosphate, and 25-hydroxyvitamin D_3 levels and raised serum alkaline phosphatase.

Figure 5.5 Rickets due to vitamin D deficiency Radiological changes in rickets include cupping and flaring of the metaphysis and broadening of the growth plate which is widened, hazy, and irregular. There is also loss of the sharp line of the zone of provisional calcification, thinning of the cortex, and an abnormal trabecular pattern in medullary bone. These changes are seen in bones around the elbow joint in (a). Histologically, the growth plate in rickets is widened, irregular, and distorted with loss of the regular columnar arrangement (b). Cartilage cells fail to mature and mineralize. Irregular masses of unmineralized cartilage extend into trabeculae in the bone metaphysis. Thick osteoid seams (arrow) cover the projections of growth plate cartilage and underlying metaphyseal bone (c, von Kossa stain).

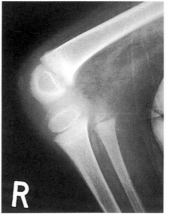
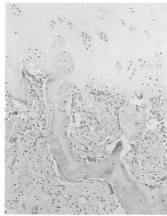

Figure 5.5

b c

a

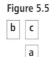
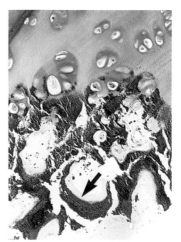

Figure 5.6 **Osteomalacia due to vitamin D deficiency** In osteomalacia, there is generalized weakness and diffuse bone pain on weight bearing and bone tenderness; pathological fractures may occur in the spine, resulting in kyphosis. Radiologically, there is generalized bone rarefaction with a blurred trabecular pattern, linear intracortical streaking, and thinning of the cortex. Typically, there are also pseudofractures (Looser's zones), which are ribbon-like areas of radiolucency lying at right angles to the long axis of the bone cortex; they are commonly bilateral and symmetrical and represent stress fractures that have healed by the deposition of unmineralized osteoid. They may be seen in any bone but most commonly occur in the pubic rami, femur (arrow), upper humerus, ribs, and scapula.

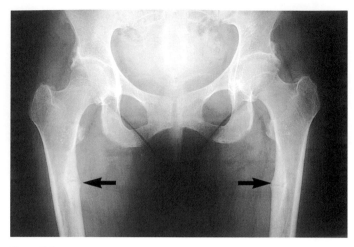

Figure 5.6

Figure 5.7 **Osteomalacia due to vitamin D deficiency** Osteomalacia is characterized by the presence of an excess of unmineralized osteoid in bone. This is seen as a thickened osteoid seam on the surface of trabecular bone and in Haversian channels (a, b, Goldner stain). Under polarized light, the thickened osteoid seams contain more than four birefringent lamellae (c, Goldner stain). Islands of non-mineralized bone matrix may be present within bone trabeculae and around osteocytes (d, Goldner stain); these features are not generally seen in high-turnover states (e.g. Paget's disease). Histomorphometry shows an increase in osteoid volume, the osteoid surface, and the mean width of osteoid seams. Tetracycline labelling shows a diffuse band of fluorescence over bone surfaces (e). Double tetracycline labelling characteristically shows a prolonged mineralization lag time.

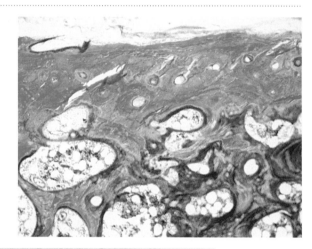

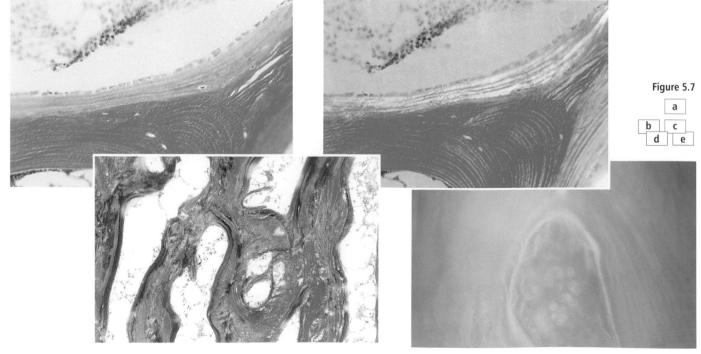

Figure 5.7

| a |
| b | c |
| d | e |

Figure 5.8 **Vitamin D-dependent rickets (VDDR)** This term describes two conditions: VDDR type I and VDDR type II; both are rare errors of vitamin D metabolism which are thought to be inherited autosomal recessive. Type I VDDR usually presents as rickets before the age of 2 years and is thought to be due to a lack or defect in the activity of the renal 1α-hydroxylase enzyme, resulting in an inability to convert 25-hydroxyvitamin D_3 into 1,25-dihydroxyvitamin D_3 ($1,25(OH)_2D_3$). Type II VDDR may present as either rickets or osteomalacia. This condition is thought to be due to end-organ resistance to the active vitamin D metabolite, resulting in inadequate calcium absorption from the gut and abnormal bone metabolism. High circulating levels of $1,25(OH)_2D_3$ are seen. Figure 5.8a shows excessive unmineralized osteoid in VDDR type II (Goldner stain); unmineralized osteoid is greater than four birefringent lamellae under polarized light (b).

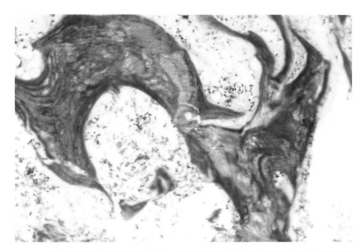

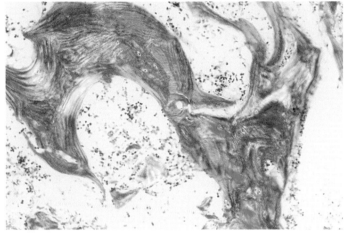

Figure 5.8

a

b

Figure 5.9 **X-linked hypophosphataemic rickets** In this condition, there is a defect in renal proximal tubular reabsorption of phosphate and increased phosphate excretion. This is the most common form of inherited rickets; it is transmitted X-linked dominant (although many cases are sporadic). There is early development of rickets which requires treatment with phosphate supplements and supraphysiological doses of $1,25(OH)_2D_3$. Radiological changes are those of rickets with bone demineralization and wide and irregular epiphyses (a). Histologically, the growth plate is wide and irregular with a decrease in the formation of mineralized bone (b, von Kossa stain). There is normal trabecular bone volume but marked hyperosteoidosis (c, von Kossa stain).

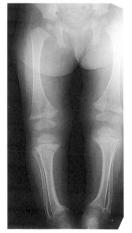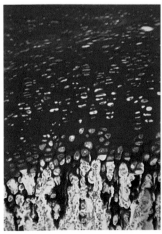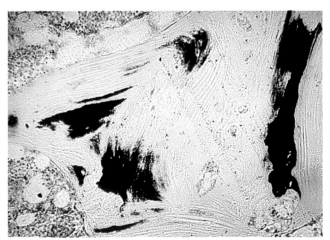

Figure 5.9

 c

Figure 5.10 Hypophosphatasia This is a very rare form of inherited rickets or osteomalacia which is characterized by deficiency of the enzyme alkaline phosphatase, resulting in deficient bone mineralization. Severe forms of the disease are inherited autosomal recessive and present in the neonatal period, infancy, or childhood, whereas milder forms, inherited autosomal dominant, present in adulthood. Prenatal diagnosis of neonatal hypophosphatasia is possible by measuring amniotic fluid levels of alkaline phosphatase. Radiological features of congenital lethal hypophosphatasia are shown. Bones of the skeleton are thin, very poorly developed and show little mineralization. The head appears globular and shows little or no evidence of ossification. Histological features are those of rickets with little evidence of mineralization of cartilage columns in the growth plate.

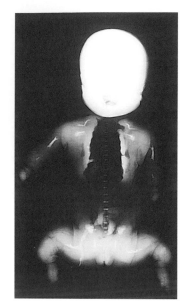

Figure 5.10

Figure 5.11 Hypophosphataemic osteomalacia Phosphate depletion may be due to a number of inherited or acquired conditions. These include phosphaturic renal tubular disorders such as Fanconi's syndrome. Hypophosphataemia may also result from low dietary intake of phosphate or overuse of aluminium-containing phosphorus-binding antacids. Hypophosphataemia and phosphaturia may also be seen in oncogenic osteomalacia, which is a rare condition that occurs most commonly in association with a number of benign and malignant mesenchymal tumours (e.g. haemangiopericytoma, giant cell tumour of tendon sheath); it has also rarely been reported in association with carcinomas, leukaemias, and myeloma. In oncogenic osteomalacia, bone changes are those of osteomalacia with thickened osteoid seams and little or no evidence of secondary hyperparathyroidism (shown here, Goldner stain). Resolution of the bone condition follows removal of the tumour. Pathogenesis is unknown but may be associated with secretion of a humoral factor that impairs phosphate reabsorption.

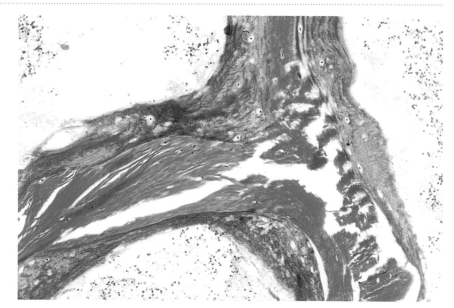

Figure 5.11

Figure 5.12 **Renal osteodystrophy** Renal osteodystrophy is the term used to describe the variety of bone changes and alterations in mineral metabolism that occur in chronic renal failure. These include secondary hyperparathyroidism (due partly to phosphate retention and lower serum levels of ionized calcium), osteomalacia (which occurs as a result of reduced 1α-hydroxylase activity, resulting in decreased production of the active form of vitamin D), osteopaenia and aluminium accumulation (see below). This may produce high-turnover renal bone disease where changes of hyperparathyroidism, including marrow fibrosis and dissecting resorption, predominate (a). In undecalcified sections, osteoid seams covering bone trabeculae may contain more than four birefringent lamellae (b, Ladewig stain). Normal or increased rates of mineral uptake may be found after tetracycline administration (c). In low-turnover renal bone disease the bone shows changes of osteomalacia or appears adynamic with normal or reduced amounts of osteoid, decreased bone cell activity and a low bone formation rate. These cases show either no tetracycline uptake or only a narrow band of fluorescence on the trabecular bone surface (d).

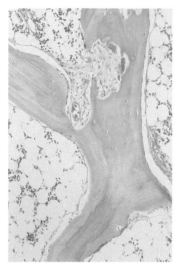 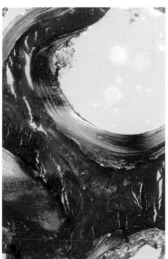 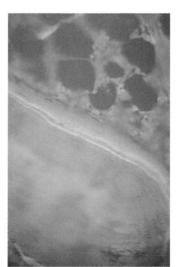 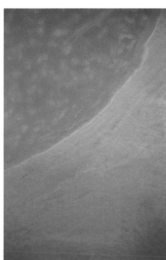

Figure 5.12

| a | b | c | d |

Figure 5.13 **Aluminium bone disease** Low-turnover renal bone disease and osteomalacia were found to occur in uraemic patients on long-term maintenance haemodialysis where a high aluminium content was present in the water supply. Deposition of aluminium at the mineralization front results in a mineralization defect and osteoid accumulation. Aluminium deposition is demonstrated by special stains such as Solochrome Azurine, (shown here), which marks the site of the aluminium deposition at the mineralization front; the osteoid seam is thickened. Aluminium deposition in bone may also result from the excessive use of aluminium-containing antacids to control hyperphosphataemia and is a complication of total parental nutrition.

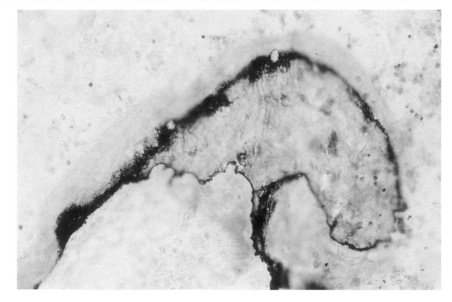

Figure 5.13

Figure 5.14 **Bone disease due to vitamin C deficiency (scurvy)** Vitamin C deficiency (scurvy) is now a rare cause of bone disease in developed countries. Vitamin C promotes hydroxylation of proline and lysine and is essential for the formation of a stable collagen molecule. All connective tissues are affected by the decrease in collagen formation. In bone, it is particularly evident in areas of increased osteoid formation such as the metaphysis in a growing child. Radiologically, the growth plate is widened and irregular (a). An area of radiolucency is present in the metaphysis; the overlying growth plate may also contain a prominent sclerotic zone. The cortex is thin and there is generalized osteopenia. Histologically, there is persistence of the provisional zone of calcified cartilage of the growth plate due to a failure to form normally mineralized osteoid. Little or no matrix formation is seen by osteoblasts at the growth plate. Bone trabeculae are thin and irregular but do not exhibit a mineralization defect. Fractures through the growth plate may occur. There is also weakening of connective tissue in the blood vessel walls and in consequence there is often subperiosteal and intraosseous (b) haemorrhage.

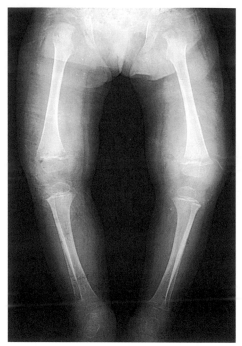

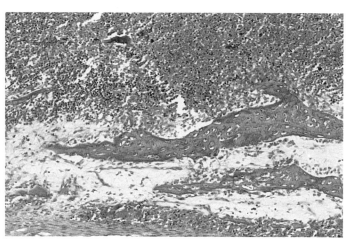

Figure 5.14

a   b

Osteoporosis

Osteoporosis is the most common metabolic bone disease and may be defined as a decrease in bone mass per unit of volume; the bone is normal in composition but there is effectively too little of it, resulting in an increased risk of fracture. Osteoporosis is classified as primary when a causal factor for bone loss cannot be identified, or secondary when it occurs as a consequence of another disease or treatment. The two most common forms of primary osteoporosis are post-menopausal and senile (age-related) osteoporosis; these are also referred to as type I and type II osteoporosis respectively. Primary idiopathic osteoporosis may rarely occur in pre-pubertal children, adolescents (juvenile osteoporosis), and young adults. Post-menopausal osteoporosis mainly affects women in the first two decades after the menopause and is manifested chiefly as a loss of trabecular bone; it thus affects those bones which contain relatively more trabecular bone such as the vertebrae and distal radius. In senile osteoporosis, a proportionally greater loss of cortical bone occurs and fractures present most commonly in the femur, humerus, tibia, and pelvis.

Figure 5.15 Osteoporosis 5.15a shows the radiological changes in the spine of a case of post-menopausal osteoporosis. The vertebral bodies show thinning of the cortex with loss of trabecular bone and prominence of the vertebral end plates; the intervertebral disc protrudes into the vertebral body resulting in the formation of biconcave codfish vertebrae (a); wedge fractures with collapse of one or more vertebral bodies are also seen. 5.15b shows a fracture of the left femoral neck occurring in a case of senile osteoporosis. The bones show marked thinning of the cortex and loss of trabecular bone. Single or dual proton energy X-ray absorptiometry (densitometry) provides a more sensitive measure of bone mass and frac-ture risk than plain radiographs. Laboratory investigations in osteoporosis usually reveal normal serum calcium, phosphate, and alkaline phosphatase.

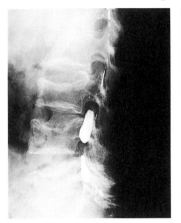
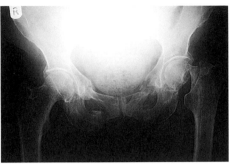

Figure 5.15

a b

Figure 5.16 Osteoporosis (low-turnover) Histologically, most cases of osteoporosis are classified as inactive or low-turnover in type with little or no evidence of osteoblastic or osteoclastic activity. There is loss of trabecular bone and thinning of the cortex (a, Ladewig stain). Osteoporotic bone remains lamellar in type and is normally mineralized. Bone trabeculae are widely separated and thin (b); as a general guide, trabecular thickness in osteoporosis is usually less than the diameter of an adipocyte in surrounding fatty marrow (c). Small islands rather than bars of trabecular bone may be present in fatty marrow (button phenomenon) (d). The bone cortex is thin and shows prominent widening of Haversian channels (e, Goldner stain) Bone histomorphometric measurements confirm that there is a decrease in the total and trabecular bone volume and a decrease in the number of bone trabeculae showing tetracycline labelling.

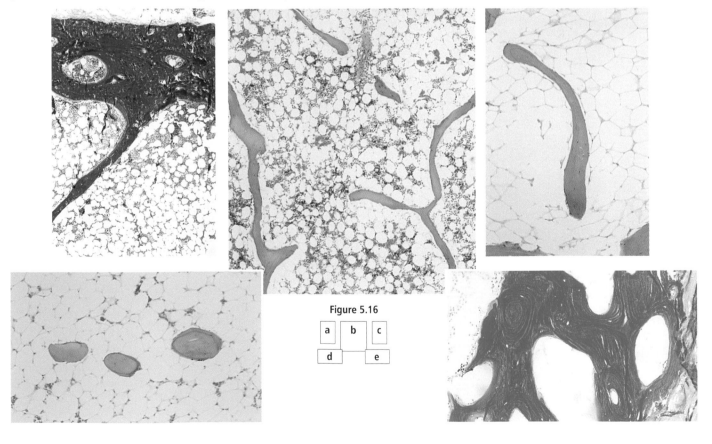

Figure 5.16

a b c
d e

Figure 5.17 **Osteoporosis (high-turnover)** About one third of osteoporotic patients have high-turnover or active osteoporosis in which there is an increase in osteoblast numbers, prominent osteoid formation, as well as increased resorptive activity. Osteoid seams are less than four birefringent lamellae in thickness (a, b, Ladewig's stain). Bone resorption with focal paratrabecular fibrosis may also be seen in some cases (c). In active osteoporosis, the fraction of trabecular surfaces exhibiting double labels is normal or increased as there is a general increase in osteoblastic and osteoclastic activity.

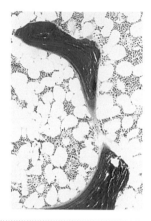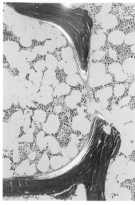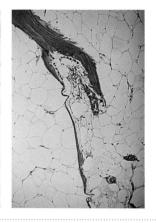

Figure 5.17

a b c

Figure 5.18 **Secondary osteoporosis** Osteoporosis may occur secondary to a large number of endocrine, genetic, or other causes. Steroid-induced osteoporosis, occurring as a complication of glucocorticoid therapy or Cushing's disease, is the most common form of secondary osteoporosis. In addition to the pathological and radiological changes of osteoporosis, there may be other complications related to steroid therapy (e.g. avascular necrosis). 5.18a shows reparative fibrous tissue and active osteoclastic resorption of thin bone trabeculae in a case of Cushing's disease with avascular necrosis of the femoral head. High-turnover and/or low-turnover bone disease may be seen histologically. Other endocrine conditions associated with osteoporosis include hypogonadism, diabetes, and thyrotoxicosis; the latter commonly shows active osteoporosis with increased osteoclastic and osteoblastic activity and prominent osteoid seams (b, von Kossa stain: polarized light).

Figure 5.18

a b

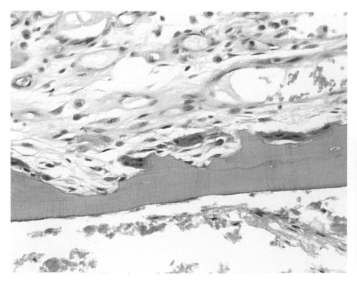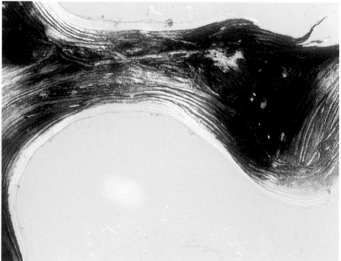

Figure 5.19 Paget's disease of bone Paget's disease is a relatively common condition which is characterized by disordered bone remodelling. It is more common in males than females and usually occurs in patients over 40 years of age. It may affect only one bone or several bones, usually asymmetrically. Patients present with bone pain, pathological fracture, deformity, and neurological complications. The pelvis, lumbar spine, femur, tibia, and skull are most often affected. 5.19a shows the radiological features of Paget's disease in the proximal femur. Bones affected by Paget's disease are enlarged, have a thickened cortex, and show coarse calcification and mottled thickening of the medullary bone. In the early stages, osteolysis dominates; later, new bone formation is seen in both the medulla and cortex, producing sclerosis, bone expansion, and coarsening of trabeculae. The sclerotic cortex contains coarse striations and there is loss of the normal corticomedullary differentiation. In the spine, vertebral trabeculae are prominent and coarse; sclerosis of the end plates produces the characteristic 'window-frame' appearance (b).

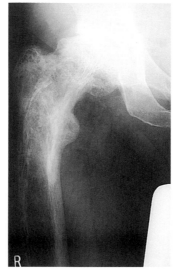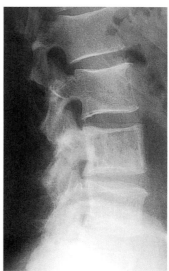

Figure 5.19

a b

Figure 5.20 Paget's disease of bone Histological features vary with the stage of the disease. Early changes include an increase in osteoclast numbers and the presence of numerous Howship's lacunae on the surface of bone which has a prominent mosaic cement line pattern (a, b). Osteoclasts are large and have more nuclei than normal; some nuclei may appear apoptotic. The bone marrow is well vascularized and contains an increase in cellular fibrous tissue (c). Under polarized light, it is evident that the bone architecture is abnormal (d); bone trabec-ulae are thickened, have a disordered lamellar pattern, and contain a variable amount of woven bone. In active Paget's disease, osteoblastic activity is evident on the surface of bone trabeculae and Haversian channels. Osteoid seams may be prominent but measure less than four birefringent lamellae in thickness (e, Goldner stain). In later stages of the disease, cellular activity is decreased and few or no osteoblasts or osteoclasts are seen. An elevation in serum alkaline phosphatase and normal calcium and phosphate are usually seen in active Paget's disease.

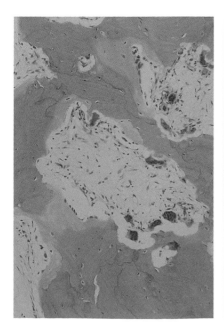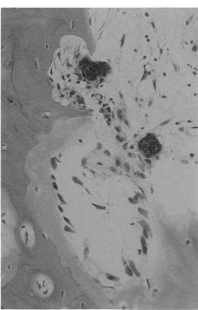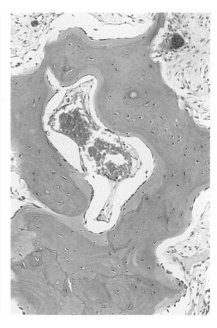

Figure 5.20

a b c

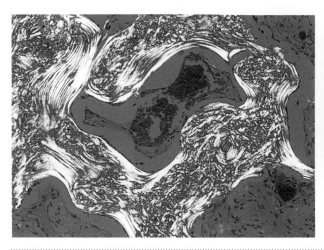
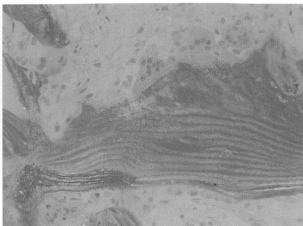

Figure 5.20
continued

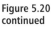

Figure 5.21 Osteomalacia in bisphosphonate-treated Paget's disease Some bisphosphonates used in high doses to treat Paget's disease (particularly sodium etidronate) may inhibit bone mineralization and lead to the development of osteomalacia. There is a marked increase in the width of the osteoid seam which contains more than four birefringent lamellae (a, b, Goldner stain). This complication may also be seen when bisphosphonates are used to treat other conditions such as ectopic ossification.

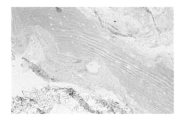
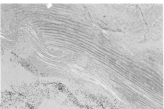

Figure 5.21

Figure 5.22 Fibrogenesis imperfecta ossium (FIO) This is a rare bone condition characterized by the production of an abnormal osteoid matrix which does not mineralize properly. Typically, the disease presents in adults with bone pain and tenderness; multiple pathological fractures occur, often in unusual sites. Serum alkaline phosphatase is often raised. 5.22a shows radiological features of FIO in the hand. Bone trabeculae appear coarse and irregular in texture and the bone cortex appears thin; there is no expansion of the bone as in Paget's disease. Vertebral collapse may occur in the spine (b). Histologically, bone trabeculae are of variable thickness but often broad with central areas composed of mineralized lamellar bone (c); the surface is covered by an eosinophilic osteoid material which is either non-birefringent or only patchily birefringent (d). A prominent cement line marks the border between mineralized and unmineralized tissue. Marrow fibrosis is not seen and there is variable osteoblastic and osteoclastic activity. A paraproteinaemia has been noted in some FIO patients. The abnormal osteoid matrix contains thin collagen fibrils which are randomly organized in a manner similar to amyloid. The course of the disease is progressive and patients die of complications associated with pathological fractures.

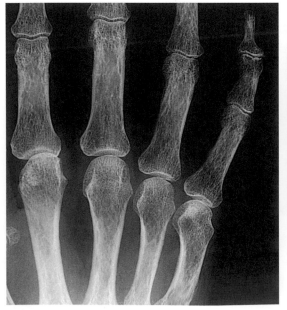
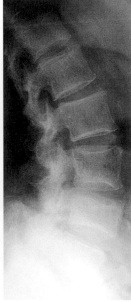

Figure 5.22

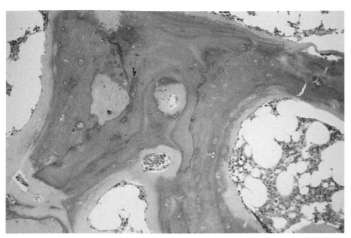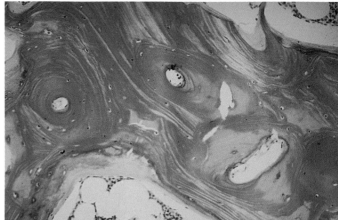

Figure 5.22 continued

| c | d |

Figure 5.23 Fluorosis Excessive fluoride ingestion may occur as a result of industrial exposure or exposure to a water supply containing a high fluoride content. The fluoride becomes deposited in the skeleton where it promotes new bone formation. This occurs within the medullary cavity, beneath the periosteum, and at points of ligament and tendon insertion, resulting in the formation of bony spurs and spinal osteophytes. Bone trabeculae appear widened and there is appositional osteoid and new bone formation. Matrix mineralization is impaired and osteoid accumulates over much of the trabecular bone surface (a, b, Ladewig stain). An increase in osteoblastic and osteoclastic activity may also be noted.

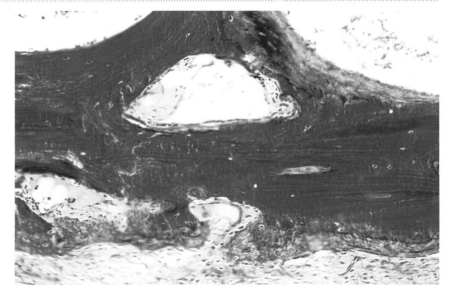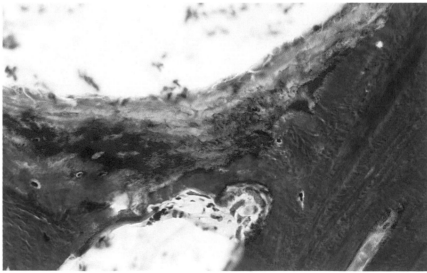

Figure 5.23

| a |

| b |

Figure 5.24 Mastocytosis An increase in the number of mast cells in marrow spaces may be seen in a number of osteolytic conditions including osteoporosis, secondary hyperparathyroidism, and Paget's disease. Patients with urticaria pigmentosa and systemic mastocytosis may also show an increase in the number of mast cells (arrowed) in the marrow (a, Goldner stain). This may lead to osteopenia. Mast cells are readily identified by the presence of metachromatic cytoplasmic granules on toluidine blue staining (b). Rarely, a discrete tumour, a mastocytoma, composed entirely of mast cells may occur in bone.

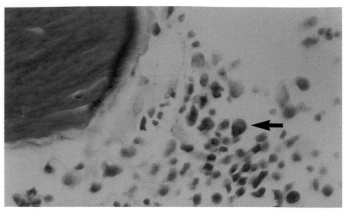

Figure 5.24

a

b

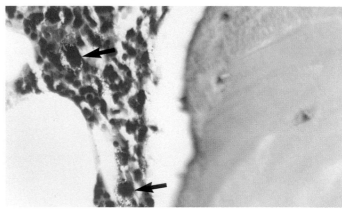

Figure 5.25 Oxalosis Primary familial oxalosis usually presents in childhood but may occasionally present in adulthood. There is deposition of calcium oxalate crystals in many tissues including bone and bone marrow. It may cause nephrolithiasis which leads to the development of chronic renal failure. Secondary oxalosis occurs more commonly than primary oxalosis and is usually due to chronic renal failure. Histological features in these two conditions are indistinguishable. Oxalate crystals are deposited in mineralized bone, articular cartilage, and bone marrow. They form star-like clusters of long, rod- or needle-shaped crystals (a, toluidine blue) that are strongly birefringent under polarized light (b). A macrophage and giant cell reaction to the deposits of crystals may be seen.

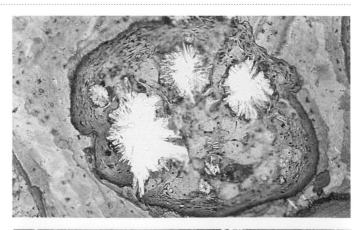

Figure 5.25

a

b

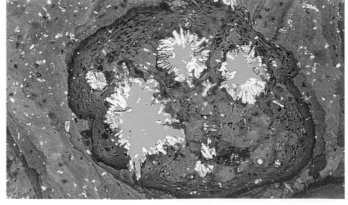

6

Diseases of joints and periarticular tissues

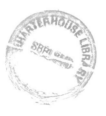

Introduction

In interpreting the pathology of joint tissues, it is important to examine changes which occur in all the osteoarticular tissues that make up the joint (i.e. the articular cartilage, subchondral bone, synovial membrane, and capsule as well as periarticular structures such as ligaments and tendons). Gross examination of joint specimens and specimen radiography are often useful in assessing changes in the articular surface and subchondral bone; the latter also aids in the selection of blocks for histolo-.gical examination. Biochemical and cytological analysis of the synovial fluid, as well as examination for crystals, is also important in determining the cause of an arthritic condition. It should be recognized that pathological changes in joint tissues do not always permit identification of a specific cause of arthritic disease.

Osteoarthritis (degenerative joint disease; osteoarthrosis)

Osteoarthritis (OA) is the commonest form of joint disease. It is characterized by the presence of degenerative changes in the articular cartilage. It mainly affects large weight-bearing joints, especially the hip and knee, of elderly individuals. OA usually develops in a previously normal joint (primary OA). In some forms of primary generalized OA, where multiple joints are affected, often symmetrically, a familial incidence has been noted; this is associated with the development of Heberden's nodes in the distal interphalangeal joints of the hand. Other patterns of primary OA involvement of one or more joints have also been described. Pathological changes of OA may also be superimposed on a previously diseased joint (secondary OA). The pathological changes of OA represent a final common pathway of many diseases affecting articular tissues.

Figure 6.1 Osteoarthritis
Degenerative changes in the articular surface are evidenced radiologically as narrowing of the joint space, sclerosis of the subchondral bone, formation of osteophytes and subchondral pseudocysts. In the hip (a), degenerative changes occur mainly in the zenith region, and in the knee joint (b), mainly in the medial compartment of the tibiofemoral joint. 6.1c shows the gross appearance of a cut surface of the femoral head. There is loss of articular cartilage, exposure of subchondral bone, osteophyte formation and several large subchondral pseudocysts opening onto the articular surface. The extent of pathological changes in OA is often best revealed by specimen radiographs. 6.1d shows a specimen radiograph of an osteoarthritic femoral head. There is erosion of the articular surface, thickening of the subchondral bone plate, pseudocyst and osteophyte formation, as well as thickening of the femoral neck and areas of rarefaction and thickening of subchondral cancellous bone.

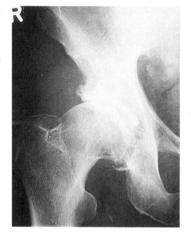
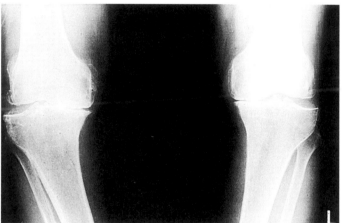

Figure 6.1

a	b
c	d

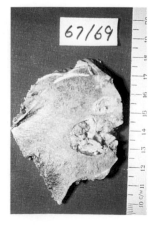
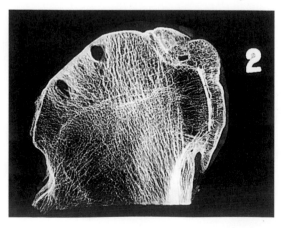

Figure 6.2 **Osteoarthritis**

Initial changes of OA are seen in articular cartilage. There is loss of matrix staining and surface fibrillation (i.e. development of numerous small cracks or splits) in the superficial zone of the articular cartilage (a). Later, deeper fissures or clefts develop in the articular cartilage which becomes reduced in thickness (b, c). These fissures are mainly oriented at right angles to the joint surface but some are oriented tangentially or horizontally. Clusters of cartilage cells which represent areas of cartilage proliferation often lie beneath the clefts and loss of matrix staining extends to the mid and deep zones of the articular cartilage. The underlying subchondral bone plate shows thickening and there is reduplication of the tidemark (arrow).

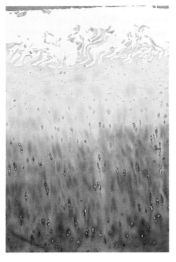 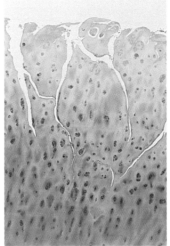 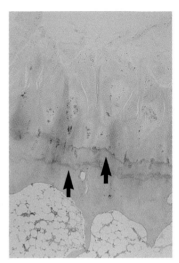

Figure 6.2

a   b   c

Figure 6.3 **Osteoarthritis**

In advanced OA, following loss and erosion of articular cartilage, the articular surface is covered by thickened sclerotic subchondral bone (a). Subchondral cysts, marrow fibrosis, and remodelling changes are seen in the underlying bone. Areas of fibrocartilaginous repair may be seen on the articular surface (b). Due to constant wear, bone covering the eroded articular surface may not only be sclerotic but also show necrotic changes with loss of osteocyte nuclei from lacunae (c). Subchondral pseudocysts have a fibrous wall of variable thickness (d). These cysts, which are usually filled with myxoid or fibromyxoid material, vary greatly in size (from millimetres to several centimetres) and communicate with the articular surface.

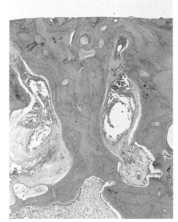 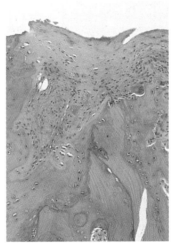 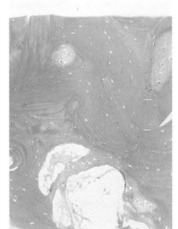

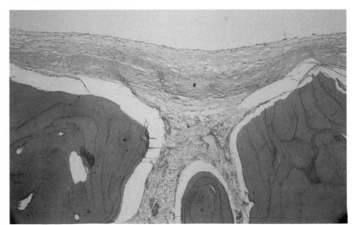

Figure 6.3

a   b   c

d

Figure 6.4 Osteoarthritis In OA, outgrowths of bone and cartilage, termed osteophytes, are formed by endochondral ossification of non-weight-bearing areas of articular cartilage. They are found most commonly at the articular margins (marginal osteophytes) (a). The articular cartilage is derived from embryonic epiphyseal cartilage from which the growth plate is formed; when it becomes vascularized, it may undergo growth-plate-like changes with proliferation of cartilage cells and endochondral ossification. Fibrous and fibrocartilaginous tissue may sometimes be seen on the surface of the osteophyte. In OA, parts of the eroded articular surface may break off and form loose bodies. Loose bodies which lie freely within the joint cavity have a central core of necrotic bone; the covering cartilage remains viable as it is nourished from the synovial fluid (b). The surface of loose bodies may become covered by fibrous tissue or fibrocartilage. 6.4c shows a loose body which has retained a blood supply by a fibrovascular pedicle (arrowed); under these conditions the central bony core remains viable.

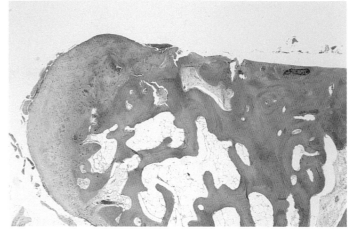

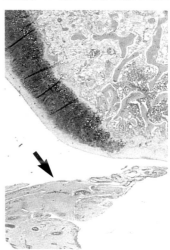

Figure 6.4

| a |
| b | c |

Figure 6.5 Osteoarthritis The synovial membrane in OA commonly shows oedema, fibrosis, and mucinous change in the subintima and patchy intimal thickening. Fragments of bone (arrow) and cartilage derived from the articular surface may become embedded in the membrane (a). A marked osteoclastic reaction in the intima and subintima is sometimes induced by deposition of bony debris derived from the eroded joint (b). Not uncommonly, the synovial membrane in OA shows marked oedema and villous thickening with intimal hyperplasia and a patchy chronic inflammatory infiltrate in the subintima; this may include scattered lymphocytes, plasma cells, and lymphoid aggregates (c). These appearances need to be distinguished from those of an inflammatory arthropathy such as rheumatoid arthritis.

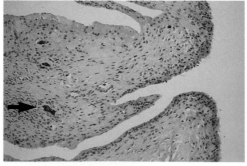
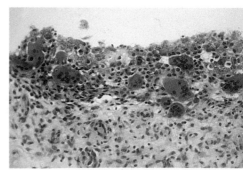
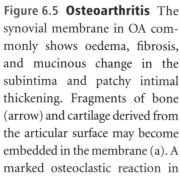
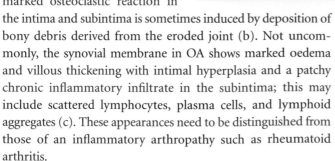
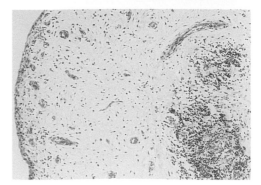

Figure 6.5

| a | b |
| c | |

Figure 6.6 **Neuropathic arthropathy (Charcot joint)** A severe form of secondary OA may develop in patients who have a sensory neuropathy. Loss of pain and proprioception lead to repetitive joint trauma and joint instability with subluxation and sometimes dislocation (a). A rapidly progressive degenerative arthritis develops with loss of articular cartilage, extensive subchondral bone sclerosis, and marked osteophyte formation. Fractures may occur and involve the joint surface. The synovial membrane is thickened and contains numerous large bone and cartilage fragments derived from the articular surface (detritic synovitis) (b).

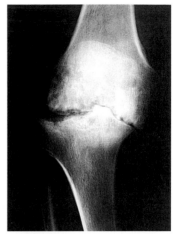

Figure 6.6

a

b

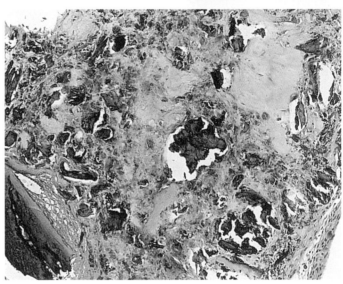

Figure 6.7 **Chondromalacia patellae** In this condition, which is seen most commonly in young adults, there is softening of the articular surface of the patella. Articular cartilage shows changes similar to those seen in early OA with loss of matrix staining in the superficial zone, fibrillation and early fissuring of articular cartilage (as shown here). The pathogenesis is unknown but may be related to trauma. Lateral subluxation of the patella is seen in some patients.

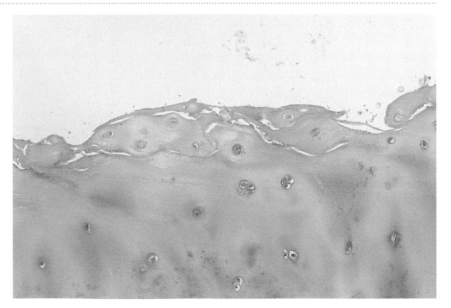

Figure 6.7

Arthritis due to deposition of crystals and other metabolic products

Figure 6.8 Gout Gout is a disorder of purine metabolism in which there is deposition of monosodium urate crystals in articular and other tissues. It is accompanied by hyperuricaemia that may be either endogenous in origin or secondary to conditions which lead to an increase in purine turnover (e.g. leukaemia, psoriasis) or a decrease in renal excretion of uric acid. Gout is much more common in males and generally occurs after the age of 40 years. An increased familial incidence has been noted. In acute gout, a single joint, usually the first metatarsophalangeal joint, becomes suddenly red, hot, swollen, and tender. Attacks recur with periods of remission between them being less complete. The condition eventually develops into one of chronic gout where there is extensive deposition of urate crystals in and around joint tissues; this is accompanied by joint destruction and secondary OA. Radiologically, there is joint swelling and punched out lesions are seen within bone, particularly at the articular margins (a). Gouty tophi, consisting of nodular aggregates of chalky white urate crystals (b), may be seen subcutaneously over bony prominences such as the olecranon.

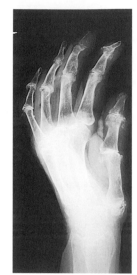
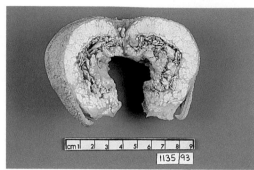

Figure 6.8

a b

Figure 6.9 Gout Deposits of urate crystals are seen in the joint cartilage, synovial membrane, and other periarticular tissues such as bursae, tendons, and ligaments. Histologically, these deposits and tophi contain a central unstained area composed of aggregates of crystals which are surrounded by fibrous tissue containing macrophages and giant cells (a). If the tissue is fixed in alcohol, feathery or 'test-tube brush' collections of crystals may be seen within the central amorphous area (b). This granuloma-like response to urate crystals (arrow) is also seen in areas of bone erosion where there is associated osteoclastic bone resorption (c). The synovial fluid in an acute attack of gout generally shows numerous inflammatory cells, particularly polymorphs, as well as abundant needle-shaped negatively birefringent crystals (d).

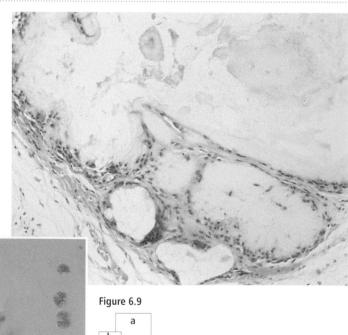

Figure 6.9

a

b

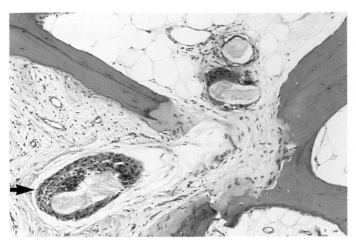

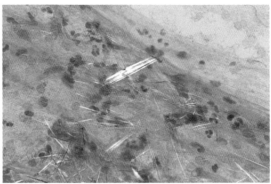

Figure 6.9 continued

Figure 6.10 Pyrophosphate arthropathy Calcium pyrophosphate dihydrate (CPPD) crystal deposition is found quite commonly in articular tissues of the knee joint, especially hyaline articular cartilage and meniscal fibrocartilage. It may also occur in other joints and in intervertebral discs. CPPD deposition is not always accompanied by clinical disease but may be associated with an acute arthritis (pseudogout) or a chronic degenerative arthritis. Radiologically, CPPD deposition in cartilage (chondrocalcinosis) is seen most commonly as a linear area of calcification in the menisci of the knee joint (a). Grossly, scattered chalky-white aggregates of pyrophosphate crystals are often found in the articular cartilage (b), menisci, and synovial tissues.

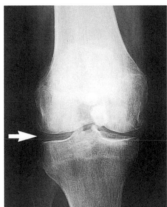

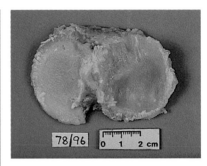

Figure 6.10

Figure 6.11 Pyrophosphate arthropathy 6.11a shows an aggregate of CPPD crystals in the meniscus; the crystals stain grey or purple with routine haematoxylin and eosin staining and under polarized light are seen to contain numerous birefringent rod-shaped crystals; these crystals show positive birefringence. There is usually little inflammatory reaction around CPPD deposits, although occasionally a histiocytic and giant cell response may be noted (b). CPPD deposits are

Figure 6.11

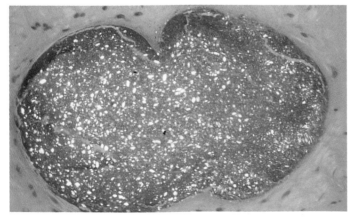

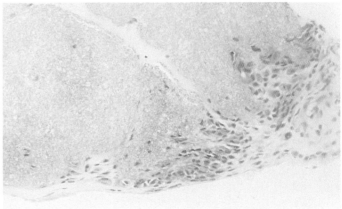

found commonly in the superficial zone of the articular cartilage where they appear as empty spaces (arrow) in histological sections of joint tissues that have been decalcified (c). CPPD deposits may also be found in the synovial membrane which may exhibit a non-specific synovitis with scattered lymphocytes, plasma cells, and macrophages in the subintima (d). In pseudogout, which presents as an acute monoarticular arthritis, rod-shaped positively birefringent crystals are seen in the synovial fluid; a number of these crystals lie within inflammatory cells.

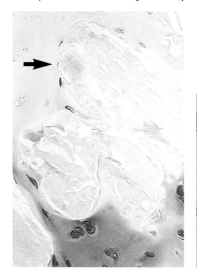
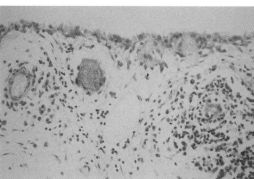
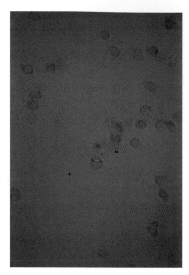

Figure 6.11 continued

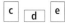

Figure 6.12 Hydroxyapatite (HAP) deposition (basic calcium phosphate) crystal deposition disease Several joint and periarticular conditions have been associated with HAP crystal deposition. Periarticular calcification with HAP crystal deposits may occur in any joint but the shoulder joint is most commonly affected. A severe erosive arthropathy associated with the Milwaukee shoulder syndrome in which there is glenohumeral joint degeneration, soft tissue calcification, and extensive lysis of the rotator cuff may rarely occur. HAP crystal deposition may also occur in chronic renal failure and 'collagen' diseases; crystals may also be found in association with degenerative and inflammatory joint disease. The crystals are too small to be seen by light microscopy. Occasional crystal aggregates in which many of the crystals are oriented along the same axis may appear birefringent under polarized light; these aggregates also stain with alizarin red S. HAP deposition is also seen in calcific tendinitis (see 2.29) and tumoral calcinosis (see 8.99).

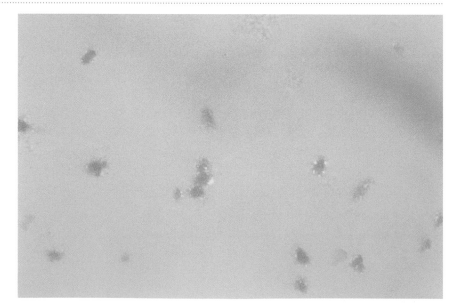

Figure 6.12

Figure 6.13 Ochronosis (alkaptonuria) This condition is due to an autosomal recessive-inherited inborn error of metabolism in which there is an absence or deficiency of homogentisic acid oxidase. This results in accumulation of homogentisic acid in connective tissues including the fibrocartilage of intervertebral discs and hyaline articular cartilage. Deposition of this product makes the cartilage more brittle and predisposes it to joint degeneration. 6.13a

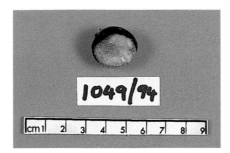

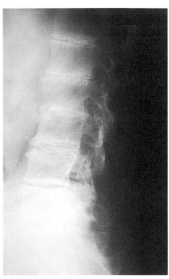

shows the articular surface of a radial head affected by ochronosis. Much of the articular surface is eroded and residual articular cartilage at the edge shows black discoloration. CPPD deposits are also seen in the articular surface and are not uncommonly present in joints affected by ochronosis. In the spine, radiological changes of ochronosis are evidenced by calcification of the intervertebral discs and narrowing of the disc space (b). Histologically, the hyaline articular cartilage shows brown pigmentation with loss and fissuring due to degenerative changes (c). Large fragments of pigmented articular cartilage are deposited in the synovial membrane (d).

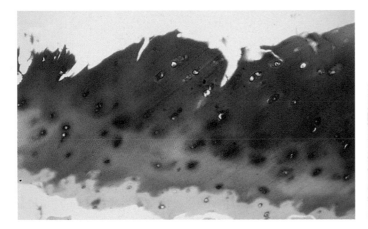

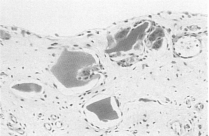

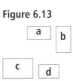

Figure 6.13

a	b
c	d

Figure 6.14 Amyloid arthropathy Joint disease associated with amyloid deposition is now most commonly seen in the context of long-term haemodialysis (or continuous ambulatory peritoneal dialysis) of uraemic patients. This results in extensive deposition of β_2-microglobulin amyloid in articular cartilage, the joint capsule, and periarticular tissues; this is associated with the development of a degenerative arthritis, a spondyloarthropathy, capsular thickening, and formation of large cysts which extend into bone. Staining of affected tissues with Lugol's iodine shows the gross extent of amyloid deposits in involved joints. 6.14a shows amyloid in intervertebral discs and paraspinal connective tissues. In synovial joints, amyloid deposition is identified by Congo red staining and is first seen on the surface of articular cartilage (b); the synovial membrane, capsule, periosteal tissues, and ligaments also commonly contain amyloid deposits. A macrophage and giant cell response may be seen around large amyloid deposits (c). Clinical disease is usually seen after many years on haemodialysis and often more than one joint is affected. Deposition of amyloid in joint tissues may also rarely occur in primary and secondary amyloidosis. 6.1d shows a case of primary (AL) amyloidosis in which there is deposition of abundant eosinophilic amyloid material in subintimal connective tissue of the synovial membrane. Focal areas of amyloid deposition in the superficial zone of the articular cartilage and capsular tissue are also commonly seen in association with ageing; this localized amyloid deposition does not have pathogenic significance.

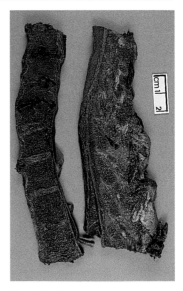

Figure 6.14

a

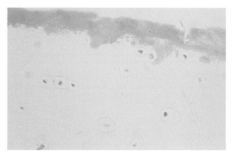 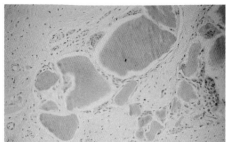 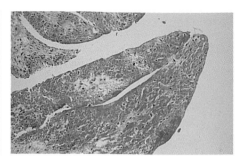

Figure 6.14

[b] [c] [d]

Figure 6.15 **Siderotic synovitis** Siderotic synovitis is a descriptive term which refers to the deposition of haemosiderin within the synovial tissues. This may be due to a number of causes including trauma to the joint, bleeding associated with degenerative or inflammatory joint disease, and avascular necrosis. It is also seen in pigmented villonodular synovitis, synovial haemangioma, and blood dyscrasias such as haemophilia. Similar features may be seen in haemochromatosis and transfusion haemosiderosis. Haemosiderin deposition within the subintima is extensive. Haemosiderin is present within subintimal macrophages and synovial lining cells. There may also be a focal giant cell reaction to haemosiderin and a patchy lymphocytic and plasma cell infiltrate in the synovial membrane.

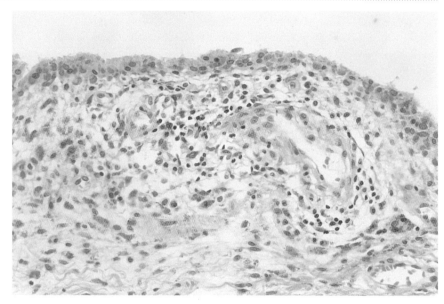

Figure 6.15

Figure 6.16 **Haemophilia** In haemophilia, repeated haemorrhagic joint effusions result in extensive haemosiderin deposition in synovial tissues. This leads to brown discoloration and thickening of the synovial membrane and the articular cartilage, which also shows erosive changes (a). There is marked synovial haemosiderin deposition (b); this is evidenced by extensive staining for iron using a Perl's stain (c). Degenerative joint disease is also seen with loss and destruction of articular cartilage and erosive changes in bone, including cyst formation (d). Extensive bleeding into soft tissues may result in the formation of a haemophiliac pseudotumour (e).

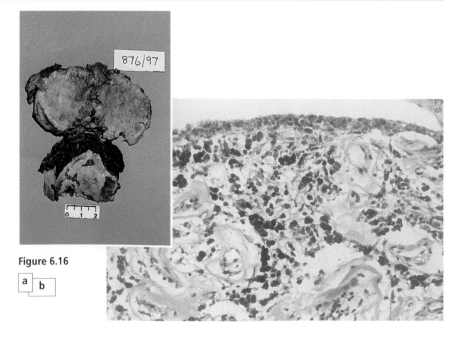

Figure 6.16

[a] [b]

Figure 6.16

c d e

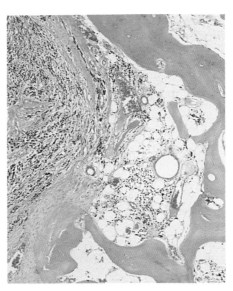
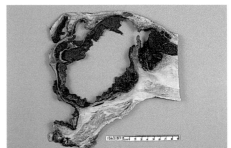

Figure 6.17 **Foreign body synovitis** A penetrating injury of the joint capsule may be followed by implantation of foreign material which may induce a non-specific inflammatory synovitis. This usually results in a monoarticular arthritis. The fingers, wrist, and knee joint are most commonly affected. Recognized causes of this synovitis include plant thorns, wood particles, silica, plastic, and sea-urchin spines. Thorn injuries usually result in a chronic non-specific synovitis with a prominent lymphocytic infiltrate in the subintima (a); occasionally a heavy acute inflammatory infiltrate may be seen (b). A granulomatous synovitis may be associated with implantation of a sea urchin spine (c).

Figure 6.17

a

b c

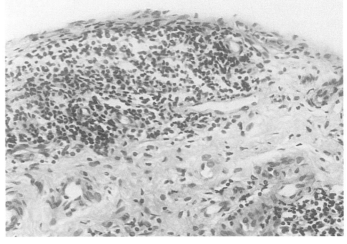
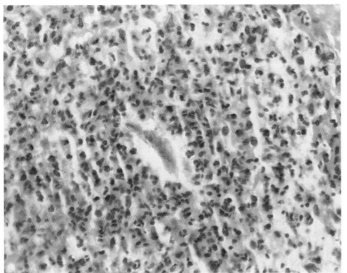
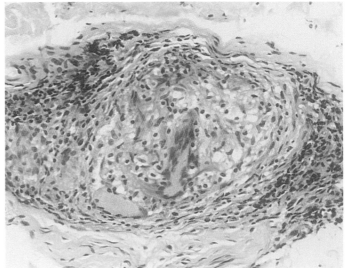

Rheumatoid arthritis

Rheumatoid arthritis (RA) is a common chronic inflammatory disease which principally affects joints but may also involve other tissues. It may arise at any age but onset is most frequent between the third and fifth decades of life. Females are more often affected than males. There is often a family history of the disease and most affected individuals are HLA-DR4 or HLA-DR1 positive, indicating a genetic predisposition. About 80 per cent of individuals have IgM autoantibodies to the Fc portion of autologous IgG (rheumatoid factor) in the serum. There is usually bilateral, symmetrical involvement of small joints of the hand, particularly the metacarpophalangeal and proximal interphalangeal joints; joints of the wrist, elbow, knee, ankle, and cervical spine are also commonly affected. Inflammatory changes begin in the synovium and extend over the articular surface; they also involve periarticular structures such as tendons and ligaments. This results in joint instability with subluxation and dislocation of affected joints.

Figure 6.18 Rheumatoid arthritis 6.8a shows the radiological changes of RA in the joints of the hands. There is narrowing of the joint space, loss of articular cartilage, juxta-articular osteopenia, and formation of marginal erosions. Grossly, rheumatoid joints have thickened tan or pale synovium. The articular surface of affected joints is covered by white inflammatory exudate and reparative fibrous tissue which extends from the articular margins, replacing articular cartilage; this becomes thicker and more fibrotic with progression of the disease (b).

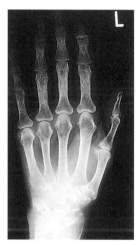
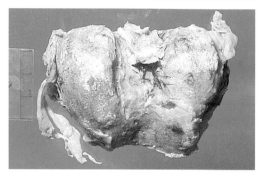

Figure 6.18

a b

Figure 6.19 Rheumatoid arthritis In early RA, the synovial membrane shows oedema, congestion, and ulceration with fibrin exudation (a). There is a mixed acute and chronic inflammatory infiltrate in which neutrophils are prominent (b). Later, the synovial membrane shows more marked villous hypertrophy and the subintima contains a heavy chronic inflammatory infiltrate composed largely of lymphocytes and plasma cells with scattered lymphoid aggregates and follicles (c); the covering synovial intima is thickened (arrow) due to recruitment of type A macrophage-like synovial lining cells (d). Eosinophilic cytoplasmic inclusions (Russell bodies) (arrow) may be seen in subintimal plasma cells which contain abundant immunoglobulin (e). Small fibrin bodies, which may contain a few inflammatory cells, may be attached to the synovial membrane or lie loose in the joint cavity (f). The synovial lining of tendon sheaths and bursae shows similar inflammatory changes to those seen in joints.

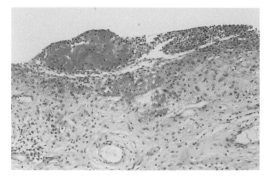
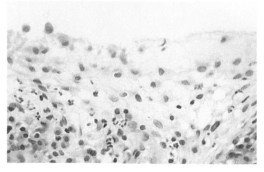
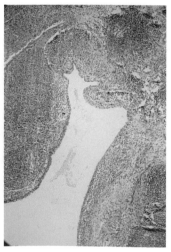

Figure 6.19

a b c

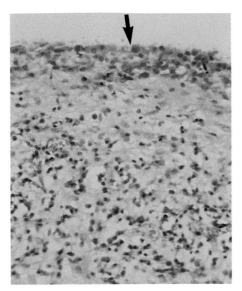
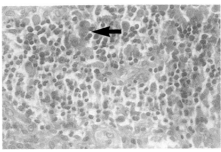
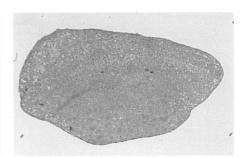

Figure 6.19 continued

d e f

Figure 6.20 Rheumatoid arthritis The inflamed synovial tissue (pannus) extends over the articular surface from the articular margin. There is destruction and replacement of articular cartilage (a, b). Articular cartilage in the vicinity of the spreading rheumatoid pannus is often covered by a fibrinous exudate (c); there is also loss of matrix staining and necrosis of chondrocytes in the superficial zone. The subchondral bone marrow commonly contains a scattered chronic inflammatory cell infiltrate including lymphocytes, plasma cells, and lymphoid aggregates (d). There is also often subchondral osteopenia due to relative disuse of the affected joint or as a consequence of steroid therapy.

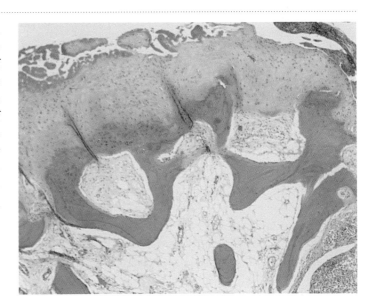

Figure 6.20

a

b c d

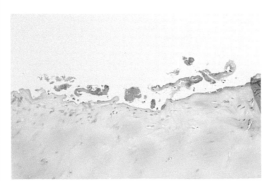
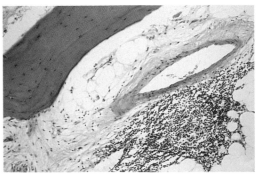

Figure 6.21 Rheumatoid arthritis Inflammatory pannus in RA extends from the synovium into adjacent bone which undergoes active resorption, resulting in the formation of marginal erosions (a). After the articular cartilage has been destroyed, inflammatory pannus is replaced by cellular and collagenous fibrous tissue. Fibrous tissue bridges the gap between the two articular surfaces and fibrous ankylosis results (b); bony ankylosis may also rarely occur. This accounts for the development of the fixed deformities characteristic of this condition.

Figure 6.21

| a | b |

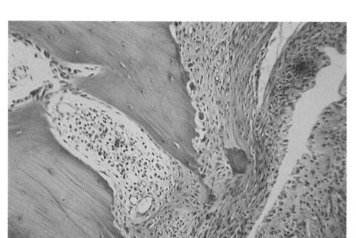
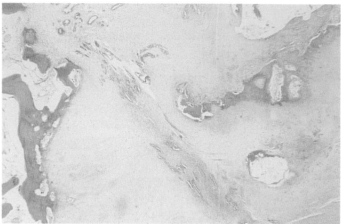

Figure 6.22 Rheumatoid nodules and vasculitis Rheumatoid nodules are found in 25 per cent of RA patients, usually those with severe seropositive disease. They are most commonly found over bony prominences, particularly around the elbow joint, the ulnar aspect of the forearm, and the occiput, but may occur elsewhere. Histologically, rheumatoid nodules consist of multiple rheumatoid granulomas, each of which is composed of a central stellate area of fibrinoid necrosis with a surrounding palisade of plump epithelioid macrophages and fibroblasts (a, b). A scattered chronic inflammatory cell infiltrate, composed largely of lymphocytes and plasma cells, is often present in

Figure 6.22

| a | b |

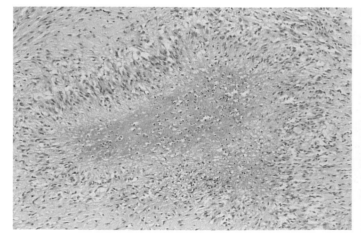
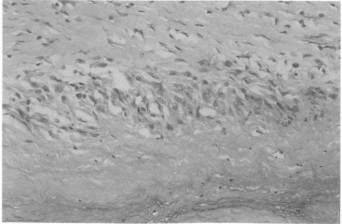

surrounding connective tissue. A focal lymphocytic and plasma cell infiltrate is often seen in extra-articular tissues (e.g. heart valve, eye) that are affected in RA. A vasculitis affecting small and medium-sized arterial vessels and venules may also occur in RA. This may be an acute vasculitis resembling polyarteritis nodosa, a leucocytoclastic venulitis (c) in which there is fibrin exudation and a heavy polymorph infiltrate in the vessel wall, or a subacute vasculitis (d) in which chronic inflammatory cells, largely lymphocytes, surround affected vessels.

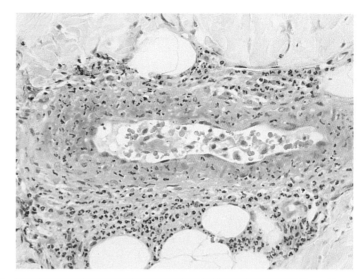

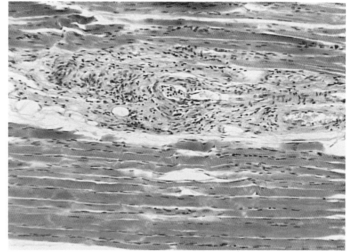

Figure 6.22

c

d

Figure 6.23 **Juvenile rheumatoid arthritis (Still's disease: juvenile chronic arthritis)**
A chronic inflammatory arthritis showing similar pathological changes to those of adult RA may occur in children less than 16 years of age. The disease tends to affect larger joints and only one or a few joints may be involved. Rheumatoid nodules and rheumatoid factor are usually absent except in those patients who exhibit severe RA-like disease. Systemic disease is relatively more frequent. The prognosis is more favourable than in adult RA; complete remission occur in 75–80 per cent of cases. Pathological changes in joints are essentially similar to those of adult RA with a chronic inflammatory synovitis, pannus formation, and destruction of joint tissues.

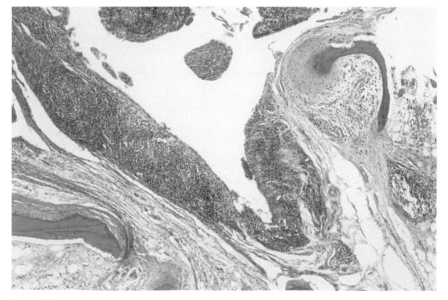

Figure 6.23

Seronegative inflammatory arthropathies

Figure 6.24 **Ankylosing spondylitis (AS)**

This is a chronic progressive inflammatory arthritis which affects mainly the fibrocartilaginous joints of the spine. AS is a seronegative (i.e. rheumatoid factor-negative) disorder which occurs much more commonly in males than females. It usually presents in late adolescence or young adulthood. HLA-B27 is present in more than 90 per cent of patients who complain of progressive back pain and stiffness. Radiological changes include fusion, sclerosis, and obliteration of the sacroiliac and other spinal joints. Calcification of the anterior and lateral spinal ligaments and fusion of adjacent discs results in the formation of a rigid 'bamboo' spine (a). The initial pathological changes are those of an enthesopathy with inflammation and congestion at sites of ligamentous attachment to bone (b) as well as intervertebral joints. Fibrous and bony ankylosis ensue with ossification across the margins of intervertebral discs between adjacent vertebrae (c). This ultimately leads to destruction of disc tissue and bony fusion of adjacent vertebrae (d, e). Unlike ankylosing hyperostosis, ossification occurs within the margins of the intervertebral disc and does not greatly extend into paravertebral ligaments. A chronic inflammatory arthritis, which pathologically resembles RA, may also occur in other joints such as the hip, knee, and shoulder.

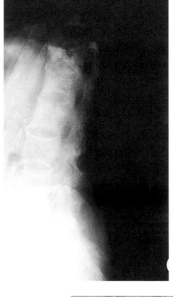
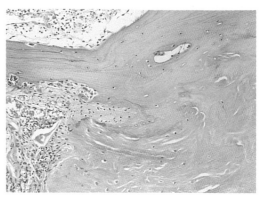
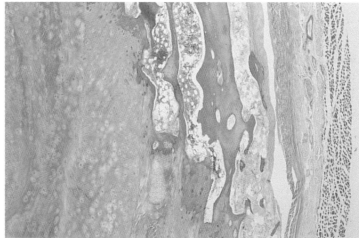
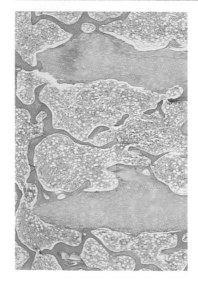
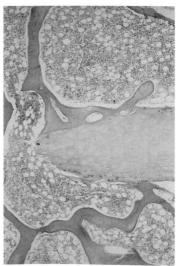

Figure 6.24

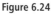

a	b
	c
d	e

Figure 6.25 Reactive arthritis Reactive arthritis is a seronegative inflammatory arthritis that may occur after an infection; organisms are not found in the joint. In Reiter's syndrome, a non-gonococcal urethritis (due to *Chlamydia trachomatis* or *Ureaplasma urealyticum*) is followed by development of a conjunctivitis and asymmetric arthritis (which usually involves only a few joints) or a spondylitis. Other lesions include keratoderma blennorrhagica and an enthesopathy. Most cases are HLA-B27 positive. A similar reactive arthritis may occur after gastrointestinal infection with *Shigella flexneri*, *Yersinia enterocolitica*, Salmonella and other organisms. Early changes are those of an acute inflammatory synovitis but later a lymphocytic and plasma cell infiltrate predominates in the subintima (as shown here). Pannus formation, joint destruction, and ankylosis uncommonly occur.

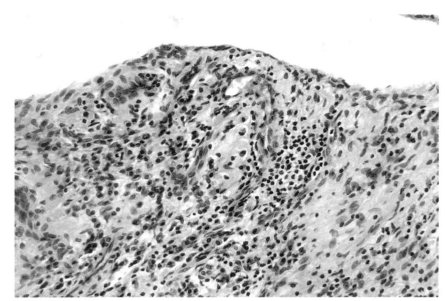

Figure 6.25

Figure 6.26 Arthritis associated with intestinal diseases A number of intestinal conditions may be associated with a seronegative inflammatory arthritis. These include ulcerative colitis and Crohn's disease, which may produce an RA-like inflammatory synovitis in large joints, or an AS-like disease; the latter occurs more commonly in patients who are HLA-B27 positive. A granulomatous synovitis may also occur in Crohn's disease. A migratory polyarthritis may occur in Whipple's disease, a rare intestinal malabsorptive disorder. In this condition numerous PAS-positive macrophages are found in the small intestine and the synovial membrane (shown here).

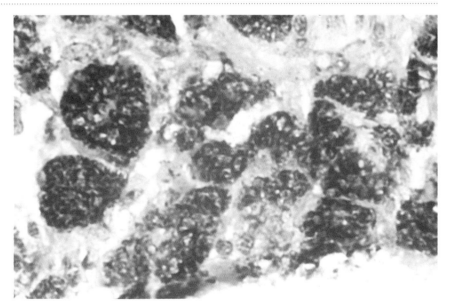

Figure 6.26

Figure 6.27 Psoriatic arthropathy Various forms of seronegative arthritis may develop in patients with psoriasis, including an AS-like disease, occurring with or without peripheral joint involvement, a symmetrical polyarthritis resembling RA, an asymmetrical oligo-arthritis, and a mutilating form of arthritis which predominantly affects the distal interphalangeal joints. Pathological features are similar to those of rheumatoid disease with villous hypertrophy, congestion, intimal thickening, and a prominent subintimal lymphocytic and plasma cell infiltrate (shown here). Pannus formation and cartilage and bone destruction may occur. Patients with spondyloarthropathy may be HLA-B27 positive.

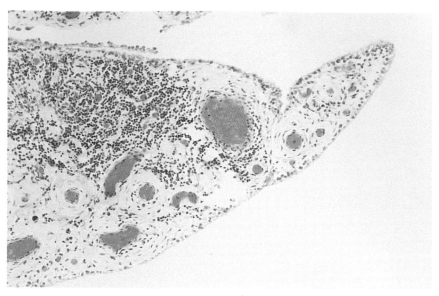

Figure 6.27

Figure 6.28 Behçet's disease This rare inflammatory arthritis of unknown aetiology is associated with oral and genital ulceration and various skin and eye lesions, particularly an iritis. Visceral involvement may also occur. It is most frequent in young males and occurs most commonly in the Eastern Mediterranean and Japan. A monoarticular or oligoarticular arthritis, affecting mainly the knees, ankles, wrists, and elbows, is usually seen. The synovium is inflamed with ulceration of the synovial lining which contains a mixed acute and chronic inflammatory infiltrate (as shown here).

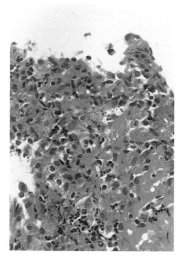

Figure 6.28

Figure 6.29 Arthritis associated with other autoimmune diseases A seronegative arthritis may also occur in other autoimmune diseases such as systemic lupus erythematosus and scleroderma. This is generally associated with an RA-like chronic inflammatory synovitis in which there is thickening and hypertrophy of the synovial membrane and a prominent lymphocytic and plasma cell infiltrate in the subintima (a). There may also be pannus formation (b). Ankylosis, however, rarely occurs. In these conditions, joint inflammation is a relatively minor feature and vasculitis affecting small and medium-sized vessels predominates. Evidence of a vasculitis may also occasionally be seen in deep synovial tissues. Blood vessel changes may also predominate in scleroderma and progressive systemic sclerosis. There is a marked increase in collagen in the dermis and occasionally superficial subcutaneous

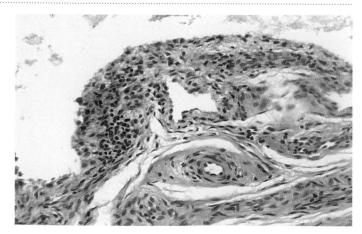

Figure 6.29

a

tissue. Systemic sclerosis patients with the CREST syndrome show focal and sometimes diffuse calcification (arrow) within this increased fibrous tissue (c).

Figure 6.29

b c

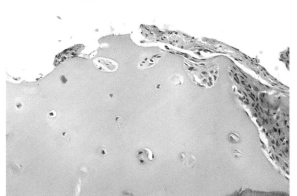

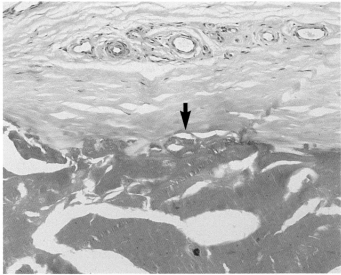

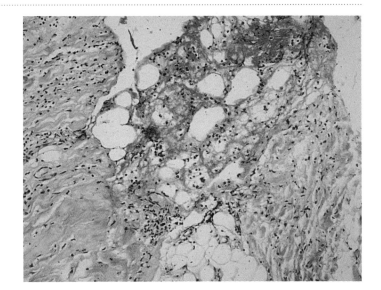

Figure 6.30 **Eosinophilic fasciitis** In this condition there is induration of the skin of the extremities, particularly in the upper limb. It occurs most commonly in young males and usually presents with pain, swelling, and tenderness. There may be marked eosinophilia and hypergammaglobulinaemia. This condition is distinguished from scleroderma by the involvement of mainly the deep subcutaneous tissue and superficial fascia (a). There is fibrosis and a variable, mixed inflammatory infiltrate which includes lymphocytes, plasma cells, and often eosinophil polymorphs (arrow) (b). These patients do not develop Raynaud's phenomenon or exhibit systemic features of systemic sclerosis.

Figure 6.30

a

b

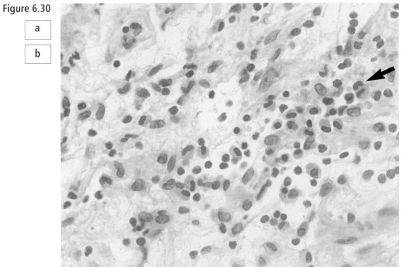

Figure 6.31 **Giant cell arteritis** This condition occurs most commonly in elderly individuals and is often associated with polymyalgia rheumatica in which there is joint stiffness, particularly of the shoulders. A vasculitis is seen in large and medium-sized arteries, especially extracranial vessels of the head and neck. This may cause headaches and visual disturbances. The temporal artery is most commonly affected. Grossly, it may be thickened and tender. Histologically, there is an arteritis that involves all the coats of the vessel wall with the media and adventitia often containing a mixed acute and chronic inflammatory cell infiltrate (a). Giant cells (arrow) and macrophages are frequently seen in relation to fragments of the internal elastic lamina (b). There is intimal thickening and occasionally thrombus formation.

Figure 6.31

| a | b |

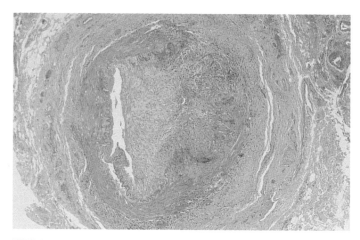 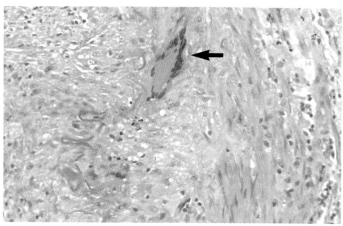

Diseases of spinal joints

Figure 6.32 **Intervertebral disc disease** Displacement of disc tissue can occur through areas of weakness in surrounding structures. Disc prolapse superiorly or inferiorly through the cartilage end plate into the vertebral body may lead to development of a Schmorl's node (a). Prolapse posteriorly or posterolaterally through areas of weakness in the annulus fibrosus may cause nerve root compression. Disc fragments may also become sequestrated, a segment of the disc flaking off and lying freely within the spinal canal. Tissue from prolapsed intervertebral discs commonly shows numerous fissures and clefts within the fibrocartilage matrix which contains areas of myxoid and cystic degeneration and clusters of cartilage cells (b). As disc tissue is avascular, prolapse may be evidenced by the presence of small areas of reparative fibrous tissue (arrow), containing fibroblasts and macrophages, that extend into or surround the degenerate fibrocartilage (c). Another not uncommon finding in disc fibrocartilage is the presence of deposits of chondrocalcinosis (arrow) containing small, birefringent rod-shaped crystals (d).

Figure 6.32

| a | b | c | d |

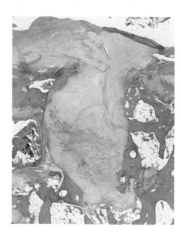 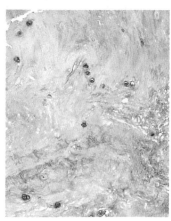 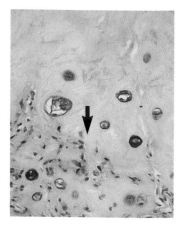 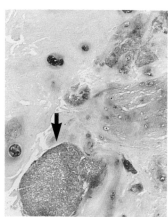

Figure 6.33 Spondylosis (osteoarthritis) of the spine This is usually seen in the more mobile segments of the spine, particularly the cervical and lumbar segments. Degenerative arthritis of the facet joints of the spine is usually progressive, leading to the formation of osteophytes which may protrude into intervertebral foramina and produce irritation of spinal nerve roots. These degenerative changes are commonly found at autopsy and are rarely seen as surgical specimens. Shown is a radiograph of the cervical spine in which degenerative changes are seen at several levels with posterior lipping. A potential complication of spondylosis is arterial insufficiency due to osteophytes impinging on the vertebral artery between C2 and C6.

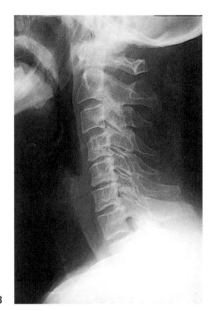

Figure 6.33

Figure 6.34 Ankylosing hyperostosis (diffuse idiopathic skeletal hyperostosis [DISH]; Forestier's disease) In ankylosing hyperostosis, beak-like outgrowths extend from the margins of adjacent vertebral bodies(a); the vertebral end plates are intact and there is no facet joint disease or sacro-ileitis. Ossification occurs in the anterior longitudinal ligament, resulting in ankylosis of the vertebral column in the absence of disc disease (b). A degree of ankylosing hyperostosis of the spine is a relatively common finding at autopsy, particularly in the thoracic and lumbar spine. The condition is usually asymptomatic and found mainly in elderly males who may also show calcification of other areas of ligamentous attachment; calcaneal spurs are commonly seen (c).

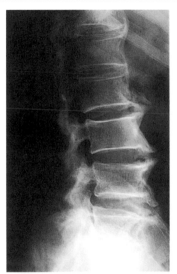 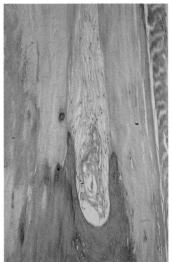

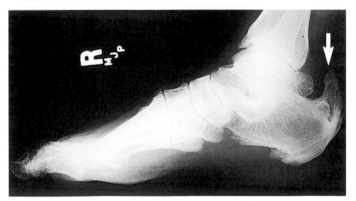

Figure 6.34

| a | b |

| c |

Pathological changes associated with prosthetic joint replacement

Figure 6.35 **Aseptic loosening** Implant components used in joint replacement surgery are usually composed of polymeric or metallic biomaterials. Wear particles derived from these implant components are commonly found in periprosthetic tissues. A fibrous membrane is usually found at the interface between the bone and the implant. In a well-fixed prosthesis, this membrane is thin and composed largely of collagenous connective tissue which contains relatively few inflammatory cells or wear particles. In an unstable prosthesis, however, this fibrous pseudomembrane is thicker and contains numerous implant-derived wear particles. 6.35a shows osteolysis, which is evident radiologically (arrow) around a loose implant; fracture may also occur. The thick fibrous pseudomembrane surrounding a loose prosthesis is often covered in part by a synovial lining and usually contains a heavy foreign-body macrophage and giant cell (macrophage polykaryon) response to implant-derived wear particles (b). This heavy mononuclear phagocyte foreign-body response to wear particles within the implant pseudomembrane may also extend for a short distance into the underlying bone (c).

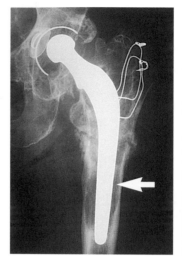
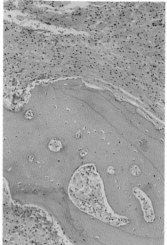

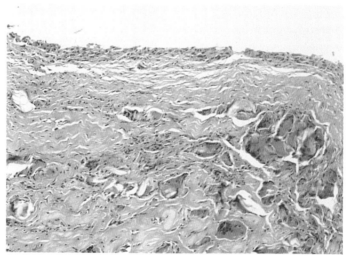

Figure 6.35

a | c
· b

Figure 6.36 **Aseptic loosening: polymethylmethacrylate (PMMA) wear particles** The pseudomembrane surrounding a loose cemented implant often contains small and large fragments of PMMA. PMMA dissolves in routine histological processing and appears in stained sections as an empty space surrounded by macrophages and macrophage polykaryons (a). These spaces often contain weakly birefringent, grey-green, granular aggregates of barium sulphate or zirconium oxide (arrow), radio-opaque markers which are incorporated into the cement (b).

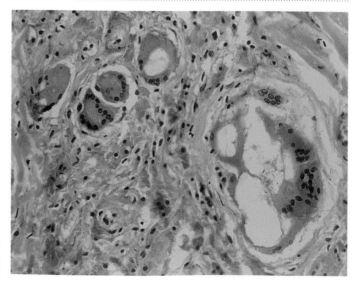

Figure 6.36

a

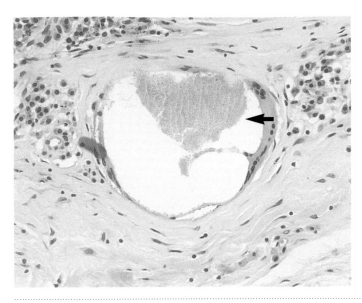

Figure 6.36 continued

b

Figure 6.37 Aseptic loosening: Ultra-high molecular weight polyethylene (UHMWP) wear particles UHMWP wear debris is mostly submicron in size and lies within the plump eosinophilic cytoplasm of the numerous macrophages and macrophage polykaryons present in the artificial joint pseudocapsule or fibrous pseudomembrane covering the implant (a). Larger fragments are visible microscopically as they are strongly birefringent under polarized light (b). Occasionally, large shards of UMHWP are deposited within periprosthetic tissues; these are surrounded by giant cells and macrophages (c).

Figure 6.37

a

b   c

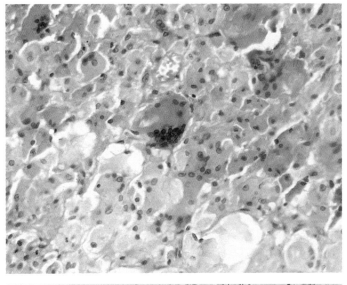

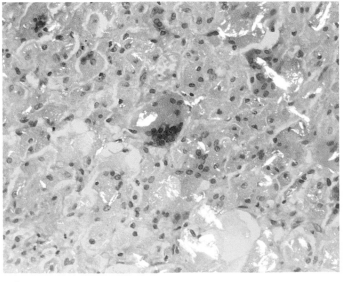

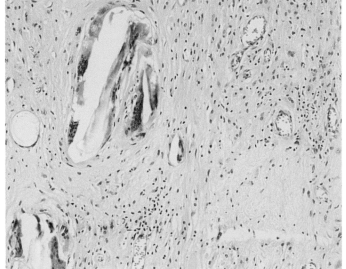

Figure 6.38 Aseptic loosening: metallic wear particles Wear debris composed of the various metallic alloys (usually stainless steel, cobalt chrome, or titanium) found in implant components is also deposited in the implant pseudomembrane. If extensive, this deposition leads to gross discoloration of the periprosthetic tissues. 6.38a show blackened fragments of the pseudomembrane surrounding a titanium alloy implant. Metallic wear particles appear as small black dots or splinters which lie within and around macrophages and giant cells in periprosthetic tissues (b); they show weakly positive dot-like birefringence (c). Corrosion products of cobalt-chrome particles may appear grey and stainless steel particles may appear yellow or brown.

Figure 6.38

a b c

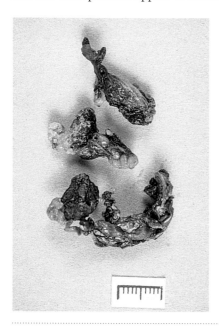
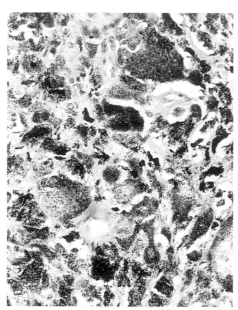
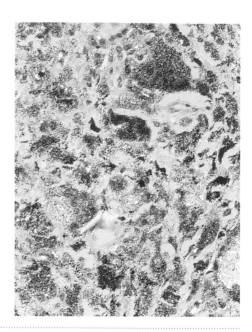

Figure 6.39 Aseptic loosening In addition to a foreign-body macrophage response to wear particles, periprosthetic tissues often contain a lymphocytic infiltrate, which is usually not prominent but occasionally may be quite florid (a). This chronic inflammatory infiltrate, which may include plasma cells and eosinophil polymorphs, is usually prominent when there is abundant wear particle deposition and presumably represents a pronounced immunological response to specific implant biomaterials. Evidence of the primary disease for which the arthroplasty was originally undertaken may also be evident in periprosthetic tissues. A heavy lymphocytic and plasma cell infiltrate is often seen in the pseudocapsule and pseudomembrane of RA patients (b). Deposits of chondrocalcinosis, containing rod-shaped birefringent pyrophosphate crystals (arrow), may also rarely be found in periprosthetic tissues (c).

Figure 6.39

a b c

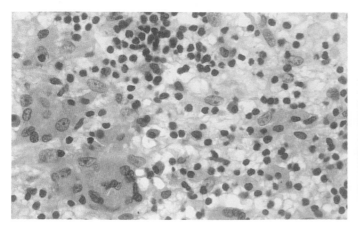
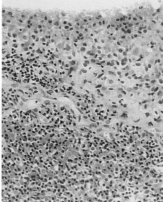
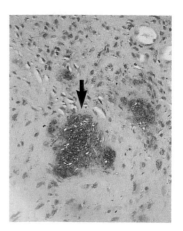

Figure 6.40 Septic loosening Infection of periprosthetic tissues is a rare cause of implant loosening. Septic loosening usually presents as early arthroplasty failure with clinical and laboratory features suggestive of infection, but less commonly it may be delayed or late onset, loosening of the prosthesis occurring several years after implantation; the latter is often difficult to distinguish from aseptic loosening in terms of clinical features, radiological and laboratory investigations, or even gross examination at operation. Organisms are often isolated with difficulty from periprosthetic tissues and histology can play a useful role in establishing the diagnosis of septic loosening. In most cases of septic loosening, periprosthetic tissues consist of abundant inflamed granulation tissue (a, b); this is covered by an inflammatory exudate and contains large numbers of neutrophil polymorphs (usually greater than one per high-power field on average after examination of at least ten high-power fields). This histological criterion is commonly employed when frozen section histology is used to decide whether a one-stage (for aseptic loosening) or two-stage (for septic loosening) revision arthroplasty procedure needs to be undertaken.

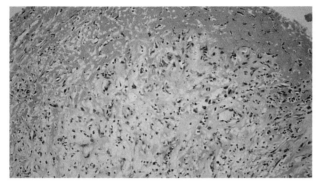
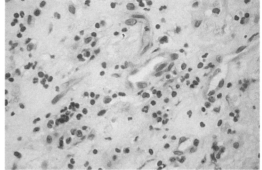

Figure 6.40

| a | b |

Figure 6.41 Reaction to other polymeric biomaterials Other biomaterial particulates which may be found in articular tissues include those derived from silicone rubber (Silastic) implants which are used to replaced carpal bones. These particulates (arrow) are usually colourless or yellow-grey, non-birefringent, and have a wrinkled appearance (a). They often evoke a heavy macrophage and giant cell response. They may be associated with the formation of a lytic pseudotumour in carpal bones (b). Carbon particles derived from carbon-reinforced polyethylene components consist of small rods or bars of black material which are distributed irregularly throughout the tissue (c); these evoke a heavy macrophage and giant cell response.

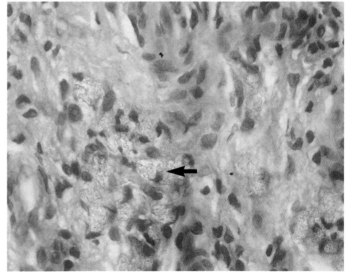

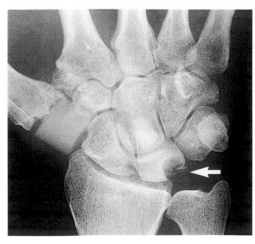

Figure 6.41

| a |
| b | c |

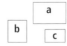
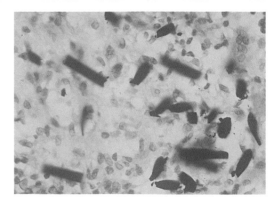

Tumours and tumour-like conditions of synovial tissues

Figure 6.42 Pigmented villonodular synovitis (PVNS) This condition occurs most commonly in young adults who complain of pain and swelling of the involved joint. The knee joint is most frequently involved but any joint may be affected; multiple joint involvement is very uncommon. PVNS may involve the joint synovium diffusely or focally in a nodular fashion. 6.42a shows an MRI of the knee in a case of diffuse PVNS. There is extensive thickening and involvement of the synovial membrane and capsule. Grossly, the synovium is yellow-brown or haemorrhagic. Histologically there is villous thickening of the synovial membrane with intimal hyperplasia and an inflamed subintima containing numerous (brown-staining) haemosiderin deposits (b). There are numerous macrophages and scattered giant cells (c). Scattered lymphocytes and plasma cells as well as occasional lymphoid aggregates may also be seen in the subintima. Macrophages often contain haemosiderin or lipid, appearing as foamy macrophages (arrow). PVNS needs to be distinguished from other causes of siderotic synovitis.

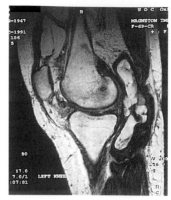

Figure 6.42

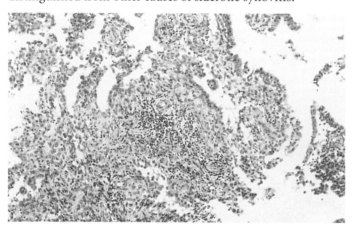

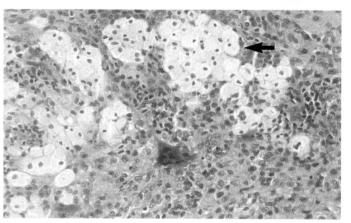

Figure 6.43 Giant cell tumour of tendon sheath This tumour may occur as either a localized (nodular tenosynovitis) or diffuse (pigmented villonodular synovitis-like) swelling of a tendon sheath. The localized type is relatively common and occurs predominantly in adults; it is slightly more common in females. It presents as a slow-growing swelling in the distal extremities (especially the fingers) but may arise elsewhere. Grossly, it is a well-defined, firm, lobulated, yellow-tan lesion (a) which is usually attached to the tendon sheath. It consists of fibrous tissue containing numerous fibroblasts and macrophages as well as scattered multinucleated giant cells (b). Haemosiderin deposition and collections of foamy macrophages as well as scattered lymphoid cells may be seen. Some tumours have abundant collagen and show hyalinization of the fibrous stroma. A prominent storiform pattern similar to that of a soft tissue benign fibrous histiocytoma may be noted in some lesions. Local recurrence occurs in up to 20 per cent of cases.

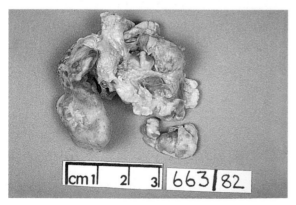

Figure 6.43

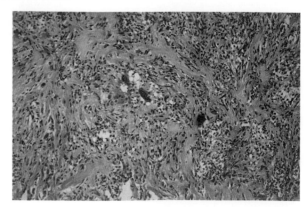

Figure 6.44 **Primary synovial chondromatosis (PSC; synovial osteochondromatosis)**

PSC is an uncommon condition in which islands of cartilage form by metaplasia within the subintimal connective tissue of the synovial membrane. It occurs over a wide age range but most commonly presents in late adolescence and early adulthood. The knee and hip joints are most frequently affected but it may occur in any joint as well as within the synovial lining of a tendon sheath or bursa. Radiographs usually show that the articular surface is normal and reveal multiple small opacities within and around the joint (a). Nodular areas of cartilaginous metaplasia are seen in the subintima (b). These nodules show an increase in cartilage cellularity; chondrocytes may appear binucleated (arrow) and show a degree of nuclear pleomorphism (c). The cartilage nodules may undergo calcification and ossification. They may also become detached to form cartilaginous or osteocartilaginous loose bodies within the joint. PSC needs to be distinguished from secondary osteochondromatosis which usually results from synovial deposition of multiple osteocartilaginous loose bodies derived from fragments of the articular surface. It should also be distinguished from chondrosarcoma which rarely arises within the synovial membrane. PSC commonly recurs after excision.

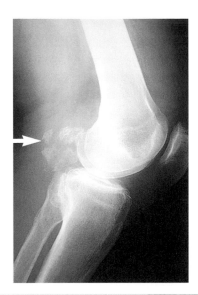

Figure 6.44

a
b
c

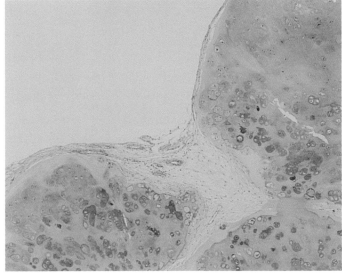

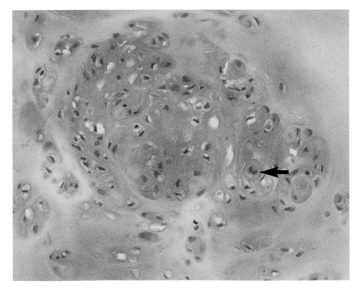

Figure 6.45 Synovial haemangioma Synovial haemangioma is a diffuse or localized benign vascular tumour which occurs most commonly in childhood and adolescence. It usually involves a single joint, most commonly the knee joint. There is often a history of recurrent joint swelling, repeated traumatic effusion, pain, and limitation of movement. Radiographs usually show thickening of the synovial membrane and osteolytic areas (arrow) in the articulating bones (a). Grossly, the synovium is red-brown and contains numerous thickened villi. Blood-filled spaces lined by endothelium are present in the subintima (b). There is often a siderotic synovitis with numerous haemosiderin-laden macrophages and abundant extracellular haemosiderin deposition.

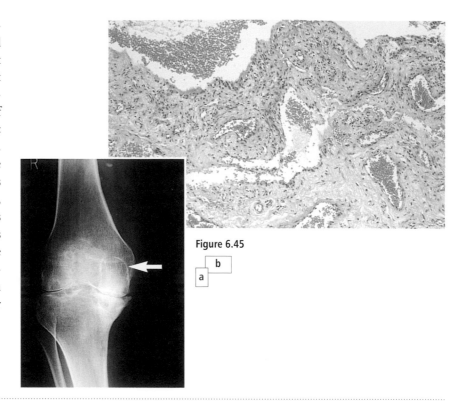

Figure 6.45

b
a

Figure 6.46 Other synovial tumours and tumour-like lesions Other benign tumours or tumour-like lesions that may rarely involve joint tissues include synovial lipomatosis in which there is diffuse lipomatous involvement of the subintima of the infrapatellar fat pad (a).

A juxta-articular myxoma may also occur in deep capsular tissue outside the synovial membrane or within a tendon sheath (b); the lesion (right) has abundant myxoid matrix and scattered stellate and spindle-shaped mesenchymal cells. (Synovial sarcoma, a malignant soft-tissue tumour which is not truly of synovial origin, is dealt with in Chapter 8.)

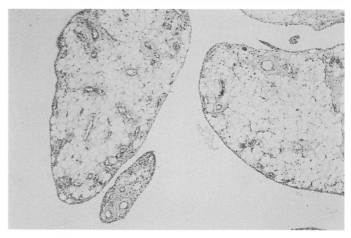

Figure 6.46

a

b

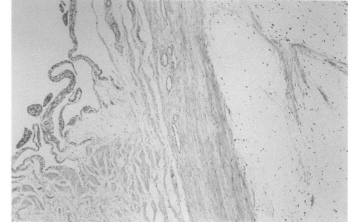

7

Bone tumours and tumour-like lesions

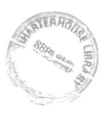

Introduction

An accurate histological diagnosis of a bone tumour is required for correct treatment and prediction of its likely behaviour. Although primary tumours of bone are more often benign than malignant, the biological behaviour of many bone tumours (and tumour-like lesions) cannot always be easily defined as benign or malignant. Some benign bone tumours, by virtue of their size or anatomical location, are difficult to treat adequately by surgical removal and consequently are prone to frequent, local recurrence. A number of tumours, usually categorized as benign, may also behave as locally aggressive lesions and some have rarely been reported to metastasize.

Bone tumours present a considerable therapeutic challenge to clinicians and their correct diagnosis and treatment requires close co-operation between the surgeon, oncologist, radiologist, and pathologist. Primary tumours of bone are relatively uncommon and many different types have been described. These tumours are generally classified on the basis of the normal cell or tissue type from which they appear to have originated; this is often evidenced by the type of matrix produced by the tumour cells. Where the histogenesis of a tumour is uncertain, it is generally classified on the basis of its specific clinicopathological features.

Most bone tumours present with non-specific clinical complaints such as pain, swelling, and limitation of movement. An increased (but generally low) risk of bone sarcoma development has been associated with a number of pre-existing conditions such as radiation, Paget's disease, bone infarction, chronic osteomyelitis, familial retinoblastoma, neurofibromatosis, osteogenesis imperfecta, and benign tumour-like lesions such as fibrous dysplasia, simple bone cyst, and aneurysmal bone cyst. With regard to diagnosis, it is important to note the age of patient (Table 7.1) and the precise location of the lesion within a particular bone (Tables 7.2 and 7.3). Bone tumours often present with a typical clinical and radiological profile. It is thus important that all the clinical and radiological information regarding a bone lesion should be assessed by the pathologist before a histological opinion is offered. In addition, the results of relevant biochemical and haematological investigations should be available. Additional histological staining to determine tissue architecture or identify cell/matrix components or immunohistochemistry is useful in some cases in establishing the histological diagnosis. Cytogenetic analysis and molecular biology are also playing an increasingly important role in determining the diagnosis, treatment, and prognosis of a number of bone tumours.

Table 7.1 Main age range at presentation of some bone tumours and tumour-like lesions

Tumour	Age in years				
	0–10	11–20	21–30	31–40	40+
Osteoma		-------------	-------------		
Osteoid osteoma	------	————	————	-------	
Osteoblastoma	---	————	————	————	----------
Osteosarcoma	----	————	————	----------	----------
Periosteal chondroma	------	————	————	----------	----------
Enchondroma	------	————	————	————	————
Parosteal osteosarcoma		----------	----------	————	————
Osteochondroma	————	————	————	----------	----------
Chondroblastoma	----	————	-----------------	-----------------	----------
Chondromyxoid fibroma	------	————	————	----------	----------
Chondrosarcoma		---------	---------	————	————
Mesenchymal/clear cell chondrosarcoma	---------	---------	————	————	----
Ewing's sarcoma	————	————	------		
Secondary neuroblastoma	————	------			
Lymphoma	-----------------	-----------------	-----------------	————	————
Myeloma				--	————
MFH/fibrosarcoma	-------------	-------------	-------------	-------------	----
Haemangioma	-------------	-------------	-------------	-------------	----
Chordoma				---	————
Adamantinoma	————	————	————	----------	----------
Paget's sarcoma				-----	————
Giant cell tumour of bone		---	————	————	————
Simple bone cyst	--	————	-----------------	-----------------	----
Aneurysmal bone cyst	---	————	----------	----------	
Fibrous dysplasia	————	————	————	-------	-------
Eosinophilic granuloma	————	————	------		
Non ossifying fibroma	————	————	————	------	
Metastatic carcinoma				-----	————

Key:

——————— Most commonly reported

-------- Less commonly reported

Table 7.2 Skeletal location of some bone tumours and tumour-like lesions

Small tubular bones	Enchondroma
	Bizarre parosteal osteochondromatous proliferation
	Subungual exostosis
	Osteoid osteoma
	Osteoblastoma
	Epidermal cyst
Long tubular bones (e.g. femur, tibia, humerus)	Most primary benign and malignant bone tumours and tumour-like lesions (excluding chordoma)
	Metastatic carcinoma
	Myeloma
Ribs/sternum	Benign/malignant cartilage tumours
	Fibrous dysplasia
	Eosinophilic granuloma
	Myeloma
	Metastatic carcinoma
Spine	Aneurysmal bone cyst
	Osteoblastoma
	Osteoid osteoma
	Haemangioma
	Chordoma
	Myeloma
	Metastatic carcinoma
Skull/facial bones	Fibrous dysplasia
	'Fibro-osseous lesions' of jaw
	Osteoma
	Giant cell reparative granuloma
	Haemangioma
	Eosinophilic granuloma
	Osteosarcoma
	Mesenchymal chondrosarcoma
	Myeloma
Pelvis	Osteochondroma
	Chondrosarcoma
	Ewing's sarcoma
	Metastatic carcinoma
	Myeloma

Table 7.3 Intraosseous location of some bone tumours and tumour-like lesions

Long bones		
	Epiphyseal (± metaphyseal)	Chondroblastoma
		Giant cell tumour of bone
		Desmoid tumour
		Clear cell chondrosarcoma
		Low-grade osteosarcoma
	Metaphyseal (± Diaphyseal)	Aneurysmal bone cyst
		Simple bone cyst
		Fibrous dysplasia
		Osteochondroma
		Chondromyxoid fibroma
		Enchondroma
		Non-ossifying fibroma
		Haemangioma
		Osteoid osteoma
		Osteoblastoma
		Chondrosarcoma
		Fibrosarcoma/MFH
		High-grade osteosarcoma
		Lymphoma
	Diaphyseal (± metaphyseal)	Ewing's sarcoma
		Adamantinoma
		Metastasis
		Myeloma
Spine		
	Vertebral body	Giant cell tumour of bone
		Chondrosarcoma
		Chordoma
		Metastasis
		Myeloma
	Vertebral arch	Metastasis
		Osteoblastoma
		Aneurysmal bone cyst
		Osteoid osteoma

Osteoid/bone-forming tumours

Figure 7.1 Osteoma This is a benign, slow-growing lesion composed of well differentiated, mature bone which has a predominantly lamellar structure. The classical ivory osteoma (ivory exostosis) is found in the skull and facial bones, especially near the external surface of the bone. Most tumours are small and asymptomatic but larger lesions may produce symptoms by growing into the orbit or, as shown in the CT scan in (a), the paranasal sinuses. Multiple ivory osteomas may occur as part of Gardner's syndrome (intestinal polyposis, multiple skin lesions, fibromatosis, and osteomas) which is inherited autosomal dominant; the gene for this syndrome is present on the long arm of chromosome 5. 7.1b shows several osteomas in the maxilla and mandible in a case of Gardner's syndrome. Osteomas are usually composed mainly, if not wholly, of compact lamellar bone containing Haversian systems (c).

Figure 7.1

a | b | c

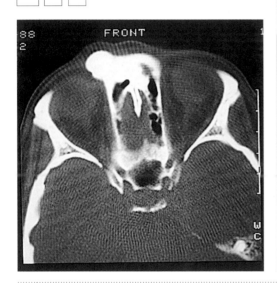
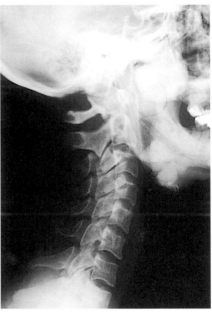
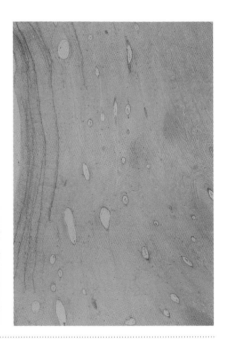

Figure 7.2 Enostosis (bone island) This is an osteoma lying in mature cancellous bone. It occurs most commonly in the femur or the tibia and is generally less than 1.0 cm in diameter. It is clinically silent and on radiographs appears as a distinct radio-opacity which needs to be distinguished from a bone-forming lesion, such as an osteoid osteoma, or an osteosclerotic bone metastasis. 7.2a shows a specimen radiograph of the femoral head showing a bone island in the epiphysis. It consists of a mass of mature lamellar compact bone which merges with surrounding cancellous bone (b). [Osteopoikilosis (multiple bone islands) is discussed in 4.22]

Figure 7.2

a | b

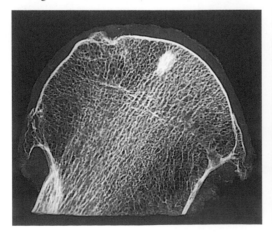
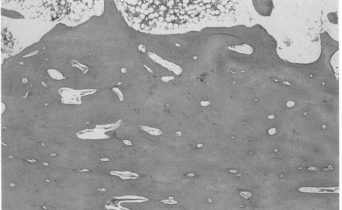

Figure 7.3 **Osteoid osteoma** This is a relatively common, benign bone-forming tumour that occurs mainly in adolescent and young adult males. It causes severe pain and tenderness, often worse at night and relieved by aspirin. It is found most frequently in the metaphysis or diaphysis of long bones, especially the femur or tibia, but may arise in any bone; in the spine it arises in the posterior elements. In long bones, it often arises in relation to the cortex which is commonly thickened. 7.3a shows the radiological features of an osteoid osteoma of the tibia. A central area of radiolucency, which may itself contain a tiny focus of increased bone density (the nidus) is surrounded by a sclerotic reaction in cortical bone. Osteoid osteomas are usually hot on bone scan. Grossly, the lesion is a well defined, richly vascularized tumour measuring up to 2.0 cm in diameter; it is surrounded by a zone of dense sclerotic bone (b).

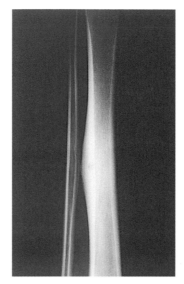
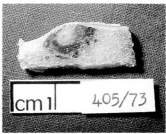

Figure 7.3

a b

Figure 7.4 **Osteoid osteoma** 7.4a shows part of the nidus of an osteoid osteoma. The lesion is well defined and surrounded by thickened cortical bone. It is composed of a haphazard arrangement of irregular sheets or strands of osteoid and/or woven bone. These are rimmed by regular, plump osteoblastic cells which often contain large hyperchromatic nuclei (b). The intervening stroma is well vascularized and also contains numerous plump osteoblastic cells (c); occasional osteoclasts lie in relation to newly formed matrix.

Figure 7.4

a

b c

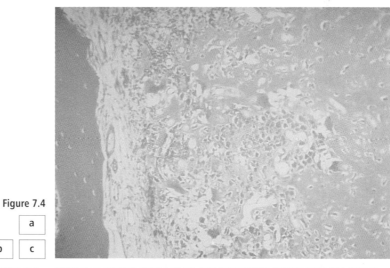

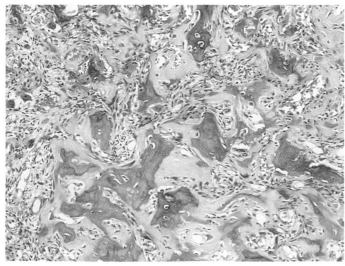

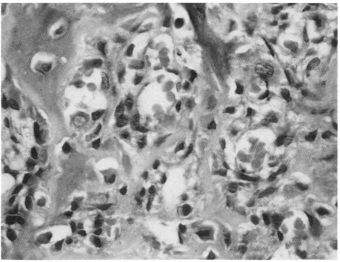

Figure 7.5 **Osteoblastoma** This uncommon benign tumour is seen predominantly in adolescents and young adult males but may occur at any age. It is found most commonly in the posterior elements of the vertebrae, the metaphysis and diaphysis of long bones, small bones of the hands and feet, and the skull and jaw. Patients usually complain of a dull pain and swelling. Radiological appearances are variable although most lesions are well defined, expansile, and radiolucent; there may also be intralesional ossification. Extensive sclerosis in surrounding bone is not seen but there may be a thin shell of reactive bone. 7.5a and 7.5b shows the radiological appearances of an osteoblastoma arising in the fourth cervical vertebra and the talus respectively.

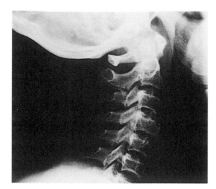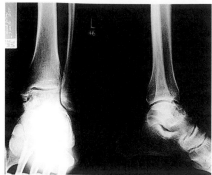

Figure 7.5

| a | b |

Figure 7.6 **Osteoblastoma** Histological appearances of osteoblastoma resemble those of osteoid osteoma. There is abundant osteoid and woven bone formation by plump osteoblasts with large hyperchromatic nuclei that may show some pleomorphism but no atypical mitotic activity (a). Secondary aneurysmal bone cyst change may occur with formation of blood-filled spaces lined by giant cells (b). An osteoblastoma which exhibits locally aggressive behaviour but does not metastasize is termed an aggressive osteoblastoma; this commonly shows broad osteoid or woven bone trabeculae surrounded by plump epithelioid osteoblasts (c). This lesion needs to be distinguished from a well-differentiated osteosarcoma. Tumours need to be removed entirely as recurrence (especially in the spine) follows incomplete removal.

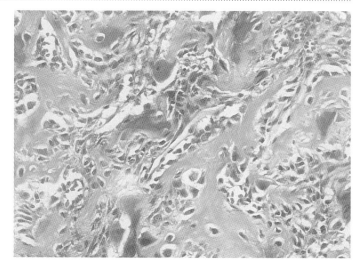

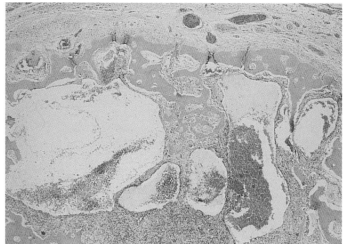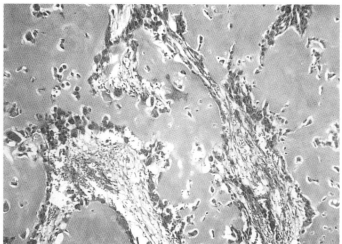

Figure 7.6

| a |

| b | c |

Figure 7.7 Osteosarcoma Excluding myeloma and other haematological neoplasms, osteosarcoma is the most common primary malignant tumour of bone. Mutations in tumour suppressor genes, such as p53 and the retinoblastoma gene, have been associated with osteosarcoma development. It occurs most commonly in adolescents and young adult males but may present at any age. Any bone may be affected but it typically arises in the metaphysis of long bones, particularly the lower end of the femur, upper end of the

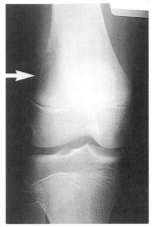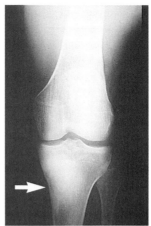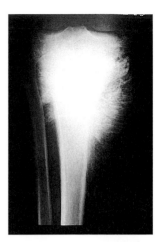

tibia, and upper humerus. Radiologically, the tumour is usually metaphyseal in location, has areas of lysis and sclerosis, infiltrative margins, and is associated with bone destruction; it commonly extends through the bone cortex into surrounding soft tissues. 7.7a shows a poorly defined, predominantly lytic osteosarcoma of the lower end of the femur (arrow). 7.7b shows a predominantly sclerotic osteosarcoma of the upper end of the tibia (arrow). Elevation of the periosteum may produce a pattern of radiating sunburst spiculation (c). Grossly, the tumour is usually large, clearly destructive, and infiltrative; it may contain identifiable areas of bone and cartilage formation and commonly contains foci of haemorrhage and necrosis (d).

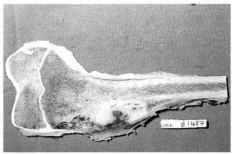

Figure 7.7

| a | b | c |

| d |

Figure 7.8 Osteosarcoma By definition, all osteosarcomas show evidence of osteoid or bone formation by tumour cells that show cytological evidence of malignancy; tumour cells are pleomorphic and have large hyperchromatic nuclei which often show mitotic activity (arrow) (a, b). Poorly differentiated tumours contain numerous highly pleomorphic cells with large abnormal hyperchromatic nuclei and tumour giant cells (arrow) (c). Tumour cells are strongly alkaline phosphatase positive (d).

Figure 7.8

| a | b | c | d |

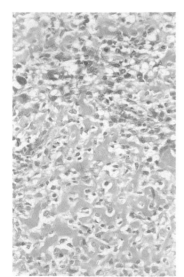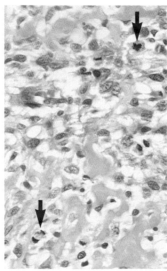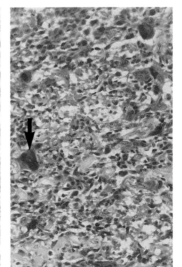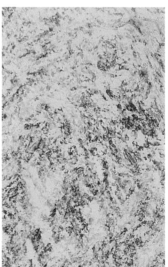

Figure 7.9 **Osteosarcoma** Several descriptive types of conventional osteosarcoma can be distinguished. Tumours showing extensive osteoblastic differentiation with abundant osteoid and bone formation are termed osteoblastic osteosarcomas (a). An osteoblastic osteosarcoma in which there is extensive formation of osteoid and woven bone by relatively few tumour cells, the tumour bone encasing host bone, is often termed a sclerosing osteosarcoma (b). A chondroblastic osteosarcoma contains, in addition to areas of osteosarcoma, abundant cartilage elements showing malignant change (c). A fibroblastic osteosarcoma contains abundant spindle-shaped tumour cells and a collagenous fibrous stroma as well as areas of typical osteosarcoma (arrow) (d). Identification of these various patterns of differentiation in a conventional osteosarcoma has not been shown to be a useful prognostic feature as more than one pattern is often present within a single tumour.

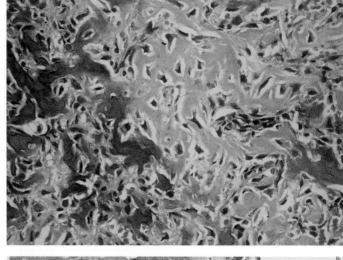

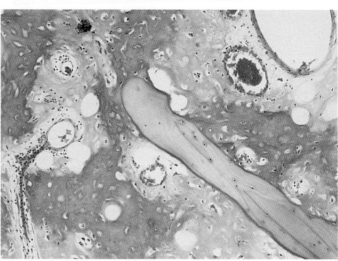

Figure 7.9

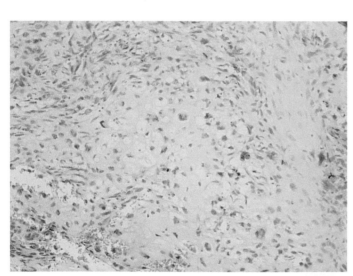

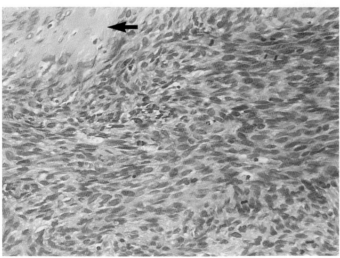

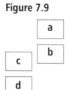

Figure 7.10 **Osteosarcoma** Osteosarcomas grow rapidly, may show evidence of vascular invasion (as shown in 7.10a), and metastasize early and widely via the bloodstream, predominantly to the lungs. In addition to surgery, osteosarcomas are usually treated by neoadjuvant and adjuvant chemotherapy. One of the effects of neoadjuvant chemotherapy is to cause extensive tumour necrosis and abundant matrix mineralization (b). A good response to chemotherapy and better prognosis has been noted when there is more than 90 per cent necrosis of the tumour following treatment.

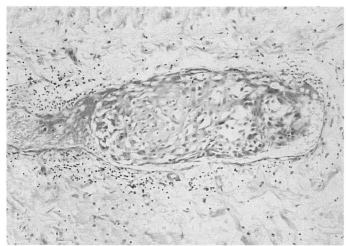

Figure 7.10

a

b

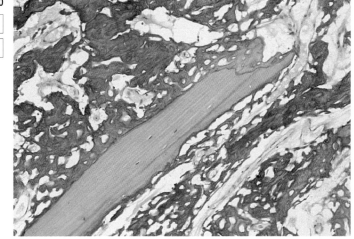

Figure 7.11 **Giant cell-rich osteosarcoma** This variant of osteosarcoma contains large numbers of benign multinucleated osteoclast-like giant cells (arrow) in addition to evidence of osteoid and bone formation by tumour cells. This variant usually behaves as a conventional osteosarcoma. It needs to be distinguished from telangiectatic osteosarcoma and giant cell tumour of bone.

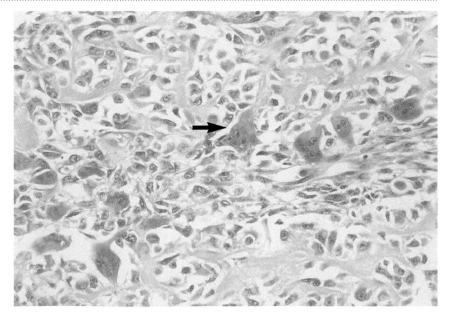

Figure 7.11

Figure 7.12 **Telangiectatic osteosarcoma** This variant of osteosarcoma superficially resembles an aneurysmal bone cyst. The tumour is often large and composed of numerous dilated blood-filled spaces separated by fibrous septa which contain abundant osteoclast-like giant cells as well as scattered malignant tumour cells forming osteoid (a, b). Tumour giant cells are also commonly seen. This variant grows rapidly and is associated with considerable bone destruction, but with modern combination therapy the prognosis is similar to that of conventional osteosarcoma.

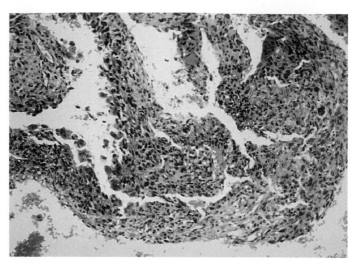

Figure 7.12

a

b

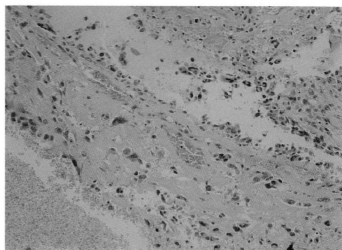

Figure 7.13 **Small (round) cell osteosarcoma** This is a high-grade form of osteosarcoma which somewhat resembles Ewing's sarcoma morphologically, being composed almost entirely of small round cells. Osteoid formation by tumour cells is usually sparse and finely distributed around the tumour cells. Some of these tumours have been reported to show the characteristic translocation between chromosomes 11 and 22 seen in Ewing's sarcoma.

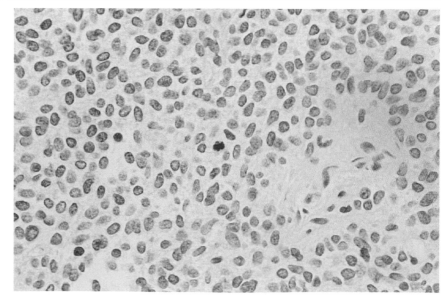

Figure 7.13

Figure 7.14 **Low-grade intramedullary osteosarcoma**
There are a number of low-grade variants of intramedullary osteosarcoma, most of which show histological features similar to fibrous dysplasia; these usually contain abundant fibroblastic tissue and foci of woven bone formation (a). Careful examination reveals that the spindle-shaped tumour cells show osteoid formation and cytological atypia (b) as well as occasional mitotic activity (arrow) (c). The tumour infiltrates between host bone trabeculae. Other low-grade forms of osteosarcoma may show features resembling desmoplastic fibroma, chondromyxoid fibroma, parosteal osteosarcoma, or osteoblastoma.

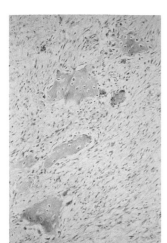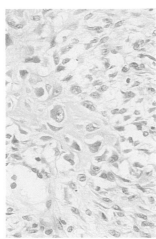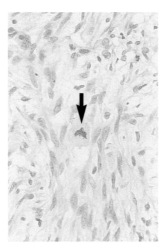

Figure 7.14
a b c

Figure 7.15 **Parosteal osteosarcoma** This is a rare, slow-growing osteosarcoma which arises on the external surface of the bone. It arises in a slightly older age group (i.e. young to middle aged adults) and has a better prognosis than conventional osteosarcoma. Sex incidence is equal. 7.5a shows the radiological features of a parosteal osteosarcoma of the lower end of the femur. The tumour is large, osteosclerotic and has a broad attachment to the underlying cortex which is also thickened and sclerotic. The tumour is composed of relatively well formed but irregular bone trabeculae that are separated by a predominantly fibrous stroma in which there may be focal areas of cartilage formation (arrow), particularly towards the growing edge 7.5b and c. The bone trabeculae contain lamellar bone and have prominent cement lines; they are of variable width and are often interconnected. The intertrabecular fibrous stroma contains spindle cells which show cytological atypia and occasional mitotic activity (arrow) (d). Early diagnosis followed by wide resection of the tumour usually results in cure.

Figure 7.15

a b c d

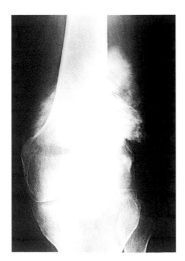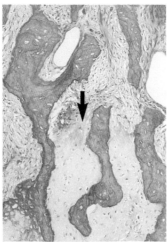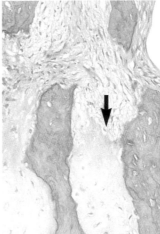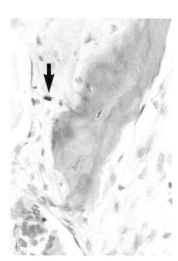

Figure 7.16 Periosteal osteosarcoma This is a very rare type of osteosarcoma which arises on the surface of the diaphysis of long bones, usually the femur or tibia. It occurs most commonly in children and adolescents; there is slight female predominance. 7.16a shows the radiological features of a periosteal osteosarcoma of the tibia. The tumour is radiolucent, contains areas of matrix opacity, and shows a periosteal reaction and a Codman's triangle. The underlying cortex is thickened and the medulla is uninvolved. The tumour is composed predominantly of lobules of low- or medium-grade chondrosarcoma in which there is commonly calcification or endochondral ossification (b). Focally, within or between cartilage lobules, there is evidence of osteoid and woven bone formation (c). The tumour may involve the underlying cortex but rarely penetrates the medullary cavity.

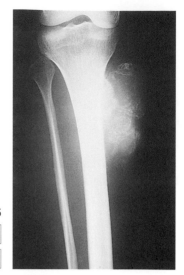

Figure 7.16

a

b c

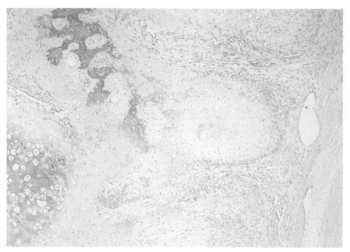

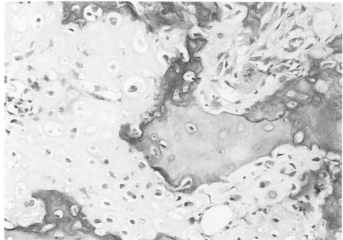

Figure 7.17 High-grade surface osteosarcoma This very rare form of surface osteosarcoma occurs most commonly in adolescents. It usually arises in the diaphysis of long bones, most frequently the femur or humerus. Radiological features somewhat resemble those of a periosteal osteosarcoma but the histological features are essentially those of a high-grade conventional osteosarcoma. There is abundant osteoid and woven bone formation by malignant tumour cells showing marked cellular and nuclear pleomorphism and increased mitotic activity. Medullary involvement is absent or minimal.

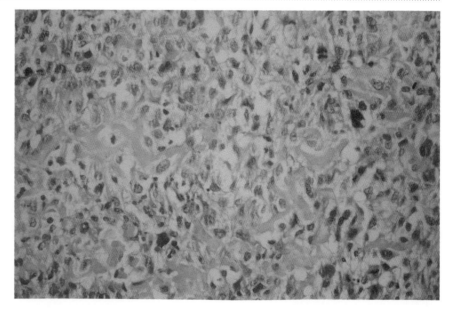

Figure 7.17

Figure 7.18 Paget's sarcoma Sarcomatous transformation occurs in less than 1 per cent of cases of Paget's disease and is more commonly seen in those with advanced polyostotic disease. It occurs generally in patients older than 40 years. The sarcoma usually arises in one of the bones affected by Paget's disease. Sarcoma development is signalled clinically by severe pain and rapid enlargement of a tumour arising in a Pagetic bone (a). The tumour is usually an osteosarcoma which is high-grade and pleomorphic (b), but chondrosarcoma, malignant fibrous histiocytoma, giant cell tumour of bone, and lymphoma may also occur. The prognosis is poor, widespread metastases occurring early.

Figure 7.18

a   b

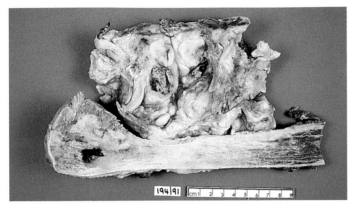
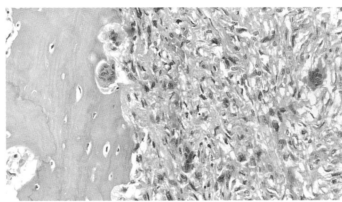

Cartilage-forming tumours

Figure 7.19 Enchondroma This is a common benign tumour which occurs mainly in children, adolescents, and young adults but it may present at any age. It arises most commonly in the medullary cavity of small tubular bones of the hands and feet. It may also be found in larger bones such as the metaphysis/diaphysis of long bones. It is usually asymptomatic. (a) The radiological features of an enchondroma of the proximal phalanx. The lesion is well defined and largely lytic, has a lobulated outline, expands the affected bone, and is covered by thin intact cortex. Punctate or ring-like areas of calcification may be present. In long tubular bones, the tumour is large, well defined, and shows frequent calcification and ossification as well as expansion of the affected bone. 7.19b shows an enchondroma of the proximal fibula.

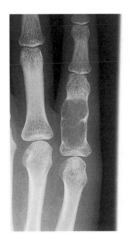
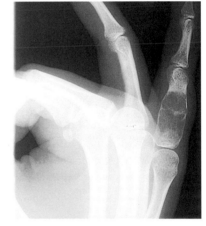

Figure 7.19

a

b

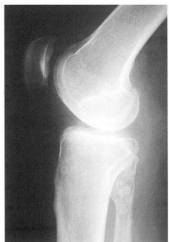

Figure 7.20 Enchondroma Enchondromas are composed of lobules of hyaline cartilage with variable numbers of chondrocytes lying in a chondroid matrix (a). The growing edge of an enchondroma is well defined and usually surrounded by lamellar bone. Rimming of cartilage lobules of an enchondroma arising in large tubular bones is often less complete (b); in contrast to low-grade chondrosarcoma there is no evidence of infiltration between bone trabeculae. Most enchondromas show little cellular or nuclear pleomorphism (c).

Enchondromas of digits are usually quite cellular and, particularly in growing children, often contain binucleated cells (arrow) (d). Binucleated cells and a greater degree of nuclear pleomorphism is seen in the enchondromas of Ollier's disease (see 4.10). There may be evidence of calcification and ossification within lobules of tumour cartilage. Malignant change rarely occurs in solitary enchondromas (especially those of the hands and feet) but occurs more commonly in Ollier's disease.

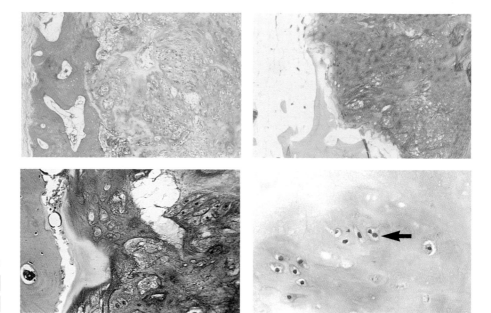

Figure 7.20

a	b
c	d

Figure 7.21 Periosteal (juxtacortical) chondroma Periosteal chondroma is a rare benign cartilaginous tumour arising from the external surface of the bone. It occurs chiefly in adolescents and young adults, presenting as a slowly enlarging, usually asymptomatic swelling. It is found mainly in the small bones of the hands and feet and the metaphysis of large tubular bones. Radiologically, it produces a large soft-tissue swelling showing focal calcification and ossification (a); the underlying cortex has a saucer-like defect with a sclerotic margin. It is composed of chondroma-like lobules of variable cellularity that are usually covered by fibrous tissue (arrow) (b). The tumour extends into the underlying bone cortex and may show minimal medullary involvement. Margins of the tumour are expansile and well defined. Binucleated cells and some cellular and

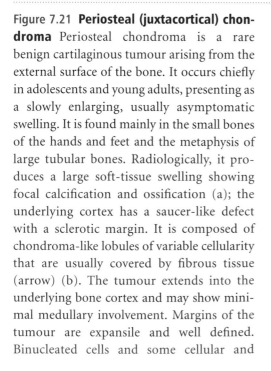
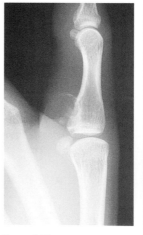
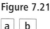
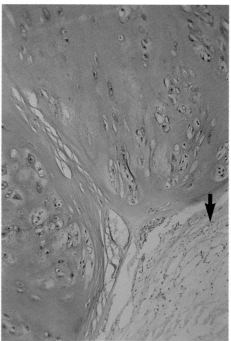

Figure 7.21

a	b

nuclear pleomorphism may be seen amongst cartilage cells (c). Lesions should be excised completely as recurrence may occur after curettage.

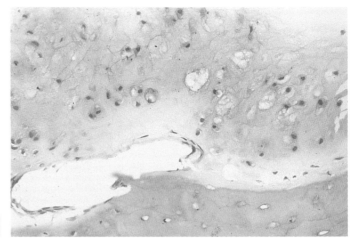

Figure 7.21

c

Figure 7.22 **Osteochondroma** Osteochondroma is the most common benign tumour of bone. It is a cartilage-capped bony projection arising from the external surface of the bone. Lesions are usually solitary; multiple osteochondromas occur in hereditary multiple exostoses (see 4.11). The tumour presents most commonly in children and adolescents as a swelling which may or may not be painful. Osteochondromas may arise in any bone formed by endochondral ossification but occur most commonly in the metaphyseal region of long bones, particularly the lower femur, upper tibia, and upper humerus. Diaphyseal migration of the lesion may occur as the patient grows older. Radiologically, the lesion lies on the surface of the bone and may have a polypoid or sessile outline. 7.22a shows a sessile osteochondroma of the upper tibia. Grossly, the tumour is covered by a cartilage cap which is usually less than 1.0 cm in thickness (b); generally, the younger the patient, the thicker the cartilaginous cap.

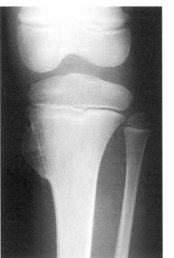

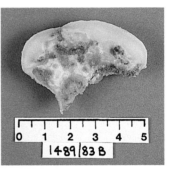

Figure 7.22

a   b

Figure 7.23 **Osteochondroma** The cartilage cap of an osteochondroma is often lobulated and, in a growing individual, shows a degree of growth-plate-like organization with endochondral ossification occurring at the base of the cap (a). In the superficial part of the cartilage cap, randomly arranged chondrocytes, often lying in groups, are covered by a fibrous perichondrium (top) (b). Degenerative changes may be seen within the cartilage matrix. At the base of the cap, during growth, there are swollen cartilage cells and endochondral ossification with remodelling of newly formed bone (c). The cellularity of the cartilage cap and the extent of endochondral ossification occurring in an osteochondroma is age-related; binucleated cells (arrow) may be present if skeletal growth is still occurring (d). Tongues of cartilage are often entrapped by lamellar and woven bone at the base of the lesion (e); this should not be interpreted as invasive malignancy. Once skeletal maturity has been reached there should be no increase in the thickness of the cartilage cap. Development of malignancy in a solitary osteochondroma is rare. Lesions are removed if they become symptomatic. Otherwise, they may be followed radiologically. Osteochondromas may recur if inadequately excised.

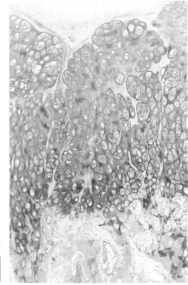

Figure 7.23

a

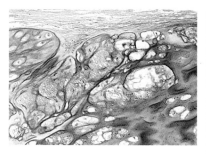
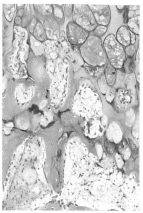
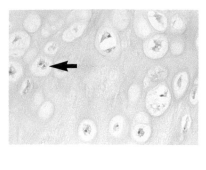
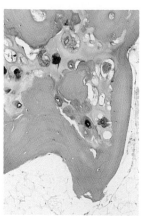

Figure 7.23 continued

b c d e

Figure 7.24 Benign chondroblastoma This uncommon benign tumour of immature cartilage cells is found most commonly in the epiphysis of long bones, particularly the humerus, femur, and tibia, but may arise elsewhere. It occurs most commonly in the second decade but may present at any age. Radiologically, the tumour usually lies eccentrically within an epiphysis (or apophysis); it may occasionally extend into the metaphysis; it is well demarcated, often has a sclerotic rim, and may show matrix calcification. 7.24a shows the radiological features of a benign chondroblastoma of the upper femur. The tumour is highly cellular and composed of mononuclear cells which have a well defined cell membrane, eosinophilic or clear cytoplasm, and a hyperchromatic or vesicular nucleus often containing a longitudinal groove (b, c). The cells lie within an amorphous, largely chondroid matrix. Focally, parts of the chondroid matrix exhibit a lace-like pattern of calcification (c). Secondary aneurysmal bone cyst formation may occur within a chondroblastoma (d). Curettage usually results in cure but recurrence may follow incomplete removal. Rarely, chondroblastomas may behave in a locally aggressive fashion. Pulmonary 'metastases' have been reported; these have generally occurred after vigorous curettage.

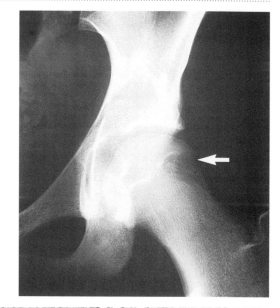

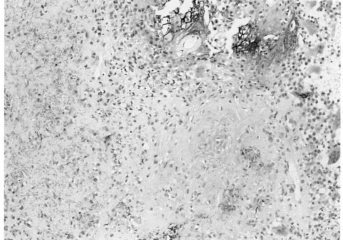

Figure 7.24

a

b

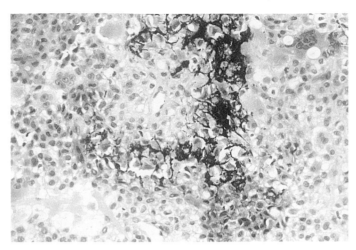

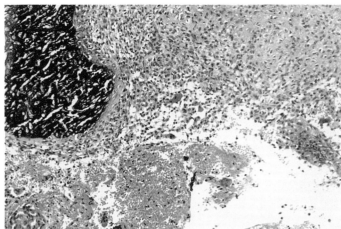

Figure 7.24 continued

c d

Figure 7.25 **Chondromyxoid fibroma** This is a rare benign cartilaginous tumour arising chiefly in young adults and adolescents. It occurs most commonly in bones below the knee, particularly in the metaphysis of the upper tibia, bones of the ankle and foot, but it may be found elsewhere. 7.25a shows a chondromyxoid fibroma of the upper tibia. The lesion is an eccentric, well defined lytic lesion with a sharp sclerotic margin; it is located in the metaphysis, does not usually involve the epiphysis, and produces expansion of the overlying cortex. The lesion is composed of lobules of myxoid or chondroid matrix containing scattered spindle-shaped or stellate cells showing some cellular and nuclear pleomorphism (b, c); the lobules are separated by more cellular areas of fibrous tissue containing similar mononuclear cells and osteoclast-like giant cells (d). The lesion is benign but commonly recurs after curettage. *En bloc* excision is recommended.

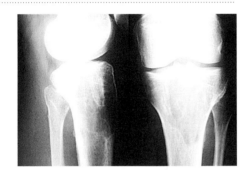

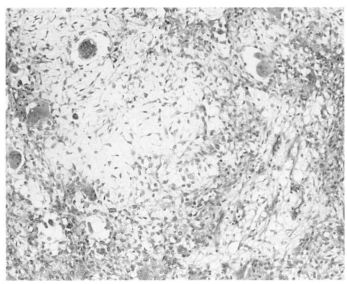

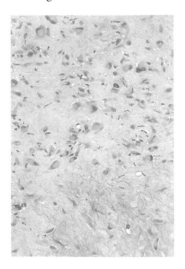

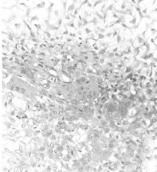

Figure 7.25

a

b

c d

Figure 7.26 Chondrosarcoma This is a relatively common primary malignant bone tumour characterized by the formation of cartilage by tumour cells. It is more common after the third decade and is usually found in the metaphysis or diaphysis of large tubular bones, the pelvis, scapula, and ribs. It rarely arises in the small bones of the hands and feet. Most chondrosarcomas arise in the medullary cavity (central chondrosarcoma) but some take origin from the external surface of the bone (peripheral chondrosarcoma). Most chondrosarcomas arise *de novo* but 10 per cent are secondary, arising in a pre-existing osteochondroma or enchondroma, usually in the context of hereditary multiple exostoses and enchondromatosis respectively. Clinically, there is swelling and often pain. 7.26a and 7.26b show the radiological features of a chondrosarcoma arising in the humerus and scapula respectively. Chondrosarcomas are often large, lytic tumours; they contain numerous areas of irregular dense or ring-like calcification. The cortex is thickened and has a scalloped inner margin; there may be cortical destruction and soft tissue extension. 7.26c shows the gross features of a large chondrosarcoma arising from a rib. The tumour is lobulated and contains translucent, firm or partly myxoid tissue with focal areas of calcification and ossification.

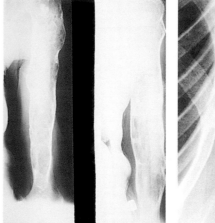
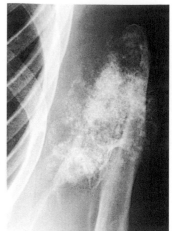

Figure 7.26

a b

c

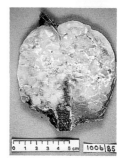

Figure 7.27 Chondrosarcoma Most tumours are low-grade and often difficult to distinguish histologically from enchondromas. Clinical and radiological features aid greatly in this distinction. Histologically, evidence of tumour invasion between host bone trabeculae (a) or marrow infiltration should particularly be sought. Myxoid change may also be seen in the cartilage matrix. In general, low-grade chondrosarcomas are usually more cellular than chondromas and show a greater degree of nuclear pleomorphism with frequent binucleated cells (arrow) (b). Grade II chondrosarcomas also have abundant matrix with scattered cartilage cells showing more marked cellular and nuclear pleomorphism and frequent binucleated cells (c). In grade III chondrosarcomas, much less cartilage matrix is usually found and tumour cells show more marked cytological and nuclear atypia (d, e). Chondrosarcomas usually cause extensive bone destruction and soft tissue involvement before metastasizing relatively late. Prognosis depends on the histological grade and stage of tumour involvement.

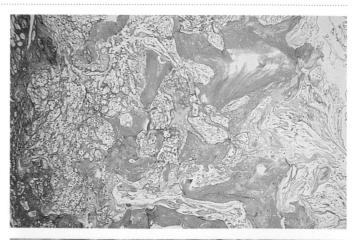

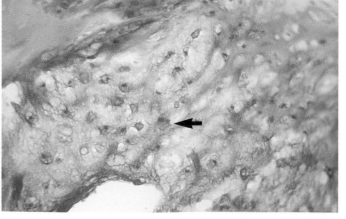

Figure 7.27

a

b

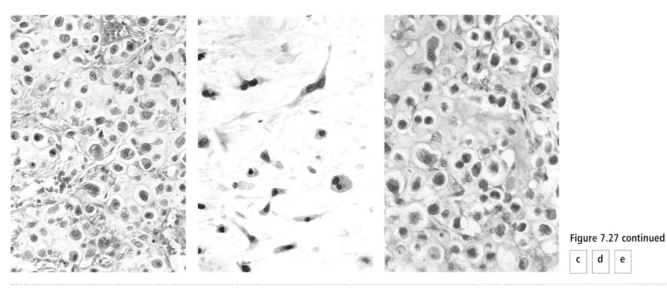

Figure 7.27 continued

c   d   e

Figure 7.28 **Dedifferentiated chondrosarcoma** In a dedifferentiated chondrosarcoma, a high-grade non-chondroid sarcoma (usually a fibrosarcoma or malignant fibrous histiocytoma) develops within a primary or more commonly recurrent well-differentiated chondrosarcoma. 7.28a shows the radiological features of a dedifferentiated chondrosarcoma of the upper femur. In addition to features of chondrosarcoma, an infiltrative lytic tumour is present and there is an associated pathological fracture. 7.28b shows the development of a malignant fibrous histiocytoma within a low-grade chondrosarcoma (arrow). The transition between chondrosarcoma and the dedifferentiated sarcoma component is abrupt (c). Pain and rapid growth often occur in dedifferentiated chondrosarcoma. Prognosis is poor.

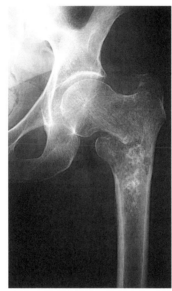

Figure 7.28

a

b   c

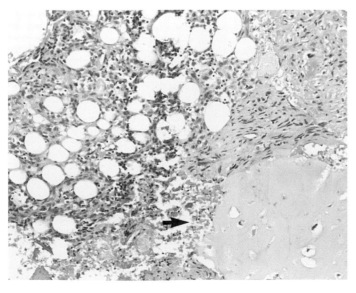

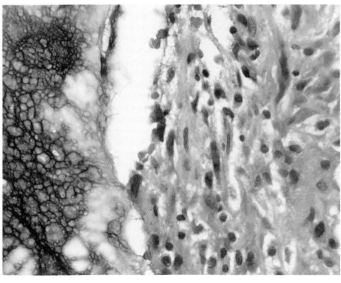

Figure 7.29 Mesenchymal chondrosarcoma This is a rare variant of chondrosarcoma which occurs most commonly in adolescents and young adults. The skull, jaw, ribs, pelvis, and long bones are most frequently affected but the tumour may also arise in soft tissues (see 8.96). 7.29a shows a mesenchymal chondrosarcoma, containing focal areas of calcification, arising in the petrous temporal bone. The tumour is composed of mesenchymal round or spindle-shaped cells amongst which lie nodules of cartilage (b, c). Areas of osteoid differentiation (d), irregular areas of calcification, and a prominent haemangiopericytomatous pattern (e) may also be seen. The lesion commonly enters into the differential diagnosis of malignant round cell tumours of bone as well as malignant cartilage and bone-forming tumours. The prognosis is poor with extensive local infiltration often preceding metastasis.

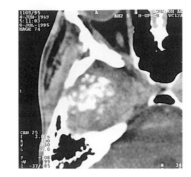
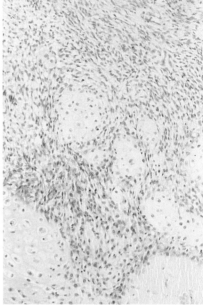

Figure 7.29

a	b

c	d	e

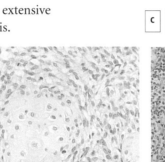
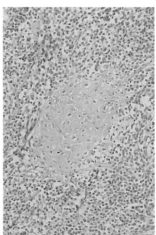
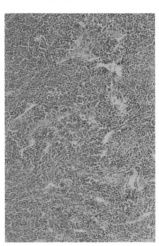

Figure 7.30 Clear cell chondrosarcoma This rare variant of chondrosarcoma is a low-grade tumour which occurs most commonly in young adults. It usually arises as a well defined lytic lesion in the epiphysis of long bones (a) and is thought by some observers to represent a malignant variant of chondroblastoma. It consists of swollen round or oval cells with abundant clear or vacuolated cytoplasm amongst which are scattered areas of cartilage matrix and small bone trabeculae (b, c). Scattered osteoclastic giant cells may be present. Areas of typical chondrosarcoma may also be found. *En bloc* excision is required for cure.

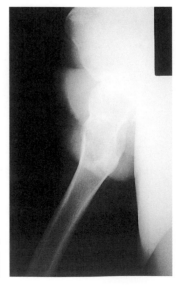

Figure 7.30

a

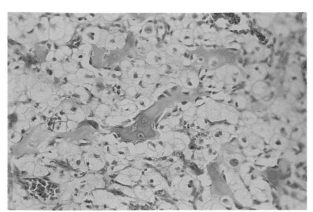 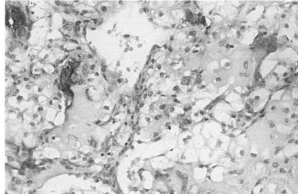

Figure 7.30 continued

b c

Figure 7.31 Juxtacortical (periosteal) chondrosarcoma This is a rare malignant cartilage-forming tumour arising on the external surface of the bone. The tumour is large, lies adjacent to the cortex, and is most likely of periosteal origin. Histologically it shows the features of a low-grade chondrosarcoma; there may be spotty calcification and endochondral ossification. Tumour osteoid or bone is absent. The tumour is usually found in a metaphyseal location. This lesion should be distinguished from periosteal osteosarcoma.

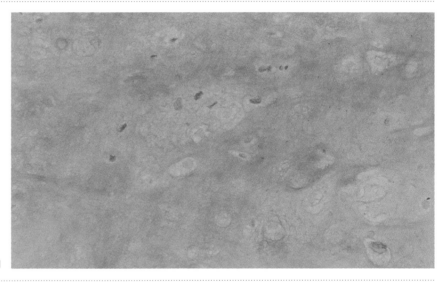

Figure 7.31

Giant cell lesions of bone

Figure 7.32 Giant cell tumour of bone This relatively uncommon but distinctive bone tumour is seen most frequently in patients who are skeletally mature. It occurs more often in females than males. Most tumours arise in the epiphysis (or apophysis) of a long bone, especially the lower end of femur and upper end of tibia/fibula, but any bone may be affected. The tumour enlarges progressively and often extends into the metaphysis and may penetrate the cortex, extending as a well-defined lesion into surrounding soft tissues. 7.32 shows the radiological features of a giant cell tumour of bone in the lower femur. It is usually a large, well defined, lytic, and often lobulated lesion, lying asymmetrically within the epiphysis. It often extends into the metaphysis and up to the articular surface. A periosteal reaction or extensive bone sclerosis is not usually seen around the tumour. Giant cell tumour of bone very commonly recurs after curettage. Complete excision is the surgical treatment of choice. Rarely, lung metastases of a giant cell tumour of bone have been reported. However, true malignant change in giant cell tumour of bone is extremely rare and usually associated with previous radiation therapy.

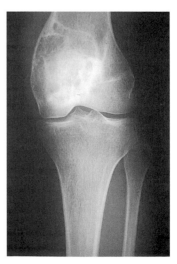

Figure 7.32

Figure 7.33 Giant cell tumour of bone The tumour contains numerous osteoclastic giant cells which are sprinkled throughout the tumour (a). The giant cells vary in size. Many are often very large and contain a large number of nuclei; no mitotic activity or nuclear atypia is seen amongst giant cells (b). The giant cells are scattered against a background of mononuclear round or spindle-shaped cells, some of which have nuclear features similar to those of the giant cells; others show a variable degree of mitotic activity and nuclear pleomorphism. Giant cell tumours are highly vascular and may contain focal areas of haemorrhage or infarction. There may be osteoid or reactive bone formation by some mononuclear cells (c). Microscopic grading of these tumours is not usually helpful in predicting behaviour. Many bone tumours and tumour-like lesions may contain areas in which there are numerous osteoclast-like giant cells and the differential diagnosis includes giant cell granuloma, aneurysmal bone cyst, fibrous dysplasia, non-ossifying fibroma, eosinophilic granuloma, osteosarcoma (telangiectatic, giant-cell rich), chondroblastoma, chondromyxoid fibroma, and non-neoplastic conditions such as brown tumour and Paget's disease. Clinical and radiological features aid in distinguishing these lesions. The giant cells of giant cell tumour of bone (and giant cell reparative granuloma of the jaw) are osteoclastic in nature and distinguished from those of other giant-cell-containing lesions of bone by expression of an osteoclast antigenic phenotype, being CD68 positive and negative for CD11/18, CD14 and usually HLA-DR (d).

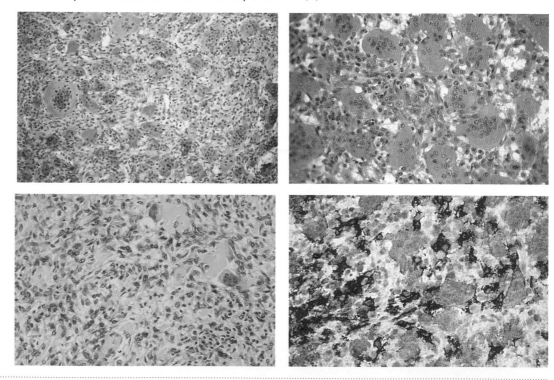

Figure 7.33

a	b
c	d

Figure 7.34 Giant cell reparative granuloma of the jaw (central giant cell granuloma) This tumour typically presents in the mandible or maxilla. Females are affected more frequently than males and patients are usually less than 30 years of age. The lesion is solitary and lytic, expanding the bone and thinning the overlying cortex (a). It contains scattered giant cells which usually lie within a prominent fibrous stroma containing small blood vessels (b, c). Giant cells express an osteoclast antigenic phenotype but are more irregularly distributed than in giant cell tumour of bone. Unlike giant cell tumour of bone, recurrence rarely occurs after curettage. Giant cell tumour of bone rarely arises in the jaw in the absence of Paget's disease.

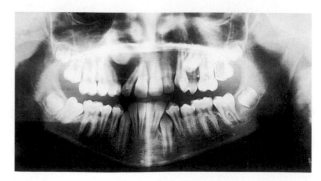

Figure 7.34

a

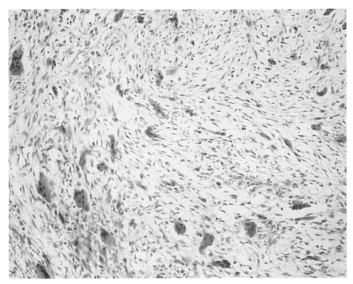

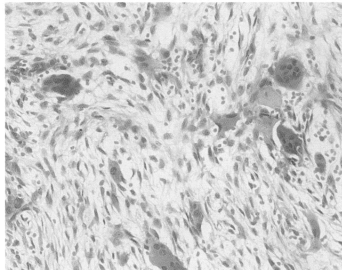

Figure 7.34 continued

| b | c |

Figure 7.35 Giant cell granuloma of small bones This is a rare, benign bone lesion which occurs over a wide age range but is seen most commonly in patients less than 30 years of age. The lesion is lytic, well defined, and usually involves the phalanges, metacarpal bones, or metatarsal bones. Focal aggregates of giant cells and scattered macrophages are seen within a cellular fibroblastic stroma which shows evidence of osteoid and bone formation (a, b). Secondary aneurysmal bone cyst formation may be noted. Differential diagnosis includes other giant cell lesions of bone, in particular the brown tumour of hyperparathyroidism.

Figure 7.35

| a | b |

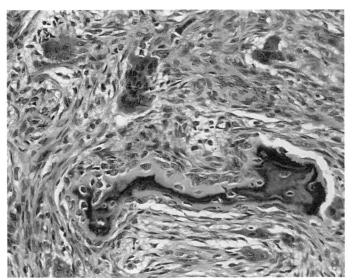

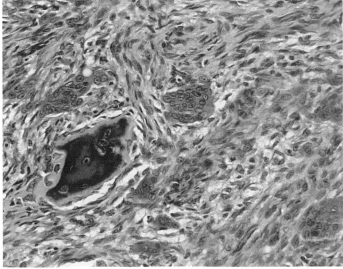

Round cell tumours of bone

Figure 7.36 Ewing's sarcoma This is a rare, highly malignant tumour of uncertain histogenesis which occurs in children or adolescents. It arises most commonly between 5 and 20 years of age and is rare in patients younger than 2 years or older than 30 years. The tumour develops within the medullary cavity in the shaft or metaphysis and rapidly spreads to involve the whole bone. There is early extension through the cortex into surrounding soft tissues. Clinically, there is often pain and swelling and sometimes systemic features such as pyrexia, anaemia, leucocytosis, and a raised erythrocyte sedimentation rate. 7.36 shows the radiological features of a Ewing's sarcoma of the upper femur. The tumour is large and there is 'moth-eaten' or permeative destruction of medullary bone. The cortex is penetrated and there is a prominent periosteal reaction. Characteristically, periosteal new bone is deposited in layers resembling those of an onion skin.

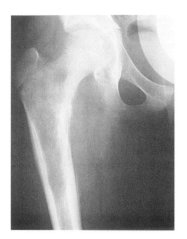

Figure 7.36

Figure 7.37 Ewing's sarcoma Ewing's sarcoma is composed of densely packed small cells with uniform round or oval nuclei which have finely dispersed chromatin (a). Tumour cells have poorly defined cell outline and scanty cytoplasm. Necrosis and areas of haemorrhage are commonly seen within the tumour (b). A filigree growth pattern (c) has been associated with a poorer prognosis than a diffuse or lobular pattern of growth. Sheets of tumour cells are commonly divided into lobules by thin fibrous strands and the reticulin network between the tumour cells is characteristically scanty (d). The tumour cells contain abundant glycogen which is PAS positive (diastase sensitive) (e); this is best determined using imprint preparations or cryostat sections of the tumour. Tumour cells are also positive for the MIC2 gene product. A small percentage of tumours (atypical Ewing's sarcoma) contain tumour cells with larger, more pleomorphic

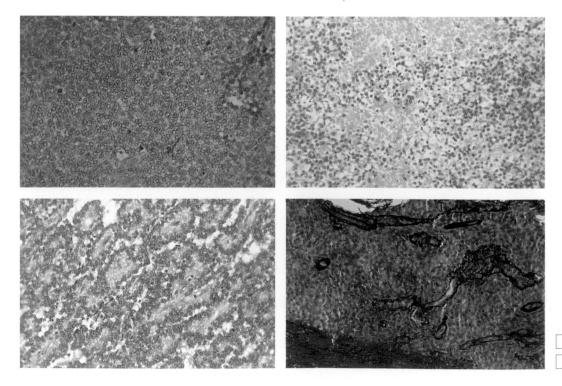

Figure 7.37

a	b
c	d

nuclei, prominent nucleoli, and increased mitotic activity (f). Ewing's sarcoma tumour cells exhibit a characteristic t(11;22) (q24;q12) chromosomal translocation. The use of combination adjuvant or neoadjuvant chemotherapy with surgery and radiation therapy has considerably improved the prognosis in Ewing's sarcoma.

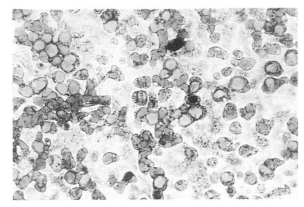
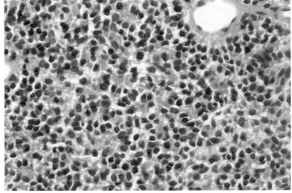

Figure 7.37

e f

Figure 7.38 Neuroectodermal tumour of bone This is a rare and highly malignant tumour that resembles the soft tissue primitive neuroectodermal tumour (peripheral neuroepithelioma) (see 8.86). It has many clinical, radiological, and pathological features in common with Ewing's sarcoma but is distinguished morphologically from the latter by the greater degree of cellular and nuclear pleomorphism exhibited by tumour cells; focally, there may be rosette or pseudorosette formation (as shown here). It also shows a greater degree of cellular and nuclear pleomorphism than typical Ewing's sarcoma. Tumour cells also commonly express neural markers such as neurone-specific enolase and Leu-7. They are positive for MIC2 and commonly exhibit the same t(11;22) chromosomal translocation seen in Ewing's sarcoma. These tumours are currently treated with the same therapeutic protocol as Ewing's sarcoma but generally show a poorer response.

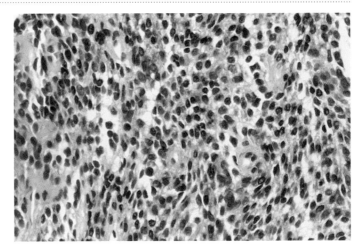

Figure 7.38

Figure 7.39 Metastatic neuroblastoma Neuroblastoma is a tumour of the sympathetic nervous system which usually arises in the adrenal medulla. It occurs in very young children, usually less than 5 years of age, and most often in the first 2 years of life. Neuroblastoma commonly metastasizes to bone and needs to be distinguished from Ewing's sarcoma and other primary round cell tumours of bone. Neuroblastomas are composed of diffuse sheets of small cells with poorly defined cell borders, indistinct cytoplasm, and round, oval, or spindle-shaped nuclei. Tumours spread diffusely through the bone (a). More differentiated tumours contain small nodules of tumour cells or exhibit rosette formation (b). Evidence of catecholamine production by tumour cells may be found in the serum or urine.

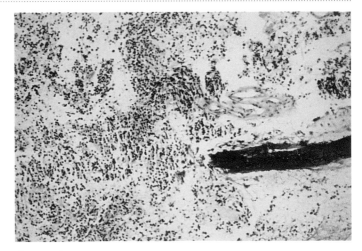

Figure 7.39

a

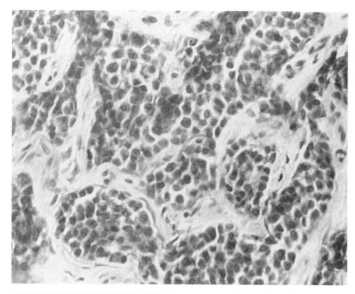

Figure 7.39 continued

b

Figure 7.40 **Malignant lymphoma** Primary lymphoma in bone occurs rarely and lymphoma in bone is usually secondary to disease involving lymphoid tissues elsewhere. Primary lymphoma is seen most often in older patients but may occasionally present in childhood. It usually involves the metaphysis or diaphysis of large tubular bones, pelvis, spine, or scapula. 7.40a shows a primary lymphoma of the proximal femur. There is 'moth-eaten' bone destruction of the medulla and cortex but little or no periosteal reaction. The tumour is usually a diffuse, high-grade B-cell lymphoma which contains identifiable lymphoid cells such as lymphocytes, lymphoblasts, centrocytes, and centroblasts (b, c). Tumour cells generally have a well-defined cell outline and large hyperchromatic or vesicular nuclei containing prominent nucleoli (c). Glycogen is usually absent. There is often a dense reticulin network around tumour cells (d). Immunohistochemical staining for leucocyte common antigen, immunoglobulins, and B-cell markers is useful in distinguishing these tumours from other round cell tumours of bone.

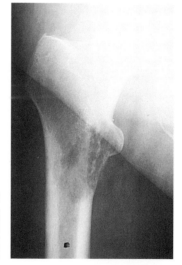

Figure 7.40

a

b c d

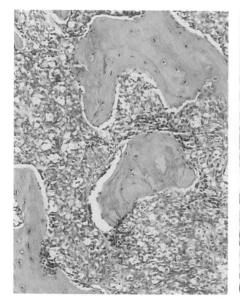

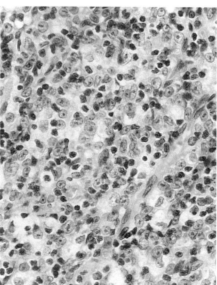

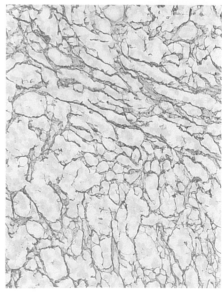

Figure 7.41 **Hodgkin's disease** Systemic Hodgkin's disease (particularly of the mixed cellularity type) can produce multifocal osteolytic or osteoblastic secondary deposits which are commonly asymptomatic. These tumours often contain a mixture of inflammatory cells and are characterized by the presence of large Sternberg–Reed cells, which have abundant cytoplasm and one or more multilobed nuclei with prominent nucleoli (arrow); these cells are CD15 and CD30 positive.

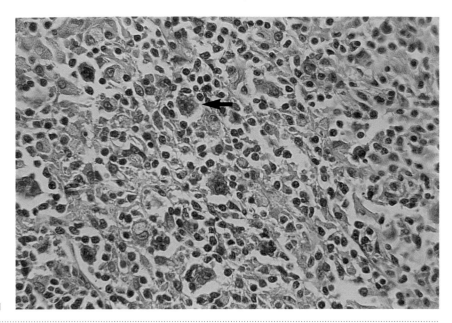

Figure 7.41

Figure 7.42 **Leukaemia in bone** Acute lymphoblastic leukaemia may rarely present as a bone tumour, producing diffuse bone rarefaction or discrete lytic lesions. A diffuse infiltrate of lymphoblasts is seen in the marrow (a). In acute myeloid leukaemia a discrete granulocytic sarcoma (chloroma) which consists of a diffuse infiltrate of myeloblasts may occur in bone or soft tissues (b). Tumour cells are chloroacetate esterase positive. These tumours are common in the orbit but may occur anywhere in the axial or appendicular skeleton. Chloromas may also occur in blastic transformation of chronic myeloid leukaemia.

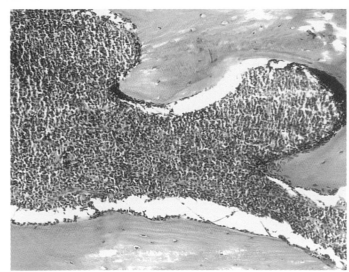

Figure 7.42

a

b

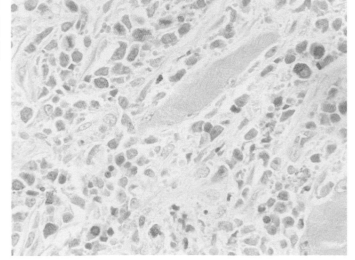

Figure 7.43 Myeloma Myeloma is the most common primary tumour of bone. Myeloma may be localized (solitary myeloma; plasmacytoma) or more commonly disseminated (multiple myeloma; myelomatosis). Almost all patients with plasmacytoma go on to develop multiple myeloma. Myeloma is associated with the production of monoclonal immunoglobulin or immunoglobulin components. It often causes disease in other organ systems. Multiple myeloma is rarely seen below 40 years of age and is more common in males. Lesions are found most frequently in bones where there is active haematopoiesis (e.g. spine, skull, pelvis, ribs, and proximal femur and humerus). Radiologically, in both solitary and multiple myeloma, lesions have a well defined 'punched out' appearance with usually little or no surrounding bone reaction. 7.43a shows a myeloma deposit in the fourth lumbar vertebra. Grossly, myeloma deposits are multiple, soft, pink, and often haemorrhagic, as in the case of myelomatosis of the skull shown in 7.43b.

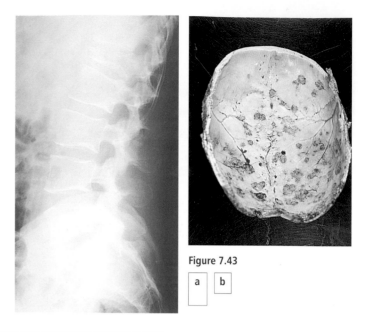

Figure 7.43

a b

Figure 7.44 Myeloma Both solitary and multiple myeloma consist of sheets of plasma cells which are usually relatively uniform and well differentiated. Tumour cells characteristically have an eccentric nucleus and peripheral 'clock face' distribution of chromatin (a, b). Tumour cells may show some cellular and nuclear pleomorphism and there may be occasional multinucleated plasma cells. Tumour cells are pyroninophilic and contain immunoglobulin of a single light chain type. There is usually little stromal connective tissue. Small deposits of amyloid may sometimes be found within the tumour. Waldenstrom's macroglobulinaemia is a rare neoplastic disorder related to myeloma in which there is production of a monoclonal high molecular weight IgM immunoglobulin. In this condition, infiltrating tumour cells in the marrow exhibit some lymphoid and plasmacytoid features (c). Multiple myeloma is a tumour of poor prognosis which is treated by chemotherapy. Radiation therapy and surgery may be employed to control the growth of lesions causing pathological fracture or spinal cord compression.

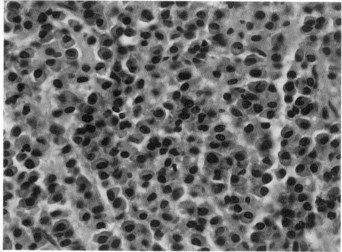

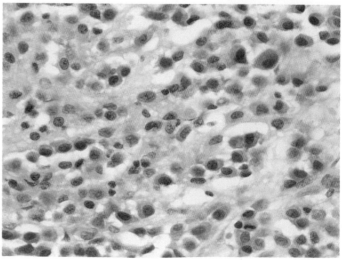

Figure 7.44

a

b

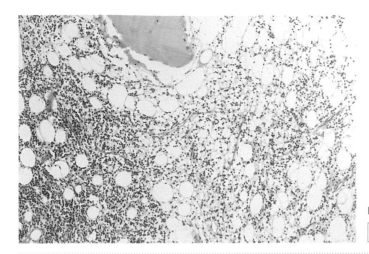

Figure 7.44 continued

c

Vascular tumours of bone

Figure 7.45 Haemangioma This benign tumour is considered to be relatively common although many reported asymptomatic haemangiomas represent areas of vascular ectasia or hamartomas rather than true haemangiomas. Haemangiomas are found most often in the calvarium, ribs, and vertebrae of adults. Radiologically, lesions are well demarcated and lytic (a), producing a prominent periosteal reaction (arrow) in skull bones (b). Grossly, lesions are well defined and composed of numerous blood-filled spaces (c). Haemangiomas are composed of numerous thin-walled vessels separated by fibrous tissue or bone trabeculae; vessels are capillary or cavernous in nature and are lined by flattened endothelium (d, e). Symptomatic lesion require excision. Haemangiomas of bone are not uncommonly multiple and may rarely be multifocal with extensive diffuse intraosseous involvement (skeletal angiomatosis); this may on occasion be associated with multiple soft tissue haemangiomas. The histology of other benign vascular tumours which may rarely arise in bone, including lymphangioma, glomus tumour, and histiocytoid haemangioma (angiolymphoid hyperplasia with eosinophilia), is similar to that of these lesions in soft tissue (see Chapter 8).

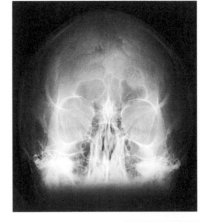
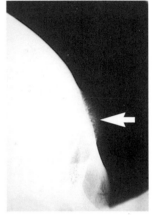

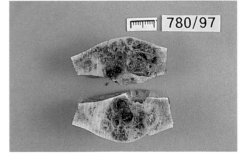

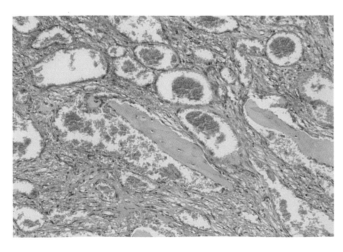

Figure 7.45

a b

c

d

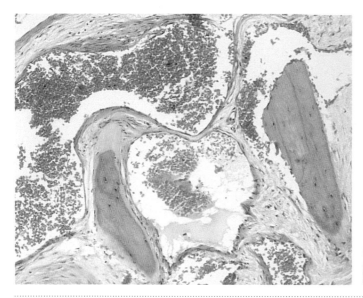

Figure 7.45 continued

e

Figure 7.46 **Gorham's disease (massive osteolysis; vanishing/disappearing/phantom bone disease)** This is a rare skeletal condition of unknown aetiology, which principally affects children and young adults. It is characterized by extensive progressive replacement of bone by fibrous tissue containing numerous thin-walled vessels and small and large vascular spaces (a, b). Vascular spaces may or may not be lined by endothelium. Any part of the skeleton may be affected and one or more (often contiguous) bones may be involved. The hip or shoulder region is most commonly affected. There is destruction of both cortex and medulla, giving rise radiologically to the 'sucked candy' appearance. Pathogenesis is unknown. Reconstitution of the bone rarely occurs.

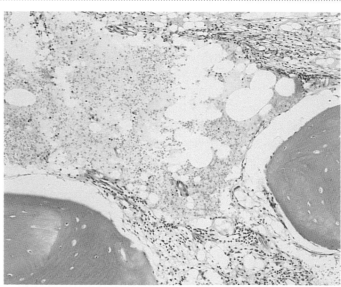

Figure 7.46

a

b

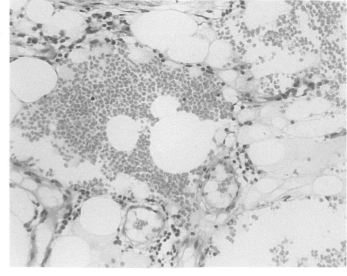

Figure 7.47 Epithelioid haemangioendothelioma This is a vascular tumour of low-grade malignancy which is usually locally aggressive. It occurs over a wide age range and may occur in any bone, particularly those of the axial skeleton or lower limb. More than one bone is often involved or several lesions may be present in one bone. Radiologically, lesions are well defined, lytic, often trabeculated, and have surrounding sclerosis. The lesions have a myxoid and fibrous stroma in which there are large endothelial cells with plump eosinophilic, often vacuolated cytoplasm and large hyperchromatic nuclei (a). Tumour cells are best identified by factor VIII staining when they can be seen to line small vascular channels (b). Local treatment alone is usually indicated; metastasis has rarely been reported. Differential diagnosis includes metastatic adenocarcinoma, angiosarcoma, and chordoma.

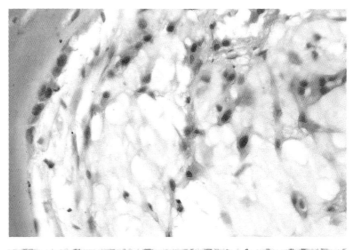

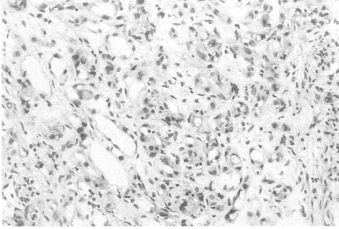

Figure 7.47

a

b

Figure 7.48 Angiosarcoma This is a rare malignant vascular tumour of bone, most frequently arising in large tubular bones of middle-aged and elderly adults. Radiologically, lesions are often large, osteolytic, and infiltrative, extending through the cortex into surrounding soft tissues. 7.48a shows the radiological features of an angiosarcoma of the lower tibia; a discrete, second vascular tumour is also present in the proximal tibia. Histologically, the tumour is composed of cords and clusters of plump endothelial cells which line vascular channels (b). Tumour cells have abundant eosinophilic cytoplasm and highly pleomorphic nuclei. Tumour cells are factor VIII positive. Radical excision is required. Prognosis is poor.

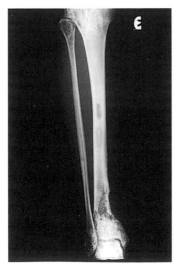

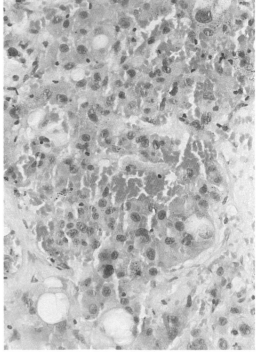

Figure 7.48

a b

Other connective tissue tumours arising in bone

Figure 7.49 Lipoma This is an uncommon benign tumour of bone which may arise in an intramedullary or periosteal location. Medullary lipomas are most frequently seen in the long bones of adults; they are often difficult to distinguish radiologically from bone infarcts as they may show extensive calcification. Radiologically, they are well defined, lytic lesions which may or may not have a surrounding zone of sclerosis. Most lie in the metaphysis or diaphysis. 7.49a shows a rare intraosseous lipoma involving the femoral epiphysis. Lesions are well defined and composed almost entirely of mature fat (b). Focal areas of calcification or a few scanty, thin bone trabeculae may be seen within an intraosseous lipoma. Periosteal lesions may be associated with new bone formation.

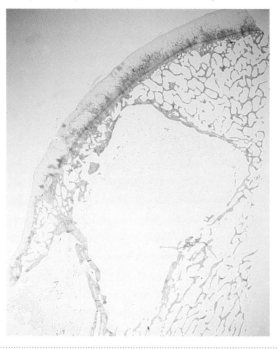
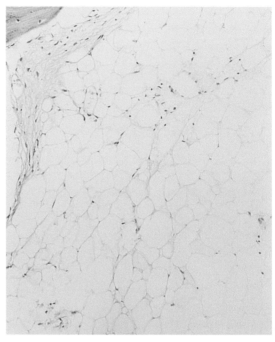

Figure 7.49

a b

Figure 7.50 Desmoplastic fibroma This is a locally aggressive tumour which is characterized by the formation of abundant collagen by fibroblastic cells. It appears to represent the intraosseous counterpart of soft tissue fibromatosis. It occurs over a wide age range but is seen most commonly in the first three decades of life. The metaphysis or diaphysis of long bones and the pelvis are most commonly affected. 7.50a shows the radiological features of a desmoplastic fibroma of the shaft of the humerus. The lesion is lytic, trabeculated, and has well-defined margins. Larger lesions are associated with cortical destruction and extension into surrounding soft tissues. The lesion is composed of mature fibroblasts and abundant collagen fibres (b). There is little or no cellular or nuclear pleomorphism or mitotic activity (c). The lesion is slow growing and locally aggressive. Recurrence is common after curettage.

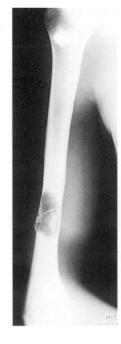

Figure 7.50

a

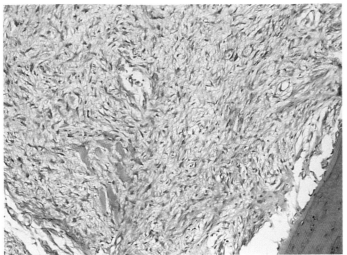

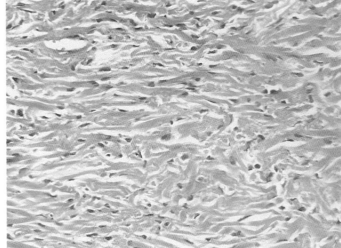

Figure 7.50 continued

b   c

Figure 7.51 Fibrosarcoma This is a rare malignant bone tumour which usually arises in the metaphysis of long bones in adults. 7.51a shows the radiological features of a fibrosarcoma of the lower femur. It is a poorly defined, largely osteolytic tumour which produces 'moth-eaten' and permeative destruction of the medulla and cortex and extends into surrounding soft tissues. It is composed of numerous fibroblast-like spindle cells that produce a variable amount of collagen (b). A herring-bone pattern may be present. Tumour cells are hyperchromatic and show some nuclear pleomorphism: there is frequent mitotic activity (c). Giant cells are not usually a feature. Prognosis is strongly related to the histological grade of the tumour.

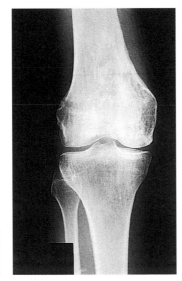

Figure 7.51

a

b   c

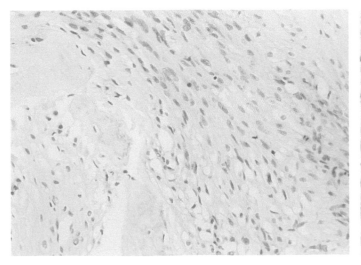

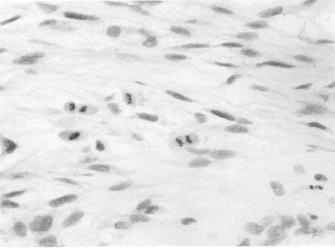

Figure 7.52 **Malignant fibrous histiocytoma (MFH)** This is an uncommon malignant bone tumour which shares some clinical, radiological, and pathological features with fibrosarcoma. It occurs mainly in adults, usually arising in the metaphysis of large tubular bones. 7.52a shows the radiological features of an MFH involving the proximal femur. The lesion is poorly defined and largely lytic; there is 'moth-eaten' and permeative destruction of bone with cortical penetration and soft tissue extension. Histologically, the tumour has a fibrous stroma and usually resembles the storiform-pleomorphic MFH of soft tissues. It is composed of spindle-shaped, round, or oval cells lying in whorls, bundles, or often in a prominent storiform arrangement (b, c). There is often prominent cellular and nuclear pleomorphism, increased mitotic activity, and occasional atypical mitotic figures (d). Scattered multinucleated osteoclast-like giant cells or tumour giant cells may be found. The lesion may arise in association with bone infarcts or after radiation therapy and is the most common form of sarcoma developing in a dedifferentiated chondrosarcoma.

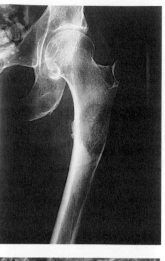

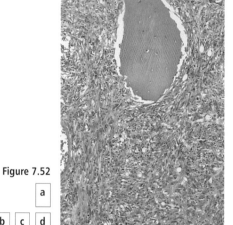
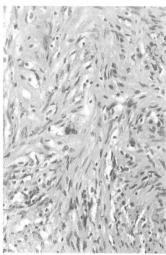
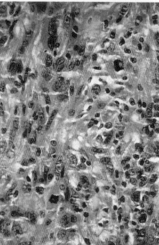

Figure 7.52

a

b c d

Figure 7.53 **Leiomyosarcoma of bone** Benign or malignant smooth muscle tumours are very rare primary tumours of bone. Most leiomyosarcomas in bone represent metastases. Primary tumours, however, may rarely occur in elderly patients, usually in large tubular bones, especially the femur and tibia. Radiological features are similar to those of a fibrosarcoma. The tumour is characterized by the presence of numerous spindle-shaped tumour cells with elongated, blunt-ended nuclei and indistinct cytoplasm (a). There is a variable degree of cellular and nuclear pleomorphism and mitotic activity is frequent. Immunohistochemistry shows that the tumour cells express desmin (b), smooth muscle actin and other muscle antigens.

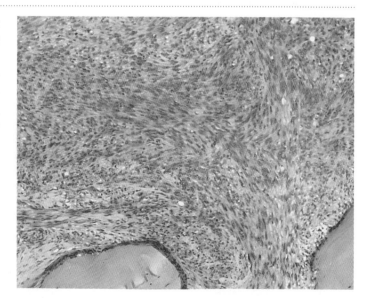

Figure 7.53

a

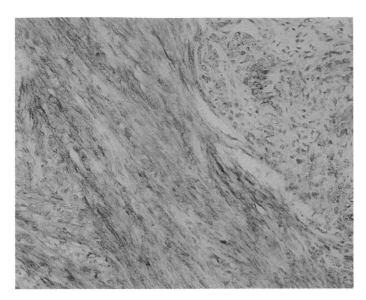

Figure 7.53 continued

b

Figure 7.54 **Myxoma** This tumour has been reported over a wide age range but occurs most commonly in young adults. It most frequently arises in the mandible and maxilla, producing a well defined, osteolytic lesion which may be trabeculated and have a sclerotic margin. The tumour contains stellate and spindle-shaped tumour cells which lie in an abundant mucinous matrix (a, b). A small amount of cellular or collagenous fibrous tissue may be present but there is no evidence of bone formation. Recurrence may occur after inadequate excision.

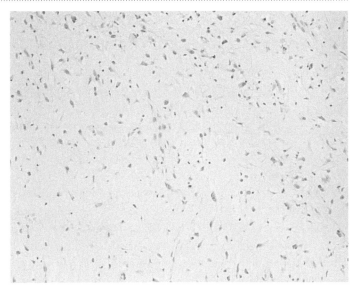

Figure 7.54

a

b

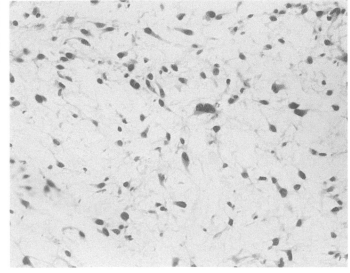

Figure 7.55 Neurilemmoma This is a very rare benign tumour of bone which has been reported over a wide age range. The mandible and sacrum are most often involved but the lesion has been reported in other bones. Histologically, the lesion contains predominantly cellular Antoni type A areas. Spindle cells with indistinct cytoplasm and wavy nuclei, often in a palisade arrangement, are present. Verocay bodies may be seen. The lesion is usually treated by curettage or excision.

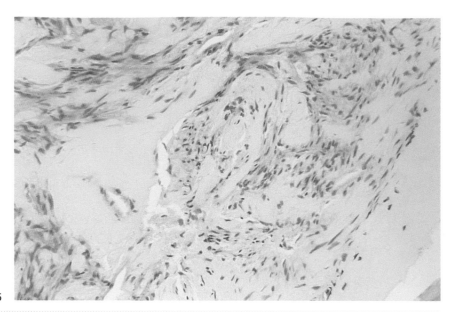

Figure 7.55

Other primary malignant tumours of bone

Figure 7.56 Chordoma This is a malignant tumour which arises from remnants of the notochord, the embryonic axial skeleton; it takes origin from within the bone substance rather than the nucleus pulposus of the disc. It arises chiefly in middle-aged and elderly adults and is more common in males than females. It is found most often in the sacral region; the spheno-occipital region and cervical and other vertebrae are also affected in descending order of frequency. 7.56 shows the radiological features of a chordoma of the sacral region. The tumour is large and causes extensive bone destruction with spread into surrounding soft tissues. Focal areas of calcification are present within the tumour. Tumours of vertebrae may be seen radiologically to take origin from the vertebral body rather than posterior elements.

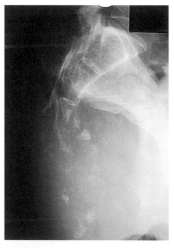

Figure 7.56

Figure 7.57 Chordoma The tumour is made up of sheets or cords of highly vacuolated physaliphorous cells that lie within an abundant mucoid extracellular matrix (a, b). Tumour cells have prominent vesicular nuclei. Mitotic activity is not prominent. Tumour cells express epithelial markers. Differential diagnosis of chordoma includes metastatic mucinous adenocarcinoma, myxopapillary ependymoma (shown in 7.57c), and chondrosarcoma. Some spheno-occipital chordomas may contain a significant cartilaginous component. These are termed chondroid chordomas and have a relatively good prognosis. Radiotherapy and surgery are required to control local growth of the lesion which eventually metastasizes in most cases.

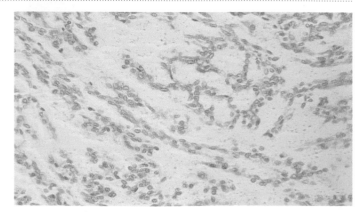

Figure 7.57

a

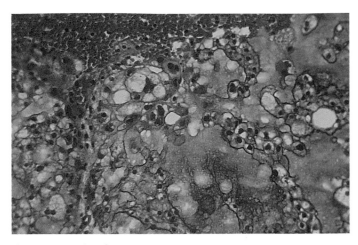
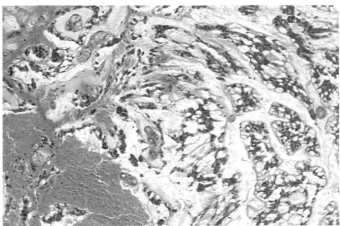

Figure 7.57 continued

b   c

Figure 7.58 Adamantinoma of long bones This is a rare, slow-growing malignant tumour of uncertain histogenesis which is found in the shaft of long bones, particularly the tibia and fibula. The tumour usually presents in young and middle-aged adults, more often males than females. 7.58a shows the radiological features of an adamantinoma of the tibia. The tumour is an eccentric, well defined, lytic lesion which is multiloculated; there is sclerosis of surrounding bone. It consists of cords and clusters of epithelial cells separated by a cellular and collagenous fibrous stroma. Small glands may be present within the tumour (b). The fibrous stroma may contain cleft-like spaces lined by plump tumour cells or contain small collections of these tumour cells (c, d). Tumour cells are positive for epithelial markers. Adamantinoma has been associated with osteofibrous dysplasia (see 7.70). The tumour grows slowly, is locally aggressive, and metastasizes late via the lymphatics and the bloodstream. It commonly recurs after curettage and should be treated by *en bloc* excision.

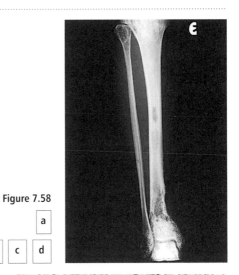

Figure 7.58

a

b   c   d

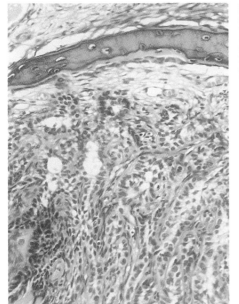
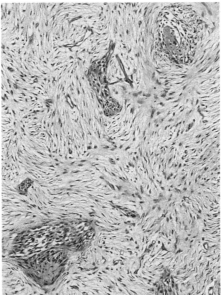
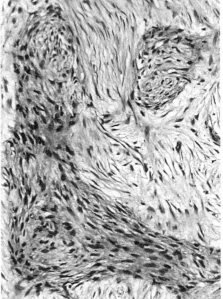

Other tumour-like lesions of bone

Figure 7.59 **Solitary bone cyst** This is a benign, non-neoplastic, solitary cystic defect which occurs most commonly in the metaphyseal region of the humerus, femur, and other long bones. It is seen most frequently in children and adolescents. Males are more often affected than females. 7.59a shows the radiological features of a typical simple bone cyst of the upper humerus. The lesion is well defined, lytic and slightly expands the bone, thinning the overlying cortex. The cyst lies directly under the growth plate and extends into the diaphysis. The cyst wall is composed largely of cellular fibrous tissue which covers the bone surface (b). The cyst wall may contain evidence of haemorrhage and areas of reparative granulation tissue, calcification, cholesterol clefts, macrophages, and other chronic inflammatory cells (c). There may also be new bone formation and thickening of bone around the cyst wall, particularly if a fracture has occurred. Abundant fibrin and occasionally amorphous calcified cementum-like material may occasionally be present within the cyst wall (d). Treatment includes aspiration of the cyst with injection of steroids or curettage and bone graft. Recurrence occurs in up to 20 per cent of cases.

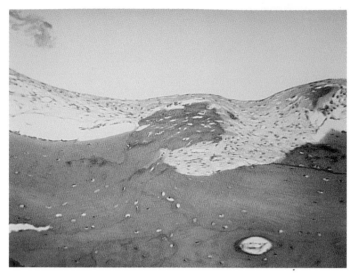

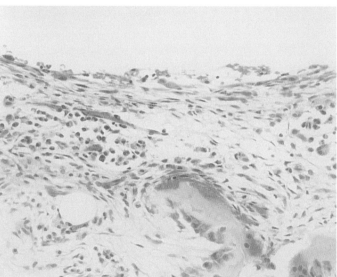

Figure 7.59

| b |
| c |
| a | d |

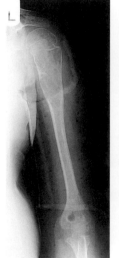

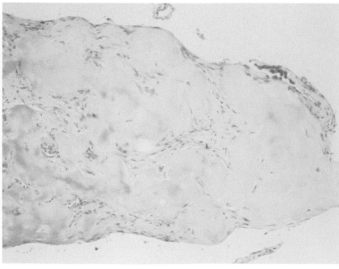

Figure 7.60 Aneurysmal bone cyst This is a solitary, often large and rapidly expanding lesion which arises most commonly in the metaphysis or shaft of long bones and the posterior elements of vertebrae. It occurs most frequently in children and adolescents. It often grows rapidly, producing an eccentric, well defined, multiloculated lytic lesion which expands the bone or balloons from the surface of the bone (a). The cyst is covered by a thin cortex or may have an indistinct outer margin. It consists of large blood-filled spaces separated by cellular and collagenous fibrous tissue (b). Osteoclast-like giant cells line blood-filled spaces and are seen within fibrous septa (c). Fibrous septa contain areas of haemorrhage and numerous haemosiderin-laden macrophages as well as reactive osteoid and woven bone formation. Some intraosseous lesions, which show features of an aneurysmal bone cyst, exhibit prominent osteoid and woven bone formation and are considered a type of solid variant of aneurysmal bone cyst (d). The lesion is benign but recurrence often follows simple curettage or incomplete excision.

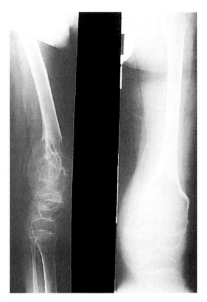

Figure 7.60

a	
b	
c	d

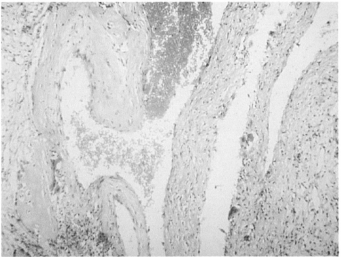

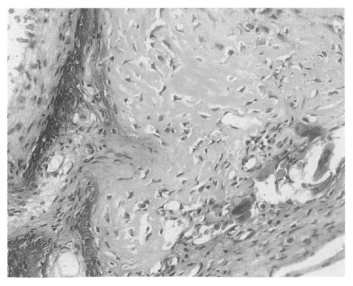

Figure 7.61 **Epidermoid inclusion cyst** This rare cystic lesion is found most commonly in the distal phalanx or in calvarial bones. Radiologically, the cyst is small, round, and purely lytic (a). The cyst wall is initially lined by stratified squamous epithelium but this is often lost and what remains is a cyst filled with keratin and part of the fibrous tissue wall of the cyst covering the bone (b); a giant cell reaction to keratin is commonly seen in the fibrous tissue wall (c). The lesion is treated by curettage or excision.

Figure 7.61

a

b c

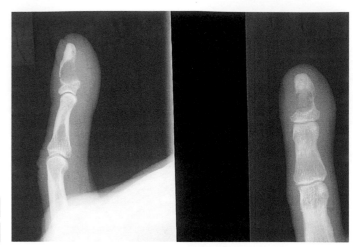

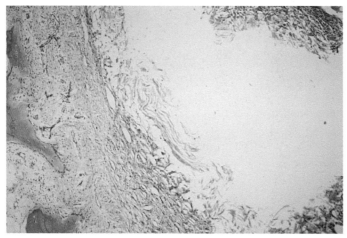

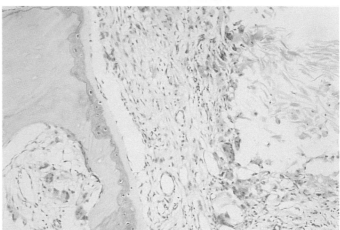

Figure 7.62 **Intraosseous ganglion (ganglion cyst of bone; juxta-articular bone cyst)** This is an uncommon cystic lesion which is found in the epiphysis of long bones, most commonly the medial malleolus of the tibia. It occurs most frequently in adults. Radiologically, the lesion is well defined, and osteolytic with sclerosis in surrounding bone (a). Histologically, it resembles a soft tissue ganglion, being composed of one or more cystic spaces that contain mucinous material; the cystic spaces lie between bone trabeculae (b). Cysts are filled with mucinous material and the cyst wall is composed of cellular collagenous fibrous tissue (c). An intraosseous ganglion may occur in association with a ganglion in overlying soft tissue. Intraosseous ganglion is distinguished from a subchondral cyst, which is usually seen in the context of joint disease (e.g. osteoarthritis), by the fact that it does not open onto the articular surface.

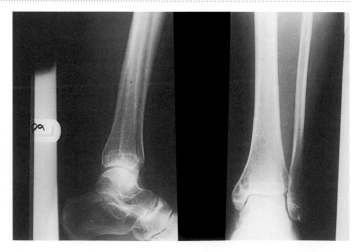

Figure 7.62

a

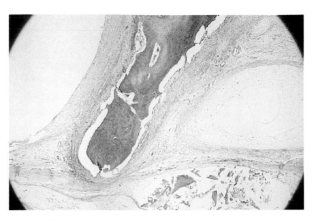
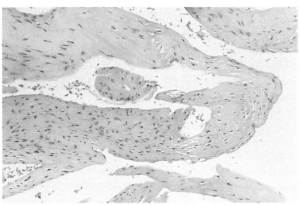

Figure 7.62 continued b c

Figure 7.63 Non-ossifying fibroma (metaphyseal fibrous defect; fibrous cortical defect) This is a relatively common lesion which is usually found in the subcortical metaphyseal region of long bones in children and adolescents. It occurs most commonly in the upper and lower tibia and lower femur. The pathogenesis is uncertain. It is not thought to be neoplastic but may be due to trauma which results in focal cortical fibrosis that extends into the medulla. Radiologically, the lesion lies in the metaphyseal region and is well defined, lytic and often multiloculated with a scalloped, sclerotic margin. 7.63 shows a non-ossifying fibroma of the distal radius. Small lesions (commonly termed meta-physeal fibrous defect) are usually asymptomatic and found incidentally on radiographs, but larger lesions (usually termed non-ossifying fibroma) may be symptomatic and cause pathological fracture. The lesion enlarges in the long axis of the bone and tends to migrate towards the diaphysis away from the growth plate.

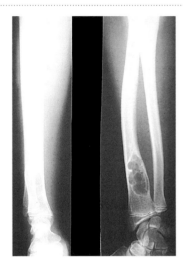

Figure 7.63

Figure 7.64 Non-ossifying fibroma Non-ossifying fibroma is composed of fibroblast-like spindle cells and round or oval macrophage-like cells arranged in a storiform pattern (a). There is a variable amount of collagen formation. Scattered collections of giant cells (b), haemosiderin deposits, and foamy macrophages (c) may be seen. Cellular and nuclear pleomorphism is not marked and there is usually little or no mitotic activity. Small lesions tend to regress spontaneously but larger lesions may require curettage. Rare lesions showing similar histological features to those of non-ossifying fibroma, which arise in other locations in the bone, particularly in adults, are now classified as benign fibrous histiocytomas of bone.

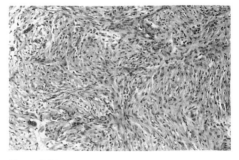
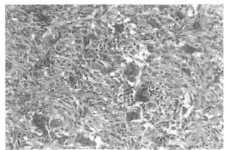
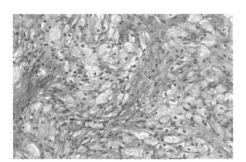

Figure 7.64

a b c

Figure 7.65 **Eosinophilic granuloma (Histiocytosis X; Langerhans cell granulomatosis)** This condition occurs most commonly in children and rarely occurs after 30 years of age. It is characterized by the formation of solitary or multiple lesions in bone, particularly in the skull, jaw, ribs, spine, and large tubular bones; there may also be systemic involvement. The terms 'Langerhans cell granulomatosis' or 'Histiocytosis X' describe the group of conditions characterized by the formation of multiple eosinophilic granuloma-like lesions in bone and other tissues. In Hand–Schüller–Christian disease, multiple eosinophilic granulomas are found in bone and there is associated diabetes insipidus, exophthalmos, lymphadenopathy, hepatosplenomegaly, and lung involvement. (Letterer–Siwe disease was formerly included amongst the conditions of Histiocytosis X but is probably best classified as a type of malignant lymphoma.) 7.65 shows the radiological features of an eosinophilic granuloma in the shaft of the tibia. The lesion is radiolucent and rather poorly defined. There is surrounding sclerosis and destruction of cortical bone with periosteal new bone formation. Radiological appearances of eosinophilic granuloma may be highly variable.

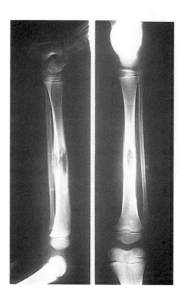

Figure 7.65

Figure 7.66 **Eosinophilic granuloma (Histiocytosis X; Langerhans cell granulomatosis)** Lesions of eosinophilic granuloma or Histiocytosis X are composed of a mixture of inflammatory cells including numerous eosinophil polymorphs (a), lymphocytes, plasma cells, macrophages, giant cells (arrow) (b), and typically large mononuclear cells (Langerhans cells) which have abundant pale cytoplasm and an indented or lobulated nucleus containing a central longitudinal groove. The lesion may extend into the cortex (c). Recently formed lesions are more cellular and contain abundant eosinophils (arrow); older lesions contain more fibrous tissue. Immunohistochemistry shows positive reaction for S-100 protein, HLA-DR and CD1 in Langerhans cells. Birbeck granules are seen on electron microscopy. Differential diagnosis includes osteomyelitis, non-ossifying fibroma, and other giant cell lesions of bone. Solitary eosinophilic granulomas may heal with time; curettage or injection of steroids is used for lesions requiring treatment. Recurrence is rare.

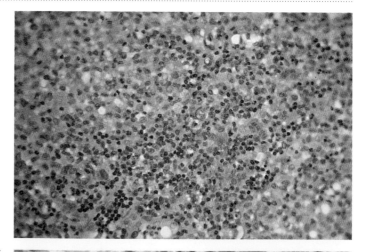

Figure 7.66

a

b

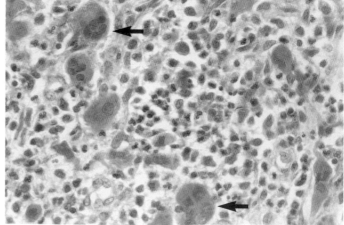

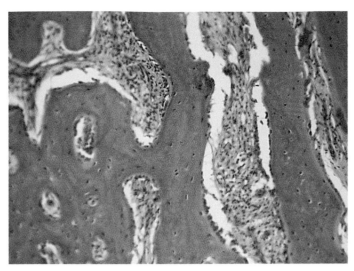
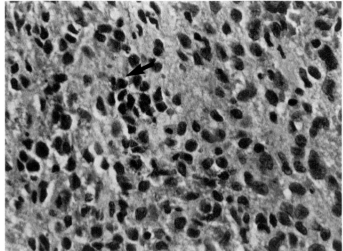

Figure 7.66 continued

| c | d |

Figure 7.67 **Erdheim–Chester disease** This condition has been included amongst the Langerhans cell granulomatosis disorders by some observers. It mainly affects elderly males and is characterized by osteosclerosis of the shaft of leg bones, predominantly the tibia (a). Affected parts of the bone usually show increased uptake on bone scan (b). A Paget's disease-like prominent, mosaic cement-line pattern is seen in cortical and cancellous bone; macrophages and mononuclear cells resembling Langerhans cells are present in the bone marrow (c, d).

Figure 7.67

| a | b |

| c | d |

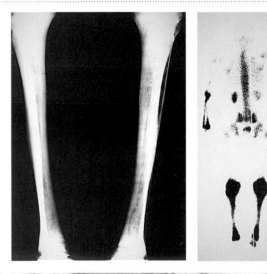

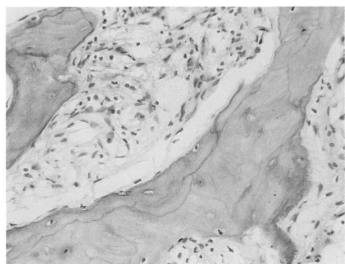
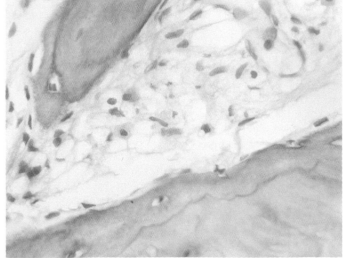

Figure 7.68 Fibrous dysplasia This is a relatively common tumour-like lesion which probably represents a developmental abnormality of bone formation. A single bone is most frequently involved but there may also be polyostotic involvement (see 4.28). Lesions usually develop within the first three decades of life but may present at any age. Any bone may be involved but the skull, facial bones, femur and tibia, ribs, and pelvis are usually affected. Most cases of monostotic fibrous dysplasia are asymptomatic, but some present with pain, swelling, or pathological fracture. 7.68 shows the characteristic radiological appearances of fibrous dysplasia in the femoral neck. The lesion is relatively well defined, has a ground glass texture, and expands the bone; there is thickening of the cortex and deformity.

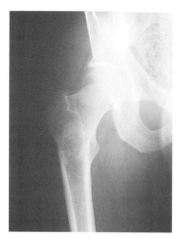

Figure 7.68

Figure 7.69 Fibrous dysplasia Fibrous dysplasia typically contains a cellular fibroblastic stroma in which there are numerous irregularly-shaped woven bone trabeculae (a). These appear to form directly by fibro-osseous metaplasia of spindle-shaped cells within the fibrous stroma; bone trabeculae do not usually show prominent osteoblastic rimming. Other features seen in fibrous dysplasia are a prominent storiform pattern (b), areas of haemosiderin deposition and collections of foamy macrophages (c) and giant cells. There may also be small calcospherites (arrowed) within fibrous tissue (d). Small islands of cartilage and extensive myxoid and cystic change as well as secondary aneurysmal bone cyst-like change may also be noted. Fibrous dysplasia often enters into the radiological and histological differential diagnosis of many bone tumours, principally those characterized by bone formation or the presence of numerous giant cells. Malignant transformation may rarely occur in fibrous dysplasia, although most reported cases have occurred after radiation treatment.

Figure 7.69

| a | b |
| c | d |

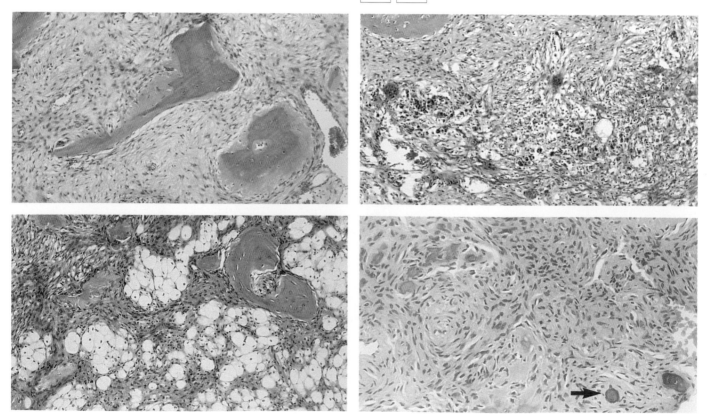

Figure 7.70 **Osteofibrous dysplasia (ossifying fibroma of long bones)** This is a benign fibro-osseous lesion which occurs in the shaft of the tibia or fibula of young children. The lesion is lytic and centred on the cortex; it grows rapidly and produces bone deformity. It contains a cellular fibroblastic stroma in which there are trabeculae of woven bone surrounded by plump osteoblasts (a, b). As trabeculae increase in size, a rim of lamellar bone is often formed over the woven bone initially formed. Other features more typical of fibrous dysplasia such as collections of giant cells and cartilage formation may also be seen. Occasional cytokeratin-positive cells have been noted in lesions of osteofibrous dysplasia and the precise relationship between this lesion and adamantinoma remains uncertain. Although osteofibrous dysplasia may continue to enlarge, particularly in the first decade, most cases behave as self-limiting lesions and further growth is not seen after skeletal maturity. Recurrence commonly occurs following surgical intervention in growing lesions.

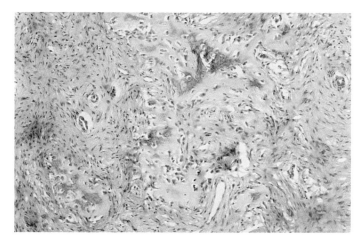

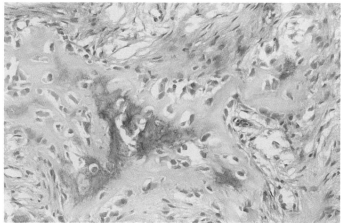

Figure 7.70

a

b

Figure 7.71 **Fibrocartilaginous mesenchymoma** This very rare lesion most probably represents a variant of fibrous dysplasia in which numerous small and large nodules of cartilage, some of which show evidence of endochondral ossification, lie in an abundant spindle cell stroma (a, b). Other features of fibrous dysplasia may be seen such as woven bone formation, giant cells, and focal collections of foamy macrophages. Lesions may be confined to the bone or extend into surrounding soft tissue.

Figure 7.71

a   b

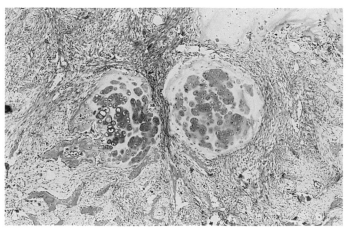

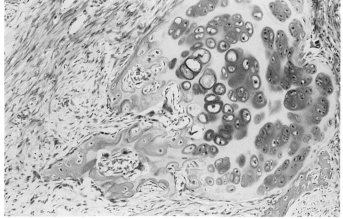

Figure 7.72 **Florid reactive periostitis (periostitis ossificans; fibro-osseous tumour of digits)** This rare benign condition occurs most commonly in children and young adults but may present at any age. Most lesions occur in the digits of the hand; digits of the foot and other bones are less often involved. There is commonly a history of previous trauma. Radiologically, a soft-tissue swelling and a prominent periosteal reaction may be evident. Histologically, there is abundant reactive fibrous tissue with collagen formation; a variable amount of osteoid or woven bone is associated with the proliferating cells (a, b). Cartilage formation may also be seen within reactive fibrous tissue. The lesion is benign and recurrence rarely occurs after excision.

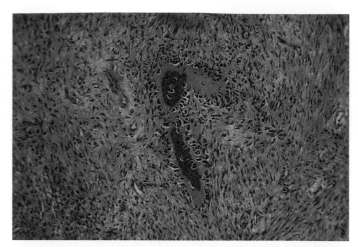

Figure 7.72

a

b

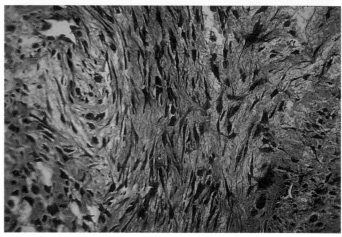

Figure 7.73 **Bizarre parosteal osteochondromatous proliferation** This rare lesion is found almost exclusively in small bones of the hands and feet, most commonly the proximal phalanges, but may rarely occur elsewhere. It occurs over a wide age range but is most common in young adults. 7.73a shows an unusual example arising in the distal radius. The lesion is well defined and is present on the surface of the affected bone but not continuous with the surrounding cortex.

The lesion is composed of a mixture of cartilage, bone, and fibrous tissue. Fibrocartilaginous metaplasia results in the formation of lobules of cartilage which are highly cellular (b, c). Chondrocytes show some evidence of nuclear pleomorphism and there is osteochondroma-like bone formation from cartilage (d). This lesion should be distinguished from other cartilaginous tumours that may involve the digits and reactive lesions such as subungual exostosis.

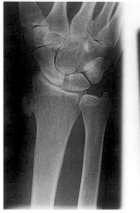

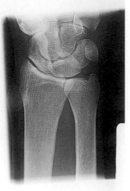

Figure 7.73

a   b

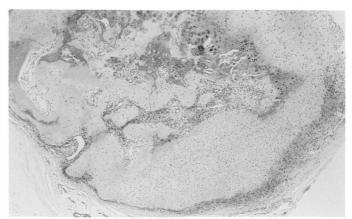

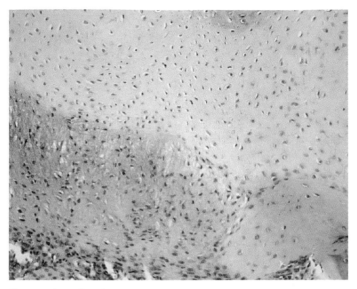
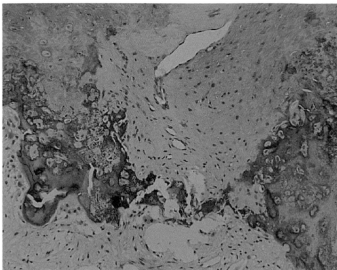

Figure 7.73 continued

c d

Figure 7.74 **Infantile cartilaginous hamartoma of rib** This very rare lesion occurs in infants and may be noted at birth. It is usually asymptomatic and presents as a solitary swelling of variable size. Radiologically, there is expansion of the rib by a lytic lesion which may show some evidence of calcification. It contains densely packed mesenchymal cells amongst which are scattered lobules of cartilage formed by fibrocartilaginous metaplasia (a, b). The lesion is benign and usually requires excision.

Figure 7.74

a b

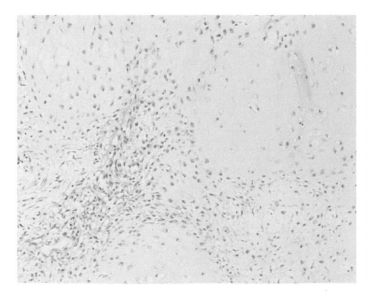
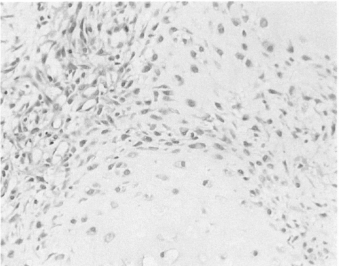

Figure 7.75 Amyloid tumour of bone An amyloid tumour in bone appears most commonly in association with multiple myeloma. It may present as multiple deposits or a single tumour-like lesion. Lesions in bone may also rarely be found in primary systemic (AL) amyloidosis and secondary (AA) amyloidosis. β_2-microglobulin amyloid deposits in bone always occur secondary to involvement of articular cartilage and periarticular tissues (see 6.14). 7.75a shows amyloid deposits in several vertebrae on MRI in a rare case of primary amyloidosis. Histologically, the amyloid deposits consist of abundant homogeneous, amorphous eosinophilic material; the amyloid is associated with a giant cell reaction (arrow) (b) or a heavy plasma cell infiltrate (c). Amyloid deposits may be identified by Congo red staining. Immunohistochemistry is employed to determine the nature of the amyloid protein.

Figure 7.75

a

b c

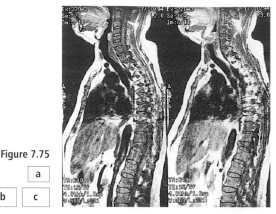

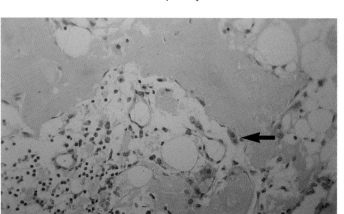

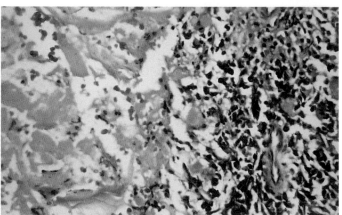

Metastases in bone

Figure 7.76 Metastatic carcinoma in bone The most common malignant tumour of bone is metastatic carcinoma. Carcinomas which most often metastasize to bone are those of the breast, lung, prostate, kidney, and thyroid. Metastatic lesions are found most frequently in bones containing relatively large amounts of haematopoietic marrow and are consequently most common in the vertebral column, innominate bones, rib and skull bones, and the proximal ends of the femur and humerus. Grossly, metastases are usually multiple, well defined. and osteolytic (a). 7.76b shows a secondary deposit of a renal cell carcinoma in the shaft of the femur. Metastatic carcinoma in bone commonly result in pathological fracture or vertebral collapse (arrow) (c). Bone scans are useful in identifying the extent of metastatic spread. Most metastases are osteolytic; metastatic prostatic carcinoma (and Hodgkin's disease) may produce osteosclerotic metastases.

Figure 7.76

a b c

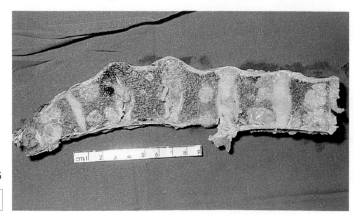

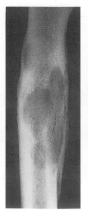

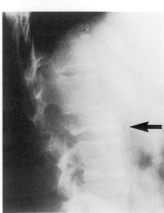

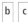

Figure 7.77 Metastatic tumour in bone Histologically, metastases in bone often recapitulate the features of the primary malignancy. Thus, metastatic prostatic carcinoma usually consists of tumour cells with abundant clear or acidophilic cytoplasm and small regular nuclei disposed in sheets, cords, or closely packed small tumour glands (a). Metastases of malignant melanoma commonly contain abundant melanin pigment (b). Metastatic renal cell carcinoma may present as a solitary, purely lytic tumour in bone. This is usually a clear cell adenocarcinoma, but in some cases may consist largely of sarcoma-like areas with numerous spindle-shaped and pleomorphic tumour cells lying in a prominent fibrous stroma (c). Mucin stains and immunohistochemical identification of cellular antigens, melanoma-associated antigen, prostate-specific antigen, and prostatic acid phosphatase) are particularly useful in determining the origin and nature of a metastatic tumour in bone. 7.77d shows cytokeratin staining in a metastatic squamous cell carcinoma.

Figure 7.77

| a | b |
| c | d |

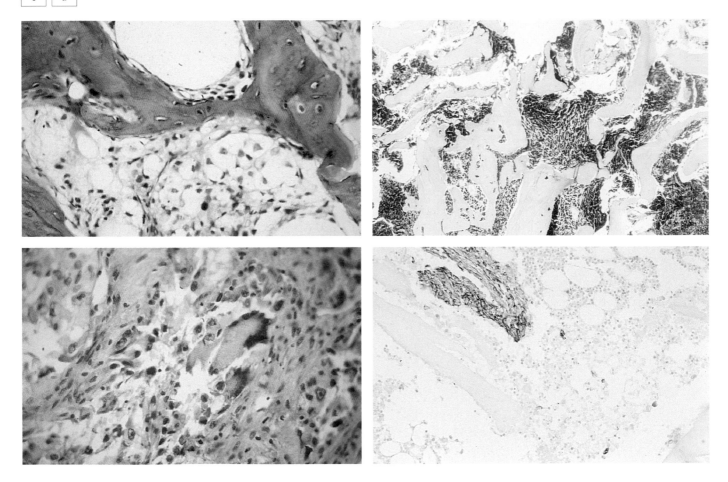

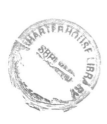

8

Soft tissue tumours and tumour-like lesions

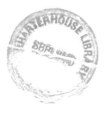

Introduction

Soft tissue tumours comprise a very heterogeneous group of neoplasms which are classified histogenetically according to the normal tissue(s) they resemble. In each of these histogenetic categories, a very large number of distinct morphological entities has been described. Apart from some benign tumours such as lipoma, benign fibrous histiocytoma, and haemangioma, most soft tissue tumours are uncommon. Malignant soft tissue tumours are particularly rare, constituting less than 1 per cent of all malignancies. The pathological diagnosis of a soft tissue tumour thus often proves difficult on account of the large number of different types described, the infrequency with which these lesions are encountered, and, often, the similar morphological appearances of the various entities.

Most soft tissue tumours present clinically as a swelling which may or may not be accompanied by pain and tenderness. It is important to take into account the age (Table 8.1) (and, to a lesser extent, the sex) of the patient as a number of soft tissue tumours have a characteristic patient profile. It is also important to note the site of the lesion, not only which part of the body (e.g. the extremities, trunk, or head and neck region) is affected but also whether the lesion arises in superficial or deep soft tissue or is closely related to a particular anatomical structure such as a peripheral nerve. Imaging techniques such as CT and MRI are useful in determining the precise anatomical compartment in which the lesion lies, the extent of the lesion, its degree of circumscription, as well as its consistency and possible composition.

As for bone tumours, histopathological examination is necessary for the precise diagnosis of a soft tissue tumour. This is aided by the use of special (e.g. mucin or connective tissue) stains to identify cell or matrix components. Immunohistochemistry, preferably using a panel of monoclonal/polyclonal antibodies, is also particularly useful in detecting the presence (or absence) of cell or tissue-related antigens known to be expressed in certain soft tissue tumours. Electron microscopy in selected cases also plays a role in identifying ultrastructural features that may establish the histogenesis of a particular tumour. Cytogenetic analysis may indicate the presence of tumour-related karyotypic abnormalities and molecular biology is also likely to play an increasing role in determining the presence of abnormal tumour-related gene products. Histological examination is also essential for establishing the grade of malignancy of a soft tissue sarcoma. This is based not only on the type of tumour but also the degree of differentiation, mitotic activity, cellularity, degree of pleomorphism, and extent of necrosis. Defining the histological grade of a soft tissue sarcoma is essential for accurate staging of these tumours.

Table 8.1 Main age range at presentation of some soft tissue sarcomas

Tumour	Age in years			
	0–20	20–40	40–60	60+
Fibrosarcoma	┈	━	━	┈
MFH (angiomatoid)	┈	━		
MFH (other)	┈	━	━	━
Liposarcoma	┈	━	━	━
Leiomyosarcoma	┈	━	━	━
Rhadbomyosarcoma (embryonal/alveolar)	━	┈		
Rhabdomyosarcoma (pleomorphic)		┈	━	
Angiosarcoma	┈	┈	━	━
Haemangiopericytoma	┈	━	━	
Malignant schwannoma	┈	━	━	
Neuroblastoma	━	┈		
PNET	┈	━	━	┈
Paraganglioma		┈	━	━
Synovial sarcoma	┈	━	━	┈
Mesothelioma		┈	━	
Chondrosarcoma		┈	┈	
Mesenchymal chondrosarcoma	┈	━	━	┈
Osteosarcoma		┈	━	━
Alveolar soft part sarcoma	┈	━	━	┈
Epithelioid sarcoma	┈	━	━	┈
Clear cell sarcoma	┈	━	━	┈

Key:

━━━━━ Most commonly reported

┈┈┈┈┈ Less commonly reported

Tumours and tumour-like lesions of fibrous tissue

Figure 8.1 Keloid A keloid is a reactive overgrowth of fibrous scar tissue within dermal and subcutaneous tissues. It consists of swollen, hyalinized, glassy collagen fibres which are separated by stellate fibroblasts (a, b). Keloids are found most commonly in the upper part of the body, particularly over the sternum and around the ear lobes. They may arise following injury or develop spontaneously. They are more frequent in blacks than whites. An increased familial incidence has been reported in some cases. They very commonly recur after excision.

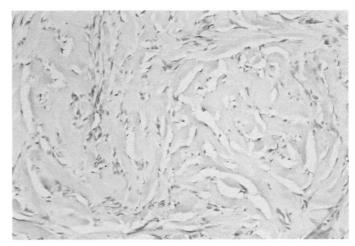
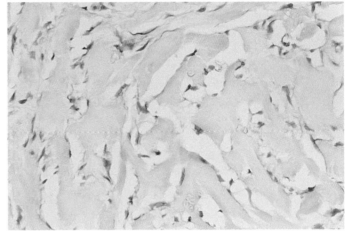

Figure 8.1

a

b

Figure 8.2 Hypertrophic scar This is a reactive overgrowth of cellular fibrous scar tissue which occurs in response to injury; it is limited to the site of injury, does not occur spontaneously, and uncommonly recurs after excision. It consists of abundant reparative cellular fibrous tissue, showing an increase in fibroblast cellularity (as shown here). There is increased collagen formation in more mature lesions. Thick keloid-like hyaline collagen fibres are not usually present and the connective tissue matrix is less mucinous.

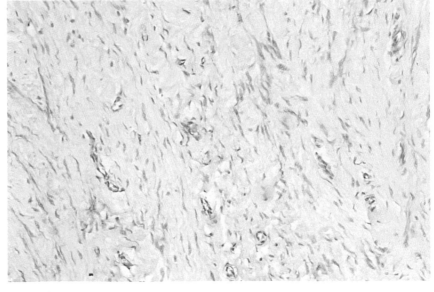

Figure 8.2

Figure 8.3 **Fibroma of tendon sheath** This benign fibrous tumour usually involves the tendons of the hands or feet of adults and is more common in males than females. It is composed of fibroma-like lobules of sparsely cellular dense collagenous connective tissue containing scattered small vessels (a, b). The lobules of fibrous tissue are separated by cleft-like spaces. More fibroblast-rich cellular areas resembling nodular fasciitis or benign fibrous histiocytoma may also be present, particularly at the edge of the lesion (c).

Figure 8.3

| a | b | c |

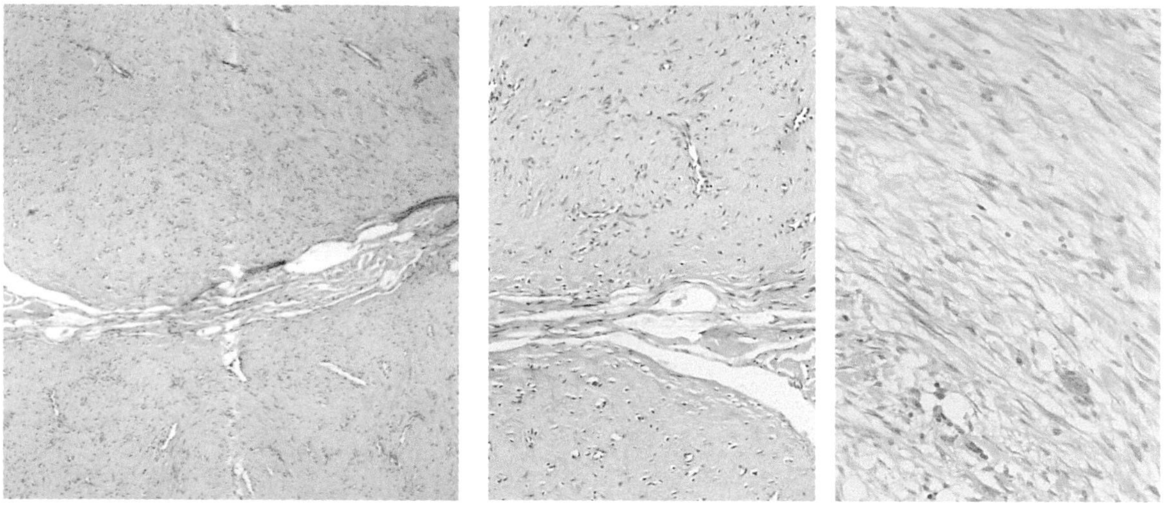

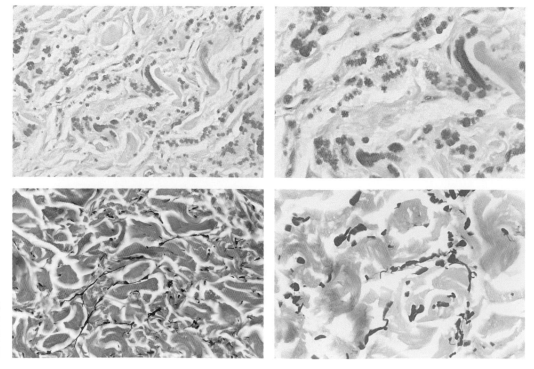

Figure 8.4 **Elastofibroma** This rare benign tumour usually arises in the subscapular region of elderly individuals. It is three times more common in females than males; the right side is more frequently affected; bilateral involvement is seen in up to 10 per cent of cases. The lesion is composed of dense collagenous fibrous tissue and numerous prominent highly eosinophilic, thickened, elastic fibres (a, b). Fibroblasts are usually scanty. Elastic stains show broad, wavy, globular or beaded elastic fibres (c, d). An increased familial incidence has been noted, possibly indicating a genetic predisposition to abnormal elastic fibre and increased collagen fibre formation after injury. Although poorly defined and not encapsulated, local recurrence is rare following surgical removal.

Figure 8.4

| a | b |
| c | d |

Figure 8.5 Calcifying (juvenile) aponeurotic fibroma This slowly enlarging fibrous tumour occurs mainly (but not exclusively) in children and adolescents. It usually arises in the hands and feet. It is a fibrous lesion containing focal areas of increased fibroblast cellularity and a heavily collagenized stroma. Areas of stellate calcification are seen within the lesion (a). These are occasionally associated with an osteoclast-like giant cell reaction (arrow) (b). Areas of cartilaginous metaplasia are present (c). The lesion commonly recurs following removal.

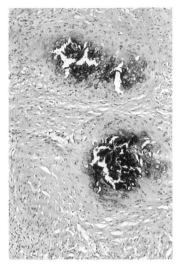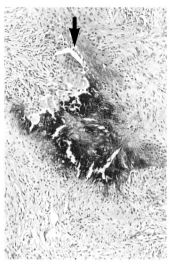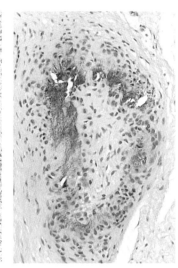

Figure 8.5

| a | b | c |

Figure 8.6 Giant cell fibroblastoma This rare fibrous tumour occurs mainly in children but may also be encountered in adults. It arises mainly in the dermal and subcutaneous tissues of the back and thigh. It consists of a densely collagenized fibrous stroma or occasionally more cellular fibroblastic tissue containing scattered multinucleated giant cells (arrow) (a); these have a floret-like arrangement of overlapping, hyperchromatic nuclei often disposed around the periphery of the cell (b). Prominent vascular spaces lined by endothelium may also be seen. Recurrence commonly occurs after excision.

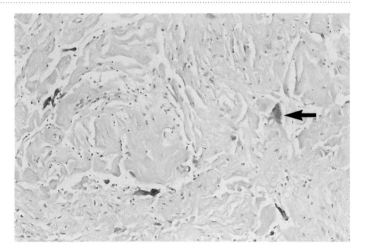

Figure 8.6

| a |

| b |

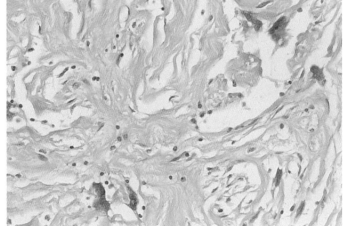

Figure 8.7 **Nodular fasciitis** This is a relatively common fibrous tumour which, on account of its rapid growth and high cellularity, is frequently misdiagnosed as a sarcoma. It occurs usually in young adults, mainly in the upper limbs, particularly the flexor aspect of the forearm, as well as the trunk and neck. It usually arises in subcutaneous tissues but may involve deeper soft tissues. The lesion has infiltrative margins and is composed of a haphazard tissue-culture-like growth of immature plump oval or spindle-shaped cells which are arranged in short or long fascicles (a). Numerous typical mitotic figures may be seen. Cells show a varying degree of nuclear pleomorphism (b). There is myxoid change and a variable degree of collagen formation as well as a patchy chronic inflammatory infiltrate and haemosiderin deposition. Giant cells are not usually seen. Extravasated red cells (arrow) often lie between proliferating cells (c). Recurrence rarely occurs following adequate excision. Similar fibroblastic proliferations may be seen in association with small and medium-sized arteries and veins (intravascular fasciitis), deep fascial connective tissues of the scalp (cranial fasciitis), and periosteal tissues (ossifying fasciitis).

Figure 8.7

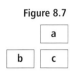

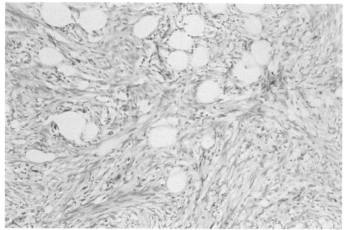

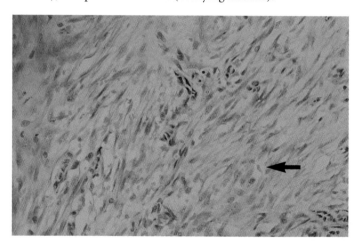

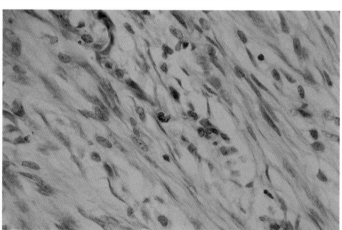

Figure 8.8 **Proliferative fasciitis** This rare fibrous tumour develops in deep fascial connective tissue or within interlobular fibrous septa in subcutaneous fat. It occurs mainly in adults, most commonly in the proximal extremities. It is composed of immature plump, polygonal or spindle-shaped fibroblastic cells amongst which are found large cells (arrow) that have abundant basophilic cytoplasm and large nuclei with prominent nucleoli (a, b). The latter, which resemble ganglion cells, may be multinucleated. Mitotic activity may be prominent but all mitotic figures are typical. Recurrence does not usually occur after adequate excision.

Figure 8.8

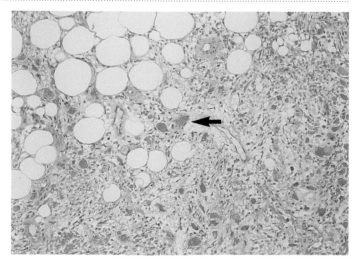

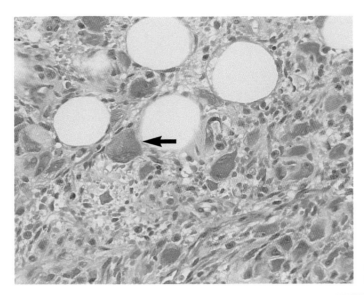

Figure 8.8 continued

b

Figure 8.9 Proliferative myositis This lesion closely resembles proliferative fasciitis, both clinically and pathologically. It occurs over a similar age range but arises in deeper soft tissues, presenting as a rapidly growing, painless mass in the muscles of the chest wall or limb girdles. It consists of a diffuse proliferation of fibroblast-like cells amongst which are found scattered large ganglion-like cells with basophilic cytoplasm and large nuclei with prominent nucleoli (a, b). This cellular proliferation extends between muscle bundles and may also separate individual muscle fibres which may be well preserved or appear atrophic. The cells lie in a fibrous matrix which may show some myxoid change or increase in collagen formation. There is a variable degree of mitotic activity but all mitoses are typical. The lesion uncommonly recurs following adequate excision.

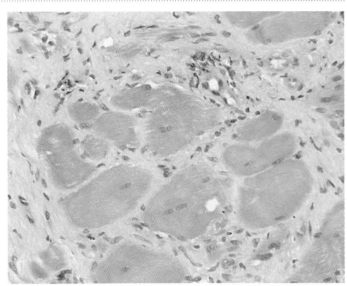

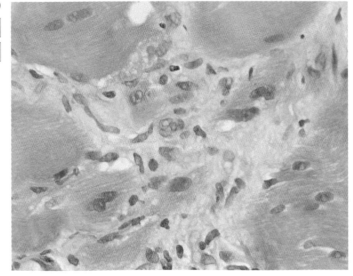

Figure 8.9

a

b

Figure 8.10 **Ischaemic fasciitis (atypical decubital fibroplasia)** This reactive lesion is seen in bed-ridden, immobilized, or debilitated patients in whom a soft-tissue mass forms over points of bony prominence (e.g. sacrum, greater trochanter). The lesion is usually located in subcutaneous tissue and is essentially composed of highly exuberant granulation tissue in which there are numerous large, proliferating plump, round, or spindle-shaped fibroblasts and thin-walled blood vessels lined by plump endothelial cells (a, b); areas of fibrin, myxoid change, and collagenous connective tissue and a variable inflammatory cell component may also be present. Nuclei are plump and hyperchromatic and there is often brisk typical mitotic activity.

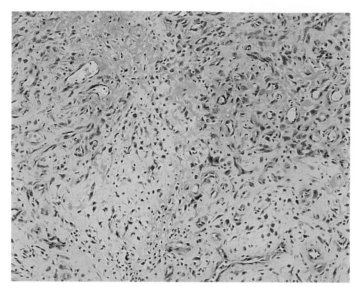

Figure 8.10

a

b

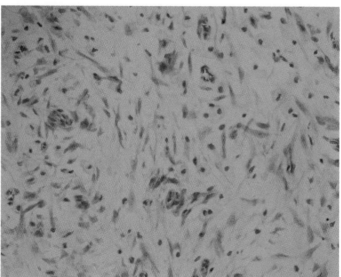

Figure 8.11 **Fibrous hamartoma of infancy** This lesion, which is most often found in the deep dermis or subcutaneous tissue of the axilla or upper arm, usually presents during the first year of life. It is more common in males than females. It has a characteristic organoid pattern (a). There are scattered areas of mature fat, fascicles of fibroblast-like spindle cells, and nests or whorls of stellate or spindle-shaped cells lying in a loose connective tissue or mucoid matrix (b, c). Local recurrence may occur following incomplete excision.

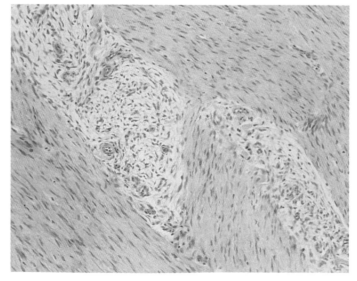

Figure 8.11

a

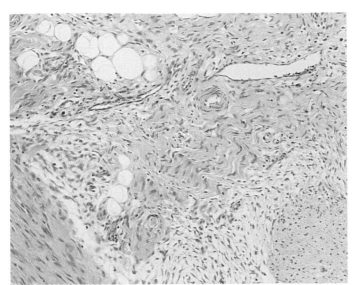

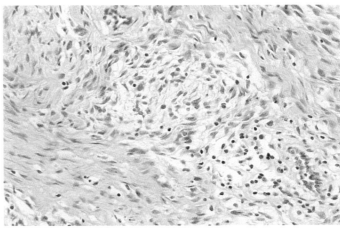

Figure 8.11 continued

b   c

Figure 8.12 Infantile myofibroma and myofibromatosis This rare condition usually presents soon after birth as a solitary lesion in the dermis and subcutaneous tissues of the trunk or head and neck. Less commonly, there may be multiple cutaneous lesions. Lesions may also arise in bone and internal organs. Each lesion is composed of a zonal arrangement of fibroblast-like cells or more plump smooth-muscle-like cells which are arranged in short fascicles or whorled bundles or nodules (a, b). Mitotic activity is variable but all mitotic figures are typical. Central areas of the lesion may contain more rounded or polygonal cells. Ultrastructurally and immunohistochemically, the cells show the characteristics of myofibroblasts. Solitary myofibroma has a good prognosis but the multicentric form with visceral involvement may cause death from pulmonary or gastro-intestinal complications.

Figure 8.12

a

b

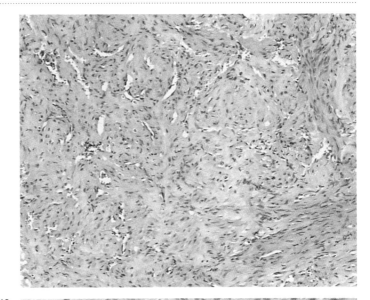

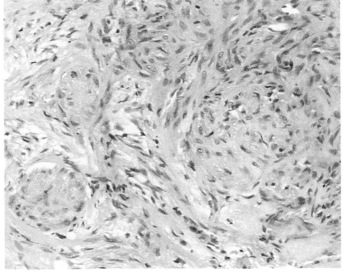

Figure 8.13 **Infantile digital fibromatosis** This uncommon benign fibrous tumour arises during infancy, producing one or more nodular lesions on the digits of the hands or feet. The lesion is poorly defined and usually located in the papillary and reticular dermis (a); it may also involve underlying superficial subcutaneous tissue. It consists of a proliferation of fibroblast-like spindle cells that contain small, round eosinophilic cytoplasmic inclusions (arrow) (composed of actin filaments) which usually lie in a perinuclear location (b); these are trichrome and PTAH positive and PAS and alcian blue negative. The lesions are commonly multiple and may cause contracture; they recur after local excision in over 50 per cent of cases but eventually regress spontaneously.

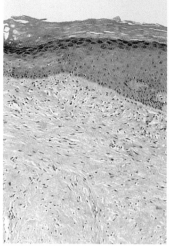
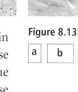

Figure 8.13

a | b

Figure 8.14 **Juvenile (nasopharyngeal) angiofibroma** This is a benign proliferation of fibrous and vascular tissue which occurs almost exclusively in adolescent males and young adults. It produces a lobulated swelling that is often firmly attached to the sphenoid or occipital bone. It consists of cellular and collagenous fibrous tissue containing scattered prominent, often dilated vascular spaces (a). These endothelial-lined vessels have a variable, often incomplete smooth muscle wall (b); vessels usually lack an elastic membrane. The lesions often grow aggressively and extend into bone; recurrence is seen in up to 60 per cent of cases.

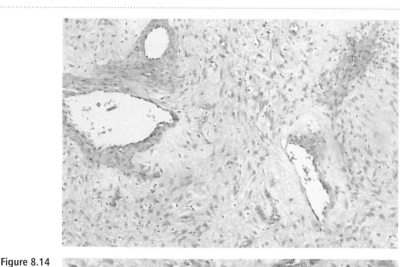
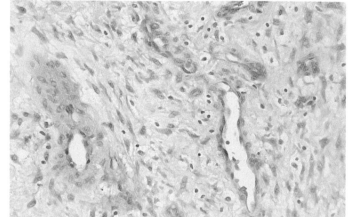

Figure 8.14

a

b

Fibromatosis

Fibromatosis is a term which is used to describe a group of disorders characterized by fibroblast/myofibroblast proliferation and increased collagen formation. A fibromatosis is characterized as either superficial or deep, depending on whether it originates respectively from the superficial fascia or from the deep fascia or connective tissues associated with large muscles. This condition may occur in a variety of locations.

Figure 8.15 Palmar fibromatosis (Dupuytren's disease/contracture) This is a common superficial fibromatosis which affects 1–2 per cent of the general population. It is more common in males than females. It is usually encountered in adults with increasing frequency as they grow older. It may affect one or both hands; the ring and little fingers are often the first and most severely involved. The pathogenesis is unknown but there appears to be an hereditary predisposition; it may occur in association with plantar fibromatosis, penile fibromatosis, and knuckle pads. Palmar fibromatosis is due to nodular thickening of the palmar fascia and overlying subcutaneous tissue (a). It consists of small fascicles or nodular areas of increased fibroblast-like spindle cells and collagenous fibrous tissue (b). The early proliferative (nodular) stage of palmar fibromatosis shows a marked increase in spindle cells and a variable amount of collagen formation; there is little cellular or nuclear pleomorphism but occasional typical mitotic activity (c). More mature lesions show less fibroblast cellularity and contain abundant intercellular collagenous connective tissue (d). Recurrence may occur after treatment. Knuckle pads are morphologically similar areas of fibrous proliferation which produce areas of fibrous thickening over the extensor surface of the interphalangeal or metacarpophalangeal joints.

Figure 8.15

| a | b |
| c | d |

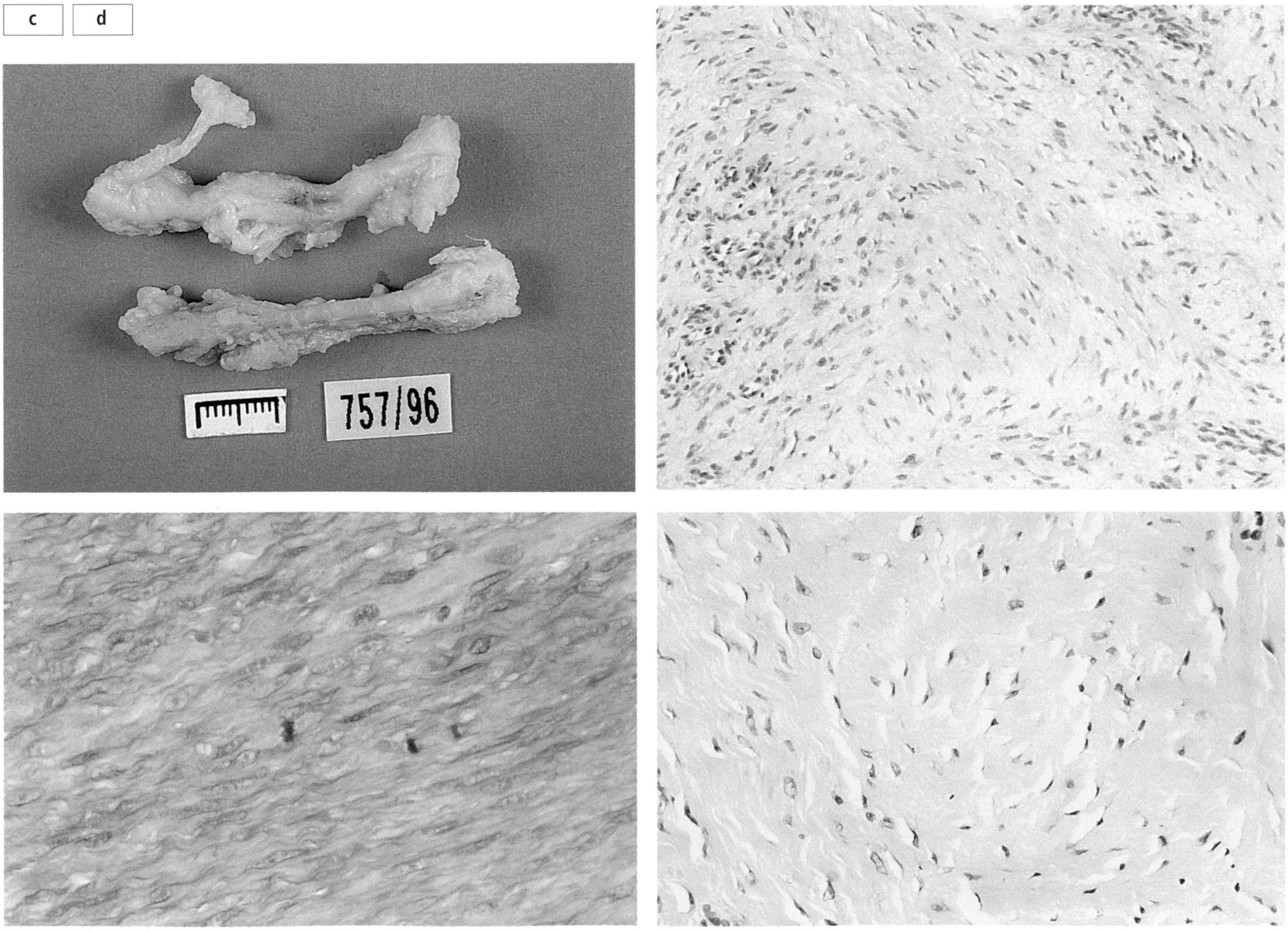

Figure 8.16 **Plantar fibromatosis** Fibromatosis of the plantar fascia of the feet is much less common than palmar fibromatosis. It is seen more frequently with advancing age but may also be encountered in children and young adults. Males are more commonly affected than females. It is bilateral in up to 25 per cent of cases but rarely causes contracture of the toes. Histologically, it resembles palmar fibromatosis. More cellular lesions may be difficult to distinguish from fibrosarcoma but, as in other forms of superficial fibromatosis, proliferating spindle-shaped cells show a degree of orientation. They also merge imperceptibly with fibroblasts in surrounding normal fascial connective tissue.

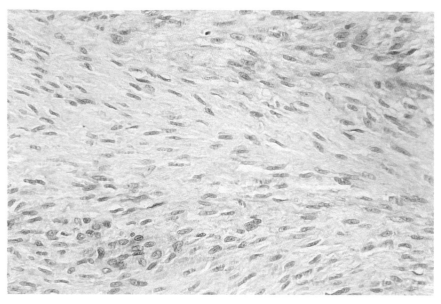

Figure 8.16

Figure 8.17 **Musculoaponeurotic (desmoid) fibromatosis** This deep fibromatosis occurs chiefly in adults, typically arising within the deep fascia and musculoaponeurotic structures of the shoulder, neck, chest wall, and thigh. There may also be involvement of deep subcutaneous tissues. Most lesions are solitary; multicentric fibromatosis uncommonly occurs. 8.17a shows the gross appearance of a fibromatosis involving the deltoid muscle; the lesion is large, firm, grey-white, and relatively well circumscribed. It consists of a uniform proliferation of fibroblasts which are surrounded by a variable amount of collagenous fibrous tissue (b). This extends into surrounding muscle. Cells are largely oriented in one direction and lie in broad fascicles; compressed thin-walled blood vessels (arrow) are often prominent amongst these bundles (c). There is little or no cellular or nuclear pleomorphism; mitoses are uncommon and always typical (arrow) (d). Recurrence commonly follows inadequate excision and is more common in lesions involving the major limb girdles.

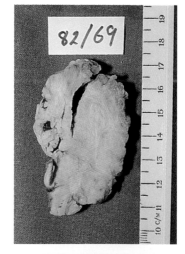

Figure 8.17

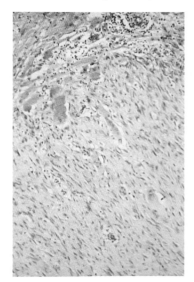
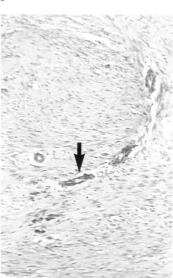
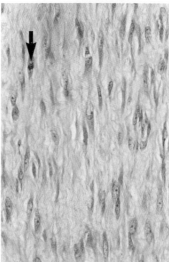

Figure 8.18 Abdominal fibromatosis (desmoid tumour) This occurs almost exclusively in parous females, developing during gestation or, more commonly, in the first year postpartum. It is classically found in the anterior sheath of the rectus abdominis muscle just below the umbilicus, but it may develop in any part of the abdominal wall. Histologically, lesions are identical to extra-abdominal desmoids and are composed of bundles showing proliferation of fibroblasts and increased collagen formation. There is extension into surrounding muscle with entrapped muscle fibres (bottom left). These lesions rarely cross the midline but may recur in up to 30 per cent of cases after excision.

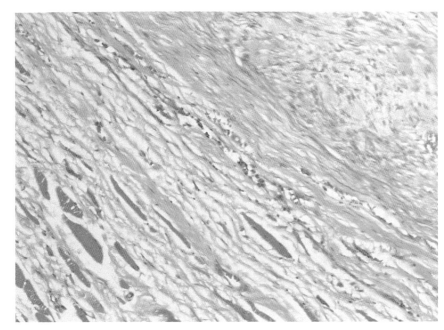

Figure 8.18

Figure 8.19 Intra-abdominal fibromatosis This deep fibromatosis may arise in the small bowel mesentery, retroperitoneum, or pelvic tissue. Mesenteric fibromatosis may be associated with Gardner's syndrome (multiple osteomas, intestinal polyposis coli, epidermal cysts, and other skin lesions) which is inherited autosomal dominant. Fibromatosis tissue extends into mesenteric fat; a perivascular lymphocytic infiltrate may be present at the advancing edge of the lesion (shown here).

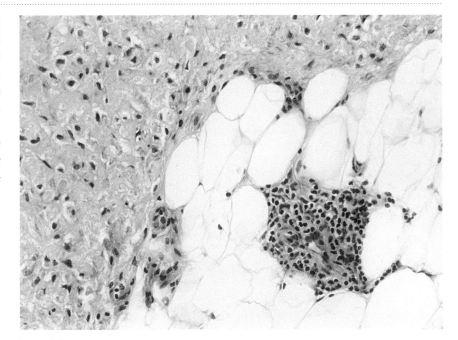

Figure 8.19

Figure 8.20 Fibromatosis colli This is a form of deep juvenile fibromatosis which occurs in the lower third of the sternocleido-mastoid muscle of infants. There is often a history of breech or forceps delivery. The lesion contains scattered fibroblasts and abundant dense collagenous connective tissue which surrounds muscle bundles and extends between atrophic muscle fibres (shown here). There is usually little associated inflammation. The lesion initially grows rapidly but, as the patient grows older, much more slowly. Most lesions regress spontaneously. Muscle resection may be required in older children with torticollis.

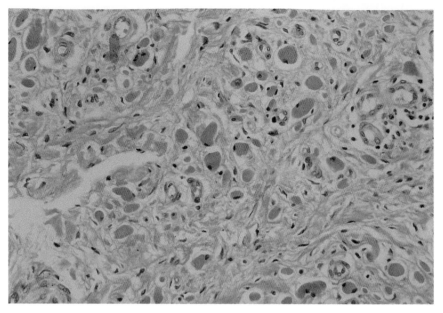

Figure 8.20

Figure 8.21 Infantile fibromatosis This condition usually presents in the first 2 years of life but may be encountered in older children as a deep-seated firm mass in the muscles of the head and neck region, shoulder, upper or lower limb. It is composed of small round or spindle-shaped cells associated with abundant collagen formation and mucoid material (a, b). There is extensive infiltration of muscle and fat and wide excision is required to prevent local recurrence. Histological distinction from infantile fibrosarcoma may be difficult but the latter is more cellular and shows more mitotic activity and nuclear pleomorphism.

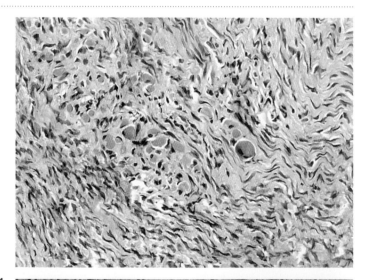

Figure 8.21

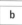

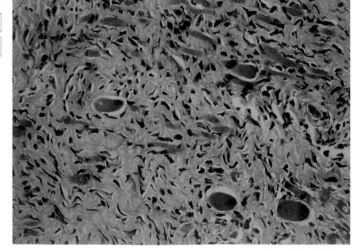

Figure 8.22 Fibrosarcoma This is an uncommon malignant tumour which arises mainly in the deep soft tissues of the extremities, trunk, or head and neck regions of middle-aged or older adults. It does not usually arise in superficial soft tissues. It may arise at the site of previous scars, burns, or radiation. It is composed of numerous spindle-shaped cells with thin, elongated, acicular nuclei; these lie in fascicles which cross each other at acute angles producing a prominent herring-bone pattern (a, b). There is variable cellular and nuclear pleomorphism and mitotic activity may be prominent. Tumour giant cells or osteoclast-like giant cells are not usually a feature.

Tumour cells are associated with a variable amount of collagen formation (c) The tumour commonly recurs and produces metastases; survival is related to the histological grade of the tumour. The uncommon congenital and infantile fibrosarcoma, which most often presents in the distal extremities, may resemble adult fibrosarcoma histologically but has a much better prognosis.

Figure 8.22

a b c

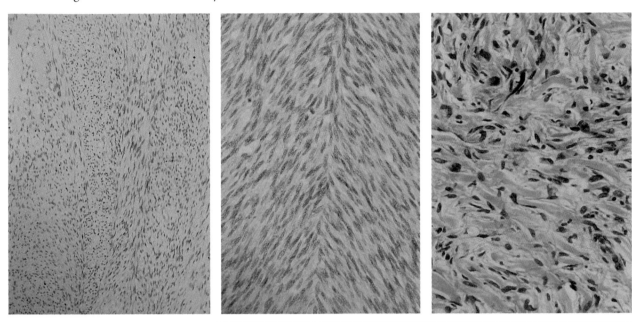

Fibrohistiocytic tumours

Figure 8.23 Benign fibrous histiocytoma This common benign soft tissue tumour usually presents as a small, firm, red, brown, or white nodule on the extremities of young or middle-aged adults. The lesion is usually located in the dermis or subcutaneous tissue but rarely may arise in deep soft tissue. Multiple lesions occur in approximately 20 per cent of cases. Most lesions are usually relatively well defined although not encapsulated and exhibit a prominent storiform pattern with short fascicles of fibroblast-like spindle cells and a varying proportion of more rounded macrophages and small capillary-sized blood vessels (a, b). Occasionally, the fibrous component is less prominent and round or oval macrophages with abundant cytoplasm and vesicular nuclei predominate (c). Mitotic activity is usually absent or scanty.

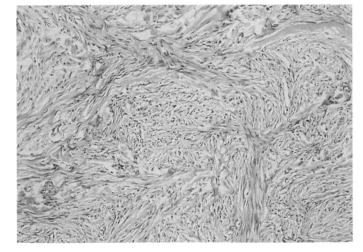

Figure 8.23

a

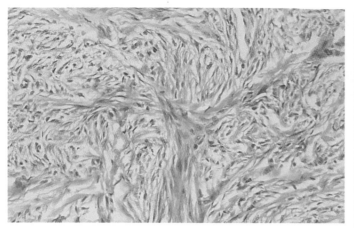

Figure 8.23 continued

| b | c |

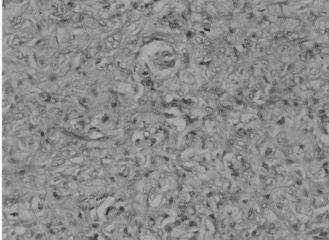

Figure 8.24 **Benign fibrous histiocytoma** Some more cellular forms of fibrous histiocytoma contain prominent small vessels (sclerosing haemangioma) (a). Variable hyalinization of the fibrous stroma may be noted (b). Other variable features include haemosiderin deposits and giant cells (arrow) (c), foamy macrophages, and a patchy lymphocytic infiltrate. Benign fibrous histiocytomas arising in deeper soft tissues often present a more monotonous storiform pattern with fewer macrophages, giant cells, and other secondary features. Superficial fibrous histiocytomas recur in about 5–10 per cent of cases. Recurrence is more common in deeper lesions which are often larger and more difficult to excise completely.

Figure 8.24

| a |

| b | c |

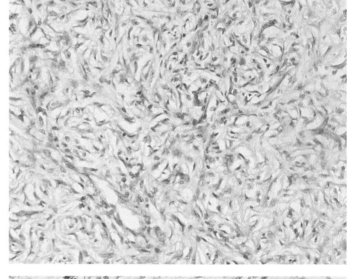

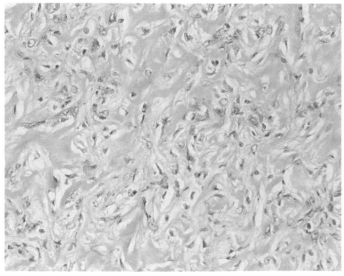

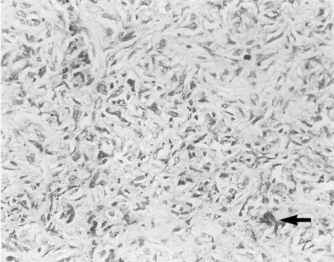

Figure 8.25 **Juvenile xanthogranuloma (naevoxanthoendothelioma)** This fibro-histiocytic lesion typically presents in infancy but may rarely occur in adults. Lesions are usually solitary but are multiple in 20 per cent of cases. They usually present as skin nodules, particularly in the head and neck region, trunk, and extremities. Infants with multiple lesions may also exhibit internal organ involvement. In the skin, lesions are usually intradermal (a) and are composed of a diffuse infiltrate of plump macrophages and scattered Touton giant cells (arrow) in which the nuclei are disposed wreath-like around the cell periphery (b). A variable infiltrate of acute and chronic inflammatory cells may also be present. In contrast to Histiocytosis X, cells do not express S-100 protein. Unlike xanthomas, there is no associated lipid or other metabolic abnormality. The lesions usually regress spontaneously.

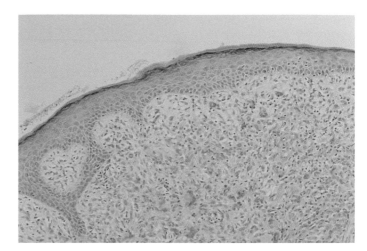

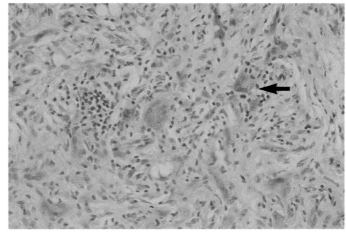

Figure 8.25

a

b

Figure 8.26 **Reticulohistiocytoma** This rare condition may present in adults either as a skin condition with one or more dermal nodules, usually in the head and neck region or trunk, or as a systemic disease (multicentric reticulohistiocytosis) in which multiple cutaneous and mucosal nodules are associated with an erosive arthritis and constitutional features such as weight loss, malaise, and pyrexia. Cutaneous lesions are similar in both forms of the disease and consist of a predominantly dermal infiltrate of macrophages having abundant eosinophilic cytoplasm and large vesicular nuclei (as shown here). Numerous scattered multinucleated giant cells with abundant glassy eosinophilic cytoplasm, large vesicular nuclei, and prominent nucleoli may also be seen. Mitotic activity is absent or scanty. The cutaneous and mucosal nodules usually regress spontaneously but the polyarthritis is progressive and irreversible.

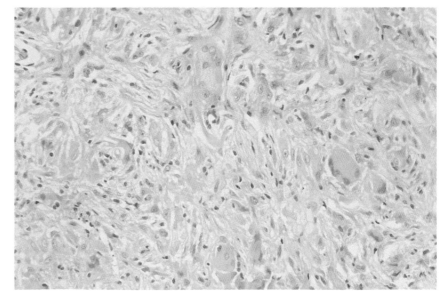

Figure 8.26

Figure 8.27 Xanthoma A xanthoma is a lesion composed of lipid-laden macrophages. It is classified grossly as eruptive, tuberous, tendinous, plane, or xanthelasma, depending on its location, and is often, but not invariably, associated with one or more forms of hyperlipidaemia. All types contain sheets of macrophages, many of which are foamy or epithelioid in type (a). In tuberous and tendinous xanthomas, macrophages and lipid-laden multinucleated giant cells are often disposed around extracellular collections of cholesterol (cholesterol clefts) (arrow) (b, c). Variable amounts of fibrosis and a chronic inflammatory infiltrate may also be present.

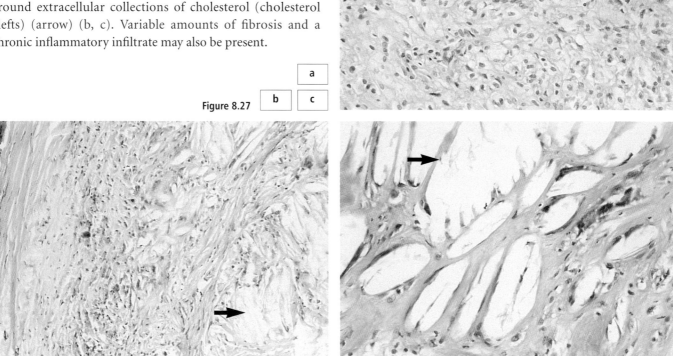

Figure 8.27

| a |
| b | c |

Figure 8.28 Atypical fibroxanthoma This uncommon fibrohistiocytic tumour usually presents as a solitary, slow-growing, small lesion arising in the dermis or subcutaneous tissue of sun-damaged areas of the head and neck region of elderly individuals, especially males. It may also occur on the limbs and trunk. It is composed of numerous pleomorphic or bizarre tumour cells (arrow), many of which are large and multinucleated (a, b). These cells contain abnormal nuclear forms and show frequent mitotic activity. Tumour cells are arranged haphazardly or lie in a vaguely fascicular or stori-form pattern. A variable degree of fibrosis is present within the tumour. The overlying or surrounding superficial dermis usually shows evidence of solar elastosis. Despite its pleomorphic appearance this tumour uncommonly recurs and rarely metastasizes.

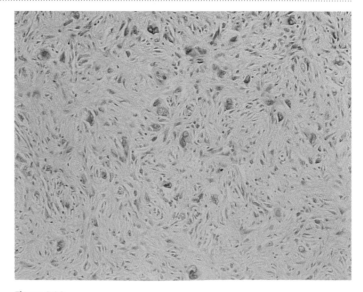

Figure 8.28

| a |

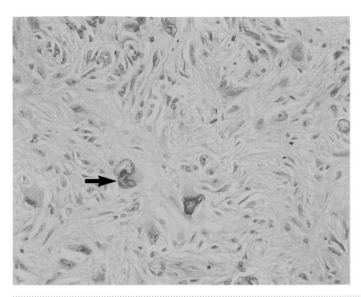

Figure 8.28 continued

b

Figure 8.29 Dermatofibrosarcoma protu-berans (DFSP) DFSP usually presents in adults as a slow-growing nodular or plaque-like lesion, arising in the dermis or subcutaneous tissue of the trunk or extremities. DFSP is generally larger than benign fibrous histiocytoma, less well defined, and composed of tightly packed cells of uniform appearance arranged in a highly regular storiform pattern (a, b). There is usually little cellular or nuclear pleomorphism or mitotic activity. Extensive collagen formation, giant cells, foamy macrophages, and haemosiderin deposition are not usually seen. DFSP is a locally aggressive lesion which commonly recurs; it uncommonly metastasizes to regional lymph nodes and may rarely produce distant metastases.

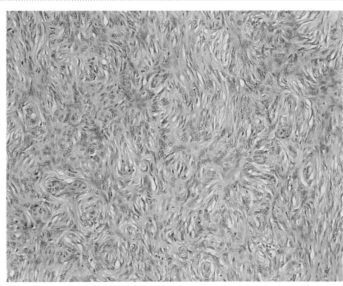

Figure 8.29

a

b

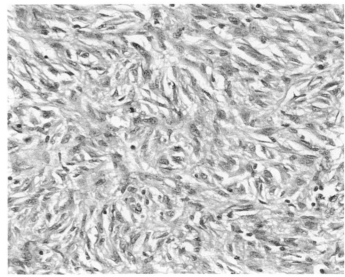

Figure 8.30 **Plexiform fibrohistiocytic tumour** This uncommon fibrohistiocytic tumour generally arises in the deep dermis and subcutaneous tissue of the extremities (usually the upper limb) of children and young adults. The lesion is composed of multiple nodules (a). These contain numerous spindle-shaped fibroblastic cells and plump macrophage-like cells amongst which are scattered occasional multinucleated giant cells (b). The nodules are surrounded by cellular or collagenous connective tissue, giving the lesion a plexiform appearance. The predominantly histiocytic cells within a nodule do not show marked cytological atypia or increased mitotic activity. The lesion is poorly defined and infiltrative and commonly recurs. Rare lymph node metastases have been reported.

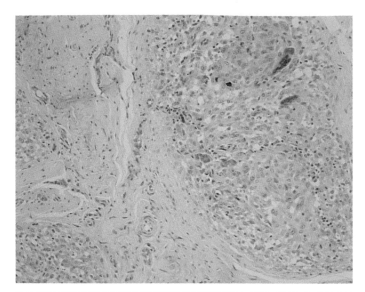

Figure 8.30

a

b

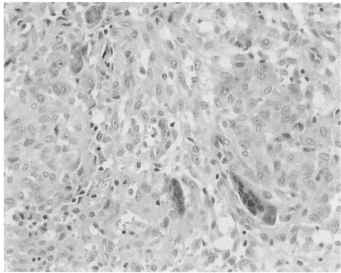

Figure 8.31 **Malignant fibrous histiocytoma (MFH)** MFH is currently the most commonly diagnosed soft tissue sarcoma in adults. The term MFH is almost certainly a misnomer as this tumour does not represent a neoplastic proliferation of histiocytes and it has not been proven that histiocytes may transform into fibroblasts (or vice versa). It is nevertheless a widely recognized diagnostic pathological entity. MFH chiefly affects the elderly and is more common in males than females. It arises mainly in deep soft tissue, especially that of the extremities and the retroperitoneum. Grossly, it is usually a large, firm, white, multilobulated tumour (as shown here). There are various morphological subtypes, all of which are characterized by the presence of fibroblast-like or histiocyte-like cells arranged in a more or less prominent storiform pattern. As a storiform pattern may be seen focally in other types of sarcoma, MFH represents a diagnosis of exclusion.

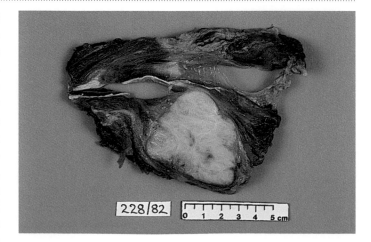

Figure 8.31

Figure 8.32 Storiform-pleomorphic MFH
This is the most common subtype of MFH and typically shows a prominent storiform pattern with cartwheel arrangement of closely packed fusiform or plump cells, amongst which are found large pleomorphic tumour cells showing cytological and nuclear atypia (a, b). Tumour cells are often large and hyperchromatic and there is a high mitotic rate. Tumour giant cells with bizarre nuclei may be seen (c). Haemorrhage and necrosis are common and there may be a variable amount of collagen formation and myxoid change. Local recurrence and metastasis commonly occur.

Figure 8.32

a

b	c

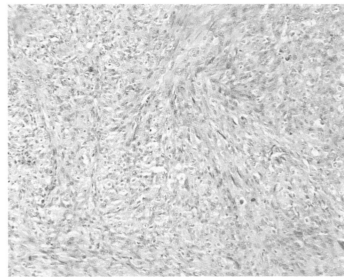

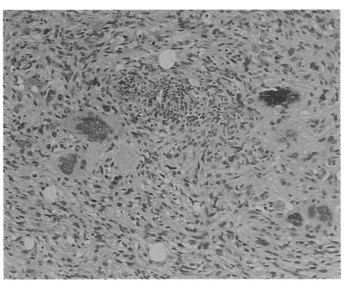

Figure 8.33 Myxoid MFH This MFH variant is characterized by the presence of conventional MFH and myxoid areas; the latter comprise more than half of the total tumour mass. There are areas of (hyaluronidase-sensitive) myxoid stroma containing hyperchromatic stellate or spindle-shaped cells, some of which may appear vacuolated (a, b). Scattered bizarre tumour giant cells as well as multivacuolated cells may also be noted. Areas containing prominent thin-walled blood vessels may be seen. Recurrence is common but metastasis is less common than in other forms of MFH.

Figure 8.33

a

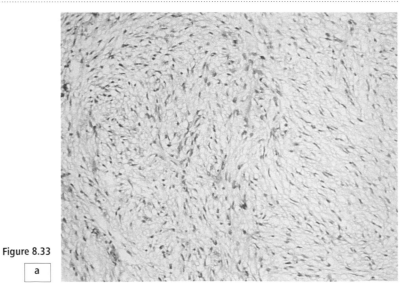

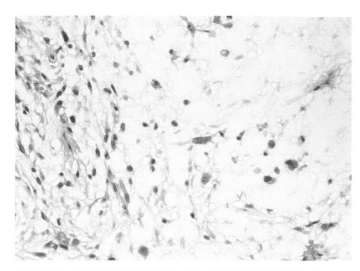

Figure 8.33 continued

b

Figure 8.34 Giant-cell-rich MFH This MFH variant may arise in superficial or deep soft tissue and commonly exhibits a multinodular pattern of growth. It is characterized by the presence of numerous large osteoclast-like giant cells which are focally or diffusely distributed throughout the tumour which otherwise shows features of a storiform MFH. Focal osteoid or woven bone formation may be seen within the tumour (arrow). Recurrence occurs commonly in both deep and superficial giant-cell-rich MFH but metastasis is much more common in tumours arising in deep soft tissue.

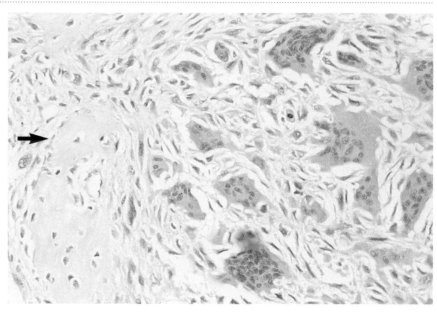

Figure 8.34

Figure 8.35 Inflammatory MFH This MFH variant most frequently arises in the retroperitoneum but may also uncommonly occur in the extremities. Retroperitoneal tumours may also be associated with systemic features such as fever and leucocytosis. It contains sheets of uniform xanthoma-like macrophages and numerous acute and chronic inflammatory cells (a). Only a few xanthoma cells show cellular or nuclear atypia and mitotic activity (b). In other areas, histiocytes contain less lipid. There are also scattered multinucleated giant cells. The tumour commonly recurs and metastasizes.

Figure 8.35

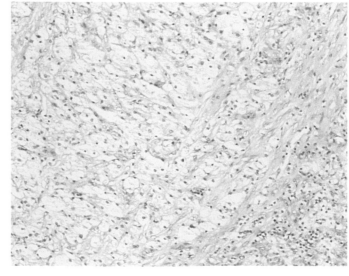

a

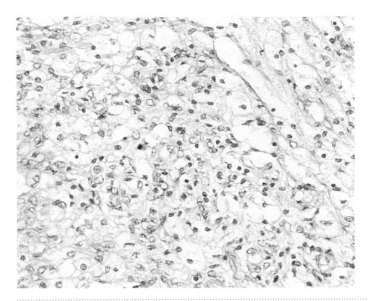

Figure 8.35 continued

b

Figure 8.36 **Angiomatoid MFH** This specific variant of MFH usually presents as a small, slow-growing, haemangioma-like lesion in the deep dermis or subcutaneous tissue of the extremities (especially the upper limb) of children and young adults. There may be associated constitutional symptoms such as fever, weight loss, or anaemia. It consists of sheets of histiocytic cells, areas of haemorrhage, and a prominent lymphoid infiltrate (a). The histiocytes are sometimes disposed in nodules, whorls, or in a storiform arrangement (b). They have abundant cytoplasm and oval nuclei which show mild to moderate nuclear pleomorphism; there is scanty mitotic activity (c). This lesion commonly recurs but only rarely metastasizes.

Figure 8.36

a

c b

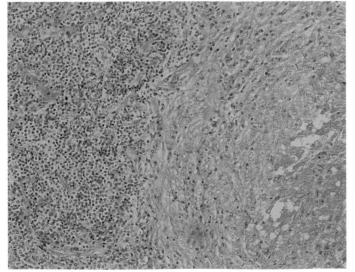

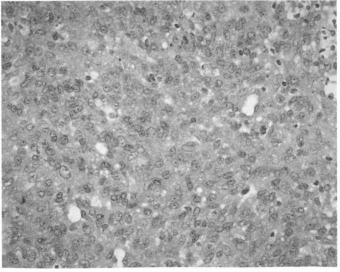

Tumours of fat

Figure 8.37 **Lipoma** Lipoma is the most common of all soft tissue tumours. Most lipomas are solitary lesions which arise in the subcutaneous tissue of the back, shoulders, neck, abdomen, and extremities; they are rarely found in deep soft tissue. Multiple lipomas may also rarely occur. A lipoma most commonly presents in middle-aged or older adults as a well defined, lobulated fatty tumour having a thin fibrous capsule. Fibrous septa separate the fat lobules which contain mature univacuolated fat cells showing only slight variation in size and shape and no nuclear atypia or mitotic activity (a). Lipomas are well vascularized, containing compressed or congested thin-walled vessels within the lobules and septa. A lipoma containing abundant dense fibrous tissue is often termed a fibrolipoma (b). Cytogenetic abnormalities, including rearrangement of the long arm of chromosome 12, are commonly found in lipomas. Lipomas may rarely recur following local excision but do not undergo malignant change.

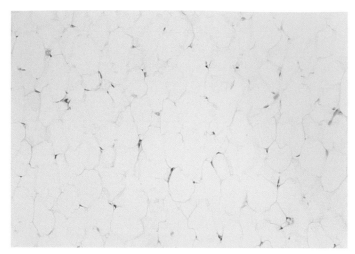
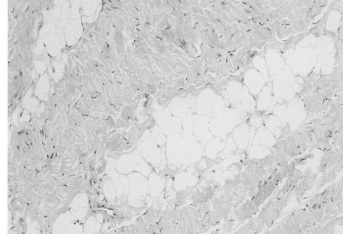

Figure 8.37

a

b

Figure 8.38 **Intramuscular lipoma** This fatty tumour produces a painless, often large swelling in large muscles of the extremities of middle-aged and older adults, more often males than females. The tumour becomes more prominent on muscle contraction and lies parallel to the long axis of the muscle in which it lies. It is composed entirely of lipoma-like mature fat cells which extend around muscle bundles and between individual muscle fibres, some of which may appear atrophic (as shown here). Lipoblasts are not seen and there is no myxoid change or plexiform vascular pattern. Local recurrence occurs in up to 15 per cent of cases.

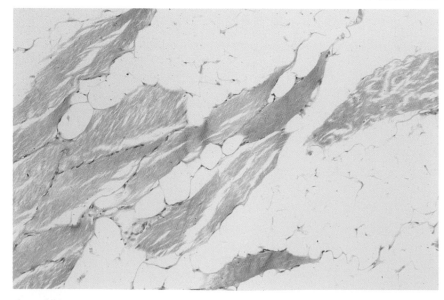

Figure 8.38

Figure 8.39 Angiolipoma This tumour arises in the subcutaneous tissue of the extremities (particularly the upper limb) or trunk of young adults, more commonly males than females. Lesions are characteristically painful and often multiple. Angiolipoma is usually well defined and (as shown here) is composed of lipoma-like mature adipose tissue amongst which can be found numerous small, branching vessels, usually of capillary size but sometimes larger; they are most often located at the edge of the lesion. Vessels may contain fibrin thrombi and there may be prominent perivascular fibrosis.

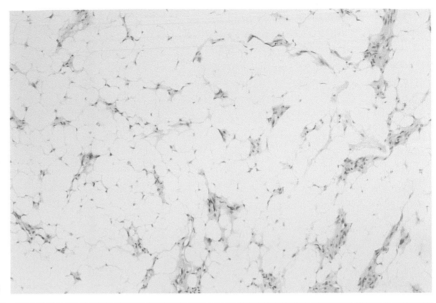

Figure 8.39

Figure 8.40 Spindle cell lipoma This is an uncommon type of lipoma which usually arises in the subcutaneous tissues of the neck, upper back, or shoulder of males who are in their fifth decade or older. It is a relatively well defined, slow-growing tumour composed of areas of mature adipose tissue and uniform bland spindle cells which lie in a variably collagenous or myxoid matrix (a, b). Either the fat or spindle cell component may predominate. Spindle cells do not show mitotic activity or marked cellular or nuclear pleomorphism but may occasionally show nuclear palisading. There is often an infiltrate of mast cells. The lesion rarely recurs locally.

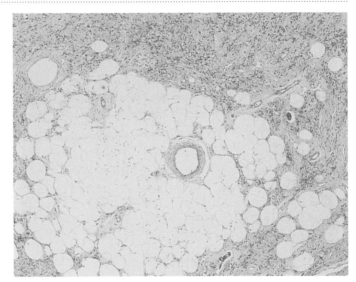

Figure 8.40

a

b

Figure 8.41 Pleomorphic lipoma This lesion is also usually found in subcutaneous tissues of the posterior neck or shoulder region of middle-aged or elderly males and may represent a pleomorphic variant of spindle cell lipoma. It is characterized by the presence of bizarre giant cells (arrow) with hyperchromatic nuclei which are often disposed peripherally (floret cells) (a, b). There is a variable amount of collagenous fibrous tissue and mature adipose tissue. There is usually little mitotic activity and no atypical mitoses are seen.

Figure 8.41

| a | b |

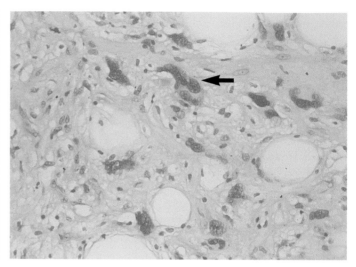

Figure 8.42 Hibernoma A hibernoma is a tumour composed largely of brown fat cells. It occurs most commonly in young and middle-aged adults in the scapular region, chest wall, neck, axilla, and groin, but may occur at other sites. The lesion is slowly enlarging, painless and yellow-tan in colour. It is composed of lobules of oval or polygonal granular eosinophilic cells with multivacuolated cytoplasm and a small round, central nucleus (a, b). Large univacuolated fat cells are interspersed amongst the brown fat cells. The lesion is benign and does not commonly recur after excision.

Figure 8.42

| b | a |

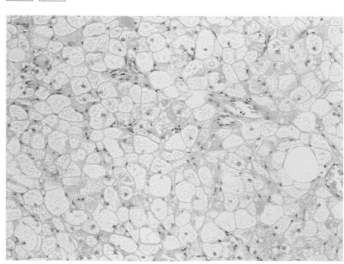

Figure 8.43 **Fibrolipomatous hamartoma of nerve (neural fibrolipoma, perineurial lipoma)** This is a fibrous and fatty overgrowth which surrounds and infiltrates peripheral nerve bundles (a). Most cases occur in the distal upper extremity and a significant proportion have macrodactyly or other bone abnormalities. The condition may be present at birth and most cases present before the age of 30 years with symptoms of nerve compression. Males are more commonly affected than females. There is an increase in fibrous tissue surrounding nerve bundles. Collagen is also present within adipose tissue which lies between nerve bundles (b).

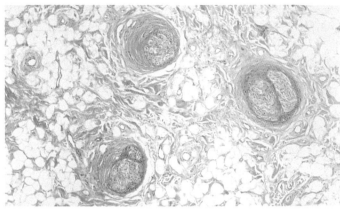

Figure 8.43

a

b

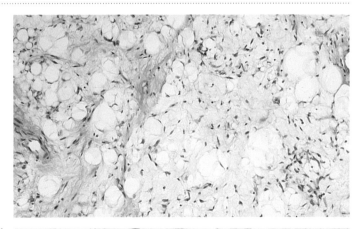

Figure 8.44 **Lipoblastoma** This rare fatty tumour presents in infancy and young children, predominantly males, as a solitary (lipoblastoma) or diffuse (lipoblastomatosis) slow-growing, painless swelling in the extremities. Localized lesions are confined to subcutaneous tissue but diffuse lesions may infiltrate underlying muscle. There is a prominent lobular pattern with proliferating immature fat cells separated by fibrous septa (a). The lobules contain small spindle-shaped or round lipoblasts containing one or more fat vacuoles as well as mature adipocytes (b). There are numerous thin-walled small blood vessels and focal myxoid change may be seen in the stroma. Recurrence rarely occurs and the lesion does not undergo malignant change.

Figure 8.44

a

b

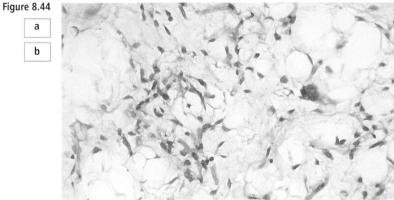

Figure 8.45 Liposarcoma This is one of the commonest soft tissue sarcomas. It is rare in children and arises chiefly in the fifth and sixth decades of life. There is a slight male predominance. Most liposarcomas are found in the extremities (especially the thigh) and retroperitoneum. Multiple tumours are found in about 10 per cent of cases. Grossly, the tumours are often large, lobulated and relatively well circumscribed with a fatty or myxoid cut surface (shown here). MRI is useful in identifying the fat composition of these soft tissue tumours. Recognition of the various histological subtypes of liposarcoma is important as these have prognostic significance.

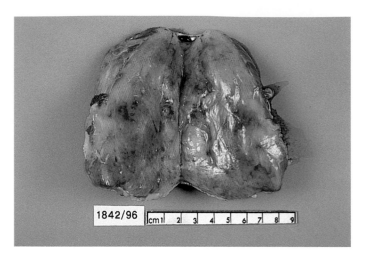

Figure 8.45

Figure 8.46 Well-differentiated liposarcoma: lipoma-like subtype Well-differentiated liposarcoma is a low-grade sarcoma which is classified into several subtypes of which lipoma-like liposarcoma is the most common. The tumour resembles a benign lipoma but shows marked variation in the size and shape of fat cells (a). Scattered lipoblasts (arrow) and hyperchromatic cells are also seen, particularly in the vicinity of areas of fibrosis or fibrous septa (b). These tumours arise most frequently in the retroperitoneum but are also commonly found in the extremities. They rarely metastasize but commonly recur. A large lipoma-like liposarcoma, usually of the retroperitoneum, may uncommonly undergo focal dedifferentiation to a more high-grade type of liposarcoma or another sarcoma type such as MFH (dedifferentiated liposarcoma). The term atypical lipoma is often used to designate a well-differentiated liposarcoma arising in superficial soft tissue as tumours in this location rarely metastasize.

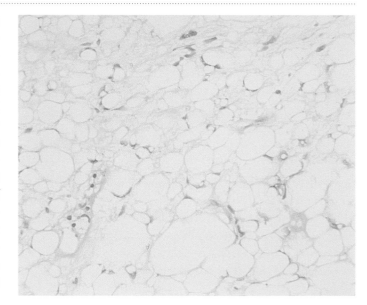

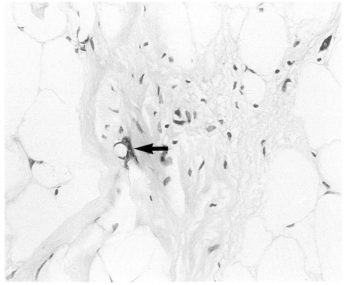

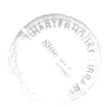

Figure 8.46

a

b

Figure 8.47 **Well-differentiated liposarcoma: sclerosing subtype** This tumour is mostly seen in the retroperitoneum and groin but may also be found elsewhere. It contains areas of lipoma-like liposarcoma and abundant fibrillary or dense collagenous fibrous tissue (a) in which may be found hyperchromatic cells. There are occasional lipoblasts (b); these are often found in the vicinity of areas of fibrosis.

Figure 8.47

| a | b |

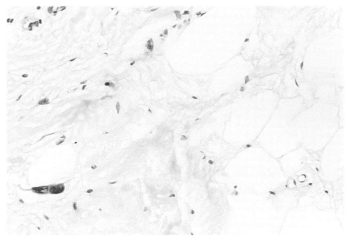

Figure 8.48 **Myxoid liposarcoma** This is the commonest histological subtype of liposarcoma, accounting for approximately 50 per cent of all cases. It contains a prominent (hyaluronidase-sensitive) myxoid matrix in which there is a prominent plexiform capillary vascular pattern and a variable admixture of small fat cells (a, b). There are numerous smooth, polygonal or round hyperchromatic mesenchymal cells and a variable number of lipoblasts (arrow) (c). Pools of myxoid material and areas of haemorrhage and cystic change may also be seen. A translocation involving chromosomes 12 and 16 is seen in most myxoid liposarcomas. This tumour commonly recurs and may metastasize but does so much less commonly than round cell or pleomorphic forms of liposarcoma.

Figure 8.48

| a | b |

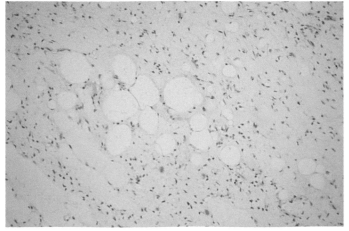

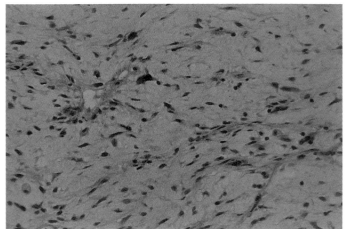

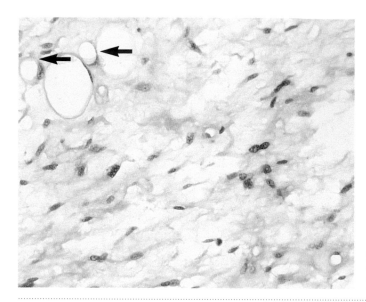

Figure 8.48 continued

c

Figure 8.49 **Round cell liposarcoma** This is an uncommon high-grade form of liposarcoma which probably represents a poorly differentiated form of myxoid liposarcoma. It contains sheets or cords of small round tumour cells with vesicular or hyperchromatic nuclei and vacuolated cytoplasm (a). Numerous lipoblasts are present (arrow) and there is prominent mitotic activity (b). Transition to areas of myxoid liposarcoma containing numerous lipoblasts may also be seen. This tumour commonly recurs and metastasizes and needs to be distinguished from other round cell sarcomas of soft tissue such as Ewing's sarcoma and lymphoma.

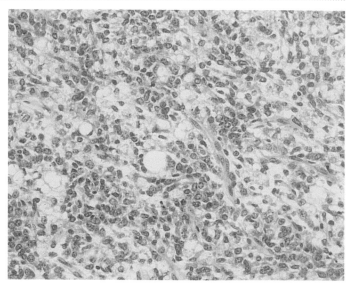

Figure 8.49

a

b

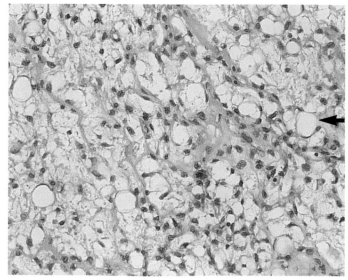

Figure 8.50 Pleomorphic liposarcoma This relatively uncommon form of high-grade liposarcoma usually develops in the deep soft tissues of the extremities. It contains bizarre mononuclear and multinucleated tumour giant cells, many of which are vacuolated and have abundant eosinophilic cytoplasm (a, b). There is increased mitotic activity and atypical mitoses. Identification of lipoblasts (arrow) permits distinction from other pleomorphic sarcomas such as rhabdomyosarcoma and MFH. Recurrence and metastases frequently occur.

Figure 8.50

| a | b |

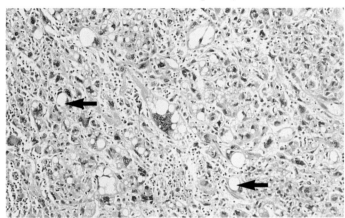
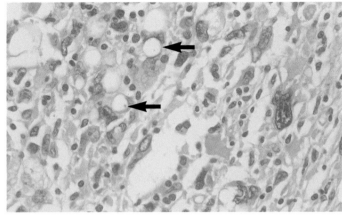

Tumours of smooth muscle

Figure 8.51 Superficial leiomyoma Benign smooth muscle tumours uncommonly develop in soft tissue. Most arise in the skin from the arrector pili muscle (cutaneous leiomyoma/leiomyoma cutis) (a), or in smooth muscle of the deep dermis and subcutaneous tissue of genital regions (genital leiomyoma). Most cutaneous leiomyomas arise in adolescents or young adults as single or multiple small painful nodules on the limbs or trunk; some lesions arise on a familial basis. Genital leiomyomas present as solitary, small painful swellings. Cutaneous leiomyomas are often separated from the overlying epidermis by an uninvolved Grenz zone (arrow) (a). Both cutaneous and genital lesions are composed of broad fascicles of fusiform smooth muscle cells with eosinophilic cytoplasm and elongated, blunt- ended nuclei which show no evidence of pleomorphism or mitotic activity. (b) Local recurrence or development of new cutaneous leiomyomas may occur but in general these lesions do not undergo malignant change.

Figure 8.51

| a |
| b |

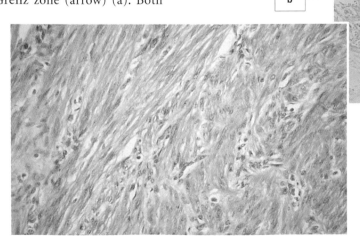

Figure 8.52 **Deep soft tissue leiomyoma**
These lesions are very uncommon, solitary, well defined, and often large tumours which are most commonly found in the extremities, abdominal cavity, and retroperitoneum of young and middle-aged adults. They resemble superficial leiomyomas histologically, being composed of bundles of smooth muscle cells (as shown here); they show no cellular or nuclear pleomorphism and little (less than one per ten high-power fields) mitotic activity. Focal hyaline fibrosis, calcification, and ossification may be seen, particularly in larger tumours.

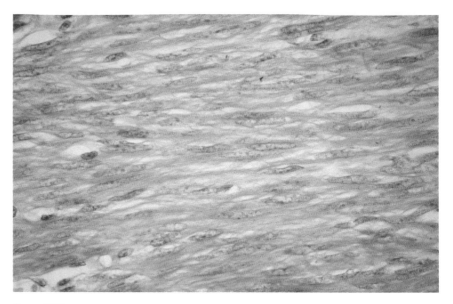

Figure 8.52

Figure 8.53 **Angioleiomyoma** This relatively common lesion arises in the deep dermis or subcutaneous tissue of the extremities, especially the lower leg of adults, more commonly females than males. The lesion is usually well circumscribed and painful. It is composed of numerous endothelial cell-lined vascular spaces which have a thick smooth muscle coat. Smooth muscle cells surrounding vessels merge with those in fascicles that lie in the interstitial tissue separating the vessels (a). Hyalinization of smooth muscle is commonly seen (b); myxoid change may also be noted. There is no mitotic activity or cytological atypia. The lesion is benign and recurrence rarely occurs.

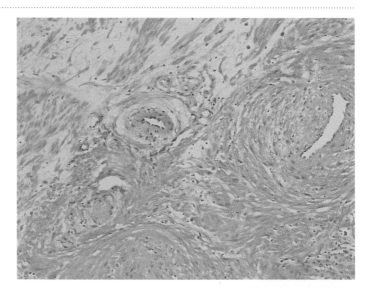

Figure 8.53

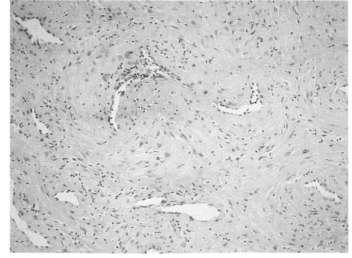

Figure 8.54 Leiomyosarcoma Leiomyosarcoma accounts for about 10 per cent of all soft tissue sarcomas. Extravisceral leiomyosarcomas mostly arise in the abdominal cavity or retroperitoneum but may also develop in superficial or deep soft tissues of the extremities. Rarely, vascular leiomyosarcomas may arise from the wall of large and medium-sized vessels (e.g. the inferior vena cava, femoral vein). Leiomyosarcoma is a tumour of late middle-aged and elderly adults and occurs predominantly in females. Grossly, superficial tumours are usually smaller than those in deeper soft tissue. Well or moderately differentiated leiomyosarcomas consist of interlacing broad fascicles composed of fusiform cells with eosinophilic cytoplasm and blunt-ended nuclei (a). Mitotic activity is variable but there are usually one or more mitoses (arrow) per ten high-power fields (b); nuclear palisading including perinuclear vacuolation may also be prominent. More poorly differentiated tumours usually retain a fascicular pattern but contain more hyperchromatic and pleomorphic cells including occasional tumour giant cells (c, d). Smooth muscle tumour cells contain glycogen and are strongly PAS positive (diastase-sensitive); trichrome or PTAH stains may demonstrate intracytoplasmic myofilaments. A dense reticulin network and basal lamina components such as collagen type IV and laminin surround individual tumour cells. Cells are also positive for desmin, smooth muscle actin, and in some cases cytokeratin. Cutaneous leiomyosarcoma commonly recurs but rarely metastasizes. Subcutaneous and intramuscular leiomyosarcomas, however, commonly recur and metastasize in up to 40 per cent of cases. Extensive local spread and metastasis is very commonly seen in intravascular and intra-abdominal leiomyosarcomas.

Figure 8.54

| a | b |
| c | d |

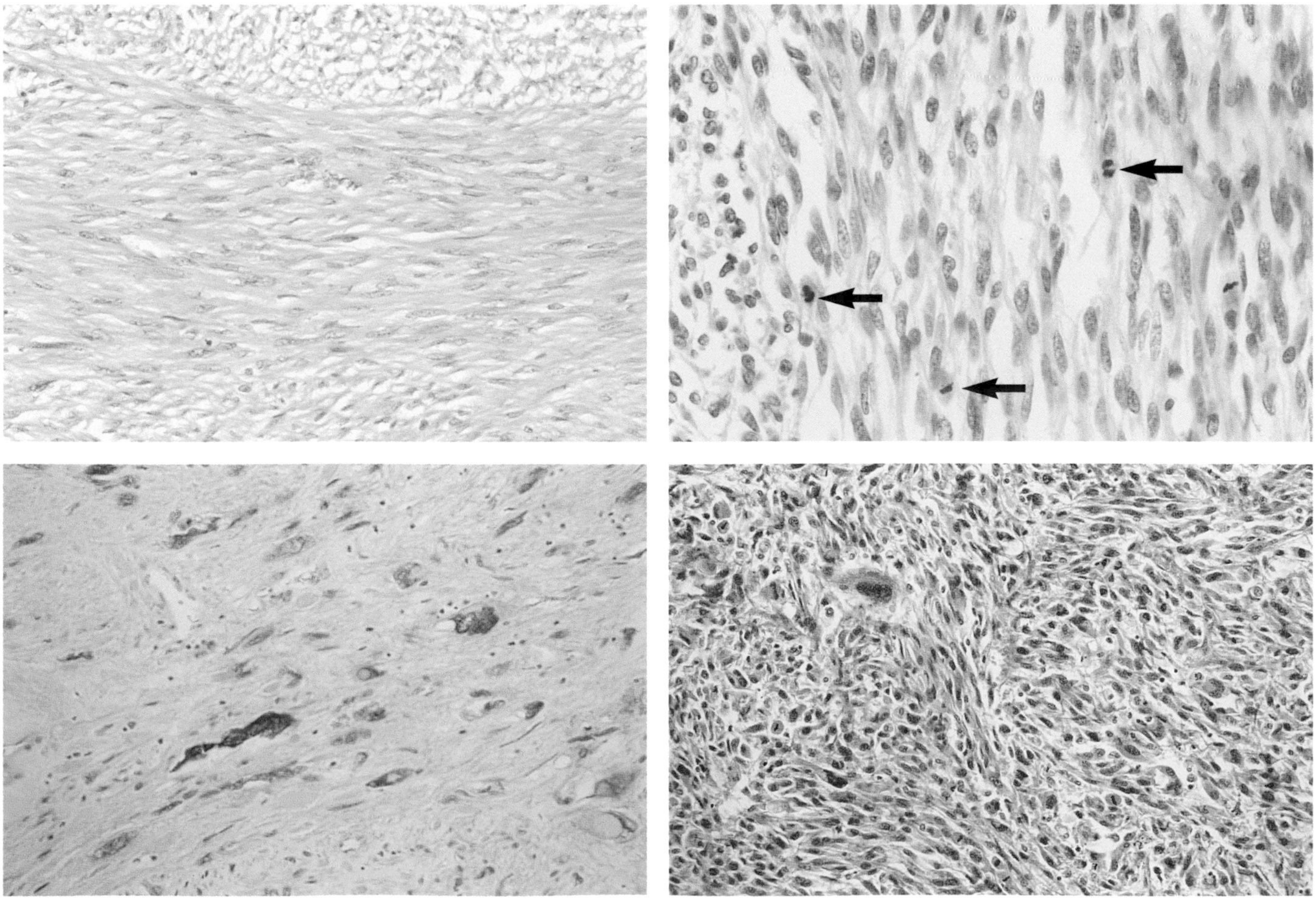

Figure 8.55 Epithelioid leiomyosarcoma (leiomyoblastoma) Epithelioid smooth muscle tumours are extremely rare in soft tissues of the extremities and develop most commonly in the stomach, mesentery, uterus, and retroperitoneum. Most epithelioid smooth muscle tumours arising in soft tissue are malignant. They consist of sheets of round or polygonal cells, with clear or eosinophilic cytoplasm (a, b). Cells show a variable degree of cytoplasmic vacuolation. Focal areas of typical leiomyosarcoma may also be present. Tumours behave aggressively and commonly metastasize.

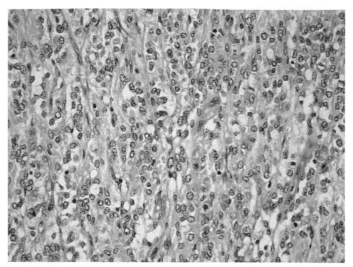

Figure 8.55

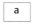
a

b

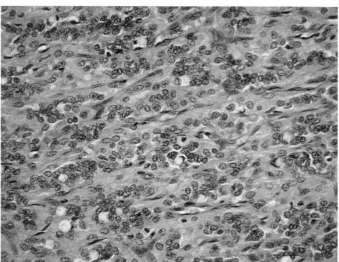

Tumours of striated muscle

Figure 8.56 Rhabdomyosarcoma Benign tumours of striated muscle (adult and fetal rhabdomyoma) are very rare. Several types of rhabdomyosarcoma, however, have been described; these arise in different age groups and their recognition is important in terms of prognosis and treatment. Skeletal muscle differentiation of tumour cells is evidenced by cross-striations which may be seen ultrastructurally or identified by PTAH staining (a). Rhabdomyosarcoma tumour cells also express muscle antigens such as desmin (b), muscle actin, and myoglobin.

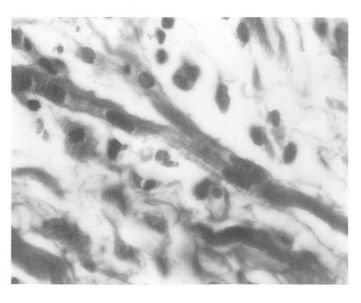

Figure 8.56

a

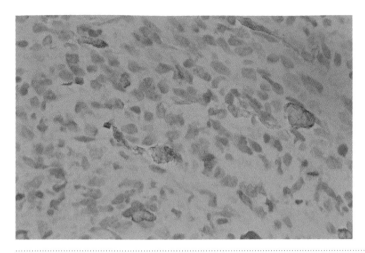

Figure 8.56 continued

b

Figure 8.57 **Embryonal rhabdomyosarcoma** This is the most common subtype of rhabdomyosarcoma, accounting for about 70 per cent of all cases. It usually arises in childhood, especially the first decade. It is uncommon after adolescence. It usually presents as a rapidly growing, painless swelling arising in the head and neck region, nasopharynx, or urogenital tract, and is relatively uncommon in the extremities or trunk. It is composed of a proliferation of round or polygonal primitive mesenchymal cells with scanty cytoplasm and oval, round, or pleomorphic hyperchromatic nuclei, some of which show mitotic activity (arrow) (a); tumour cells lie in a loose connective tissue or mucinous stroma. There are also scattered pleomorphic round or spindle-shaped tumour cells containing a variable amount of cytoplasm and abnormal, hyperchromatic nuclei (b, c). The finding of myofibrils or cross-striations in tumour cells on PTAH staining or expression of muscle antigens is usually required to confirm the histological diagnosis. Although an aggressive tumour which metastasizes early, embryonal rhabdomyosarcoma is highly responsive to combination chemotherapy.

Figure 8.57

a

b c

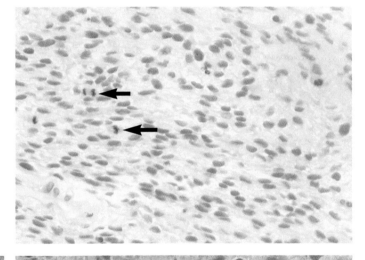

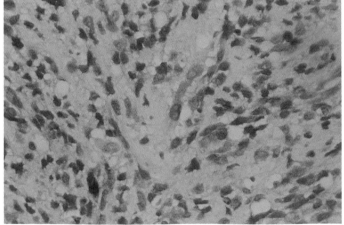

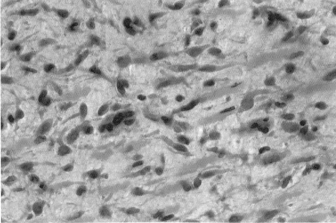

Figure 8.58 **Alveolar rhabdomyosarcoma** This subtype accounts for about 25 per cent of rhabdomyosarcomas. It usually presents as a deep soft-tissue mass involving the limbs or trunk of adolescents and young adults. It contains fibrous septa which outline alveolar spaces lined by small round pleomorphic tumour cells with scanty or abundant cytoplasm and hyperchromatic, often abnormal nuclei (a, b). Papillary proliferation of these tumour cells is seen on the surface of fibrous septa. Due to loss of cellular cohesion, groups of tumour cells often lie freely in the alveolar spaces. Multinucleated giant cells having a wreath-like arrangement of nuclei may also be seen. A solid variant of alveolar rhabdomyosarcoma may predominate in some tumours where the alveolar spaces are filled with masses of tumour cells (c). Alveolar rhabdomyosarcoma commonly shows a translocation between chromosomes 2 and 13 [t(2;13)(q37;q14)]. This tumour behaves aggressively, metastasizing early via the lymphatics and the bloodstream.

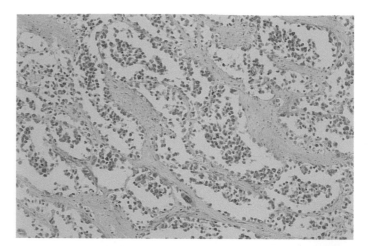

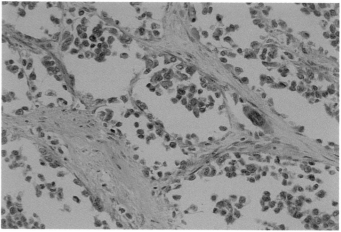

Figure 8.58

a
b

c

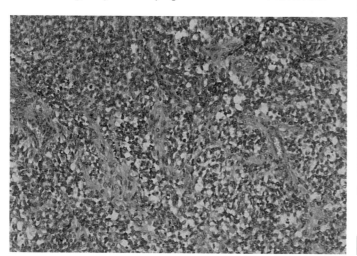

Figure 8.59 **Pleomorphic rhabdomyosarcoma** This rare form of rhabdomyosarcoma usually arises in large muscles of the extremities (especially the thigh) of middle-aged and older adults. It is a highly cellular tumour containing numerous large, round, polygonal, or spindle-shaped cells with abundant eosinophilic cytoplasm and highly pleomorphic nuclei (a). There are numerous bizarre tumour giant cells with abnormal, hyperchromatic nuclei; mitotic activity is frequent and often atypical (b). Cross-striations are rarely seen. This tumour should be distinguished from other pleomorphic sarcomas such as liposarcoma, leiomyosarcoma, malignant peripheral nerve sheath tumour, and MFH. The tumour grows rapidly and metastasizes early.

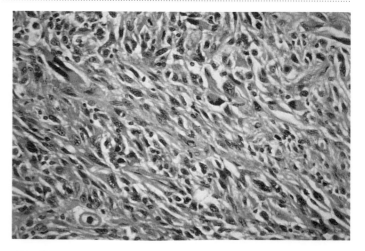

Figure 8.59

a

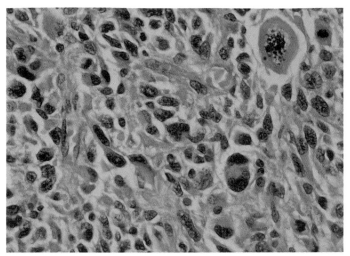

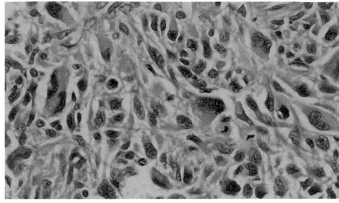

Figure 8.59 continued

b c

Tumours of vascular origin

Figure 8.60 **Capillary haemangioma** Haemangiomas are common soft tissue tumours. Most are capillary haemangiomas composed of capillary-sized vessels. These lesions usually arise in infancy or childhood, most commonly in the skin or mucous membrane of the head and neck region. The immature capillary haemangioma (strawberry naevus) is often very cellular, containing numerous proliferating plump endothelial cells, some of which line vascular spaces (a); they may exhibit numerous typical mitotic figures (arrow) (b). These lesions enlarge rapidly and often regress spontaneously. More mature capillary haemangiomas appear less cellular and contain numerous capillary-sized channels lined by flattened or round endothelial cells.

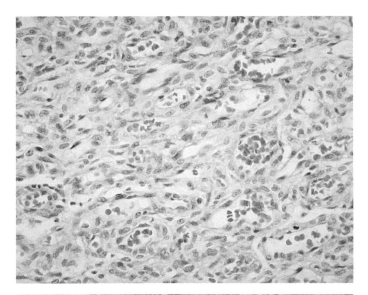

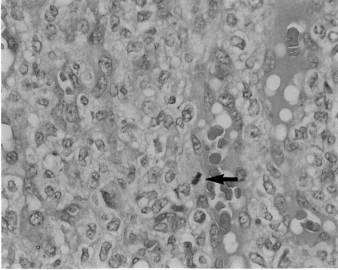

Figure 8.60

a

b

Figure 8.61 **Cavernous haemangioma** This type of haemangioma arises chiefly in childhood and involves mainly the superficial or deep soft tissues of the upper part of the body. It is composed of dilated vascular channels lined by flattened endothelial cells (a, b). The lesion has a lobulated outline and cellular or collagenous connective tissue lies between the vascular channels. Cavernous haemangiomas less frequently undergo spontaneous regression than capillary haemangiomas. When very large these lesions may be associated with thrombocytopenic purpura (Kasabach–Merritt syndrome). In Mafucci's syndrome, multiple haemangiomas, usually of cavernous type, are associated with the development of multiple enchondromas.

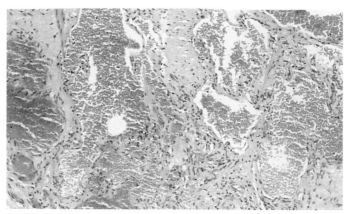

Figure 8.61

a

b

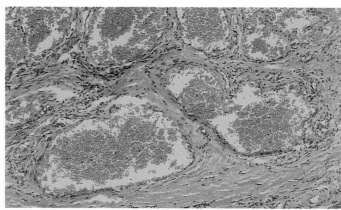

Figure 8.62 **Arteriovenous haemangioma** These uncommon lesions are found mainly in the superficial or deep soft tissues of the head and neck or extremities of young patients. They consist of medium- to large-sized arteries or veins which often lie close to each other and may contain areas which resemble a capillary or cavernous haemangioma (arrowed) (a). The vessels have a thickened muscular wall and the lumen is often dilated and of irregular outline (b). These lesions, especially deep-seated ones, may show clinical features of arteriovenous shunting.

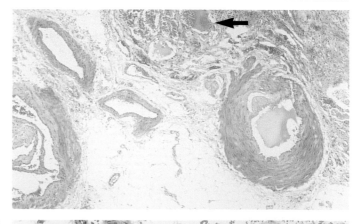

Figure 8.62

a

b

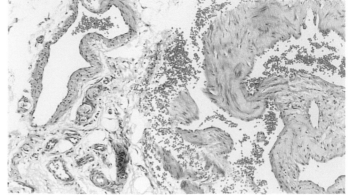

Figure 8.63 **Epithelioid haemangioma (angiolymphoid hyperplasia with eosinophilia)** This rare lesion typically involves the skin and subcutaneous tissues of the head and neck region of middle-aged females. Lesions are usually red, poorly defined, and may be single or multiple. They consist of vascular channels which are surrounded by a prominent mixed inflammatory cell infiltrate including lymphocytes, macrophages, plasma cells, lymphoid aggregates, or follicles and eosinophils (arrow) (a, b). The capillary-sized vascular channels are lined by plump endothelial cells. The lesions commonly recur after excision. Some patients exhibit regional lymphadenopathy and peripheral blood eosinophilia. Kimura's disease, in which there is also a prominent eosinophil and lymphoid infiltrate but only minor vascular proliferation, is an unrelated condition.

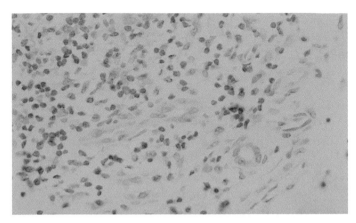

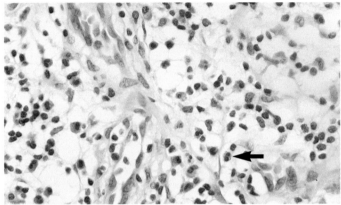

Figure 8.63

a

b

Figure 8.64 **Pyogenic granuloma** This is a common form of haemangioma which arises in skin or mucosal surfaces. It occurs most commonly around the mouth or on the hands and fingers. The lesion may present at any age; sex incidence is equal. The lesion is composed of numerous capillary-sized channels, amongst which are scattered numerous acute and chronic inflammatory cells (a, b). Endothelial cells lining blood vessels are often plump and may show typical mitotic activity. A gingival granuloma of similar appearance may arise during pregnancy. The lesion may recur after excision.

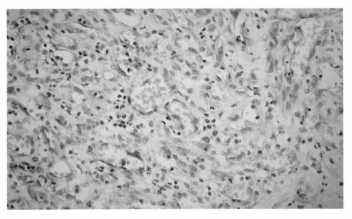

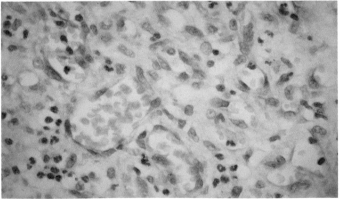

Figure 8.64

a

b

Figure 8.65 **Intramuscular haemangioma** This is an uncommon form of haemangioma which is found most commonly in the muscles of the extremities (especially the lower limb). It may arise at any age but is seen chiefly in adolescents and young adults. The lesion is poorly defined and infiltrative. Individual muscle fibres are separated by proliferating vessels which may be of large diameter (a, b). Lesions composed of vessels of small diameter may show numerous closely packed capillary channels lined by plump endothelial cells (c). When vascular channels are indistinct and the lesion appears highly cellular, it can be confused with a malignant vascular tumour. Mixed capillary and cavernous forms may be seen. The large vessel type tends to predominate in the extremities and the small vessel type is seen mainly in the head and neck region. Although benign, these lesions commonly recur after excision.

Figure 8.65

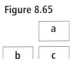

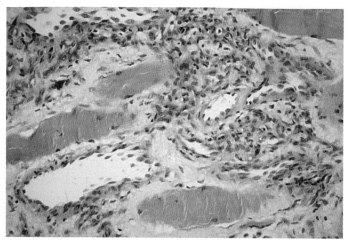

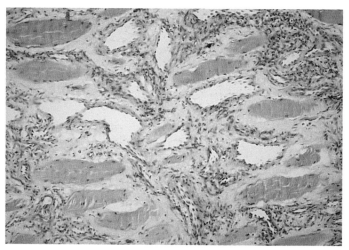

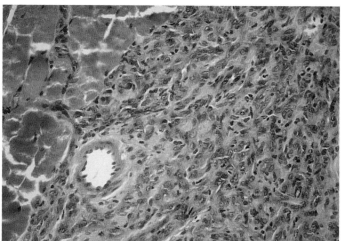

Figure 8.66 **Papillary endothelial hyperplasia (Masson's tumour)** This is an uncommon benign intravascular proliferation which occurs in an organizing thrombus. It may occur at any age and usually presents on the head or extremities as a raised, superficially located, nodular lesion less than 2.0 cm in size. The lesion is often well defined and surrounded by part of a blood vessel wall containing a thrombus or areas of haemorrhage. The lesion is composed of numerous branching and anastomosing vascular channels and contains projections of fibrous or fibrinous tissue covered by plump endothelial cells which have large, hyperchromatic nuclei (shown here). There is cellular and nuclear pleomorphism but mitoses are not usually seen. This lesion needs to be distinguished histologically from angiosarcoma. It is benign and rarely recurs after excision.

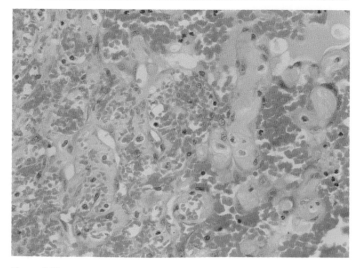

Figure 8.66

Figure 8.67 Glomus tumour The normal glomus body is an arteriovenous anastomosis that regulates blood flow in the distal extremities. A glomus tumour is an uncommon lesion which presents as a small solitary, exquisitely painful lesion. It occurs most commonly in a subungual location but may also be found in the hand, upper and lower extremities, trunk, and rarely other sites. The classic glomus tumour is composed of sheets of cells of uniform appearance with central round nuclei and pale eosinophilic cytoplasm (a, b). Numerous compressed, thin, capillary-sized channels are seen in the tumour. Myxoid change is often prominent in the stroma (c). Glomus tumours containing dilated vascular spaces similar to those of a cavernous haemangioma are termed glomangiomas (d); these lesions are usually multiple, poorly circumscribed, and found in the dermal tissues of the extremities, particularly the arms. Glomus tumours are benign but may recur after excision.

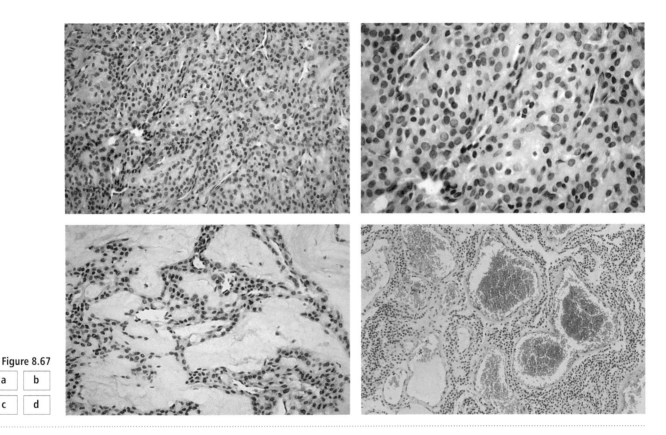

Figure 8.67

a	b
c	d

Figure 8.68 Haemangiopericytoma Haemangiopericytoma is an uncommon soft tissue tumour, usually arising in the deep soft tissues of the extremities, retroperitoneum, head and neck, and trunk of adults. It contains numerous gaping irregular branching 'stag-horn' vascular spaces lined by flattened endothelial cells (a). Short spindle-shaped cells with round or oval nuclei and poorly defined cytoplasm are disposed around these vessels and there may be perivascular hyalinization (b). Reticulin lies around individual tumour cells and outlines the blood vessels (c). Histological distinction of benign from malignant haemangiopericytoma is difficult, although mitoses are unusual in benign tumours (generally less than four per ten high-power fields). In addition, malignant tumours containing areas of haemorrhage and necrosis are usually more hypercellular and show nuclear atypia. Tumour cells are negative for factor VIII-related antigen and alpha smooth muscle actin but stain

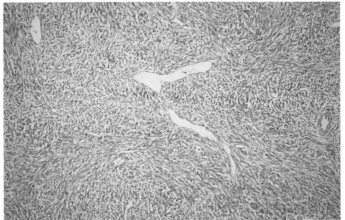

Figure 8.68

a

for CD34. Behaviour is difficult to predict; recurrence and metastasis may occur many years after the original lesion has been excised.

Figure 8.68

b   c

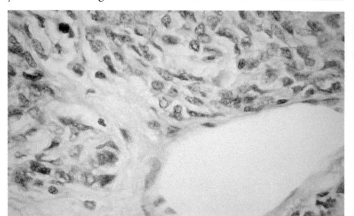

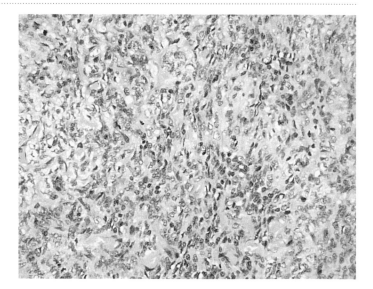

Figure 8.69 Spindle cell haemangioendothelioma This is a rare low-grade malignant tumour arising in adolescents and young adults, chiefly in the superficial soft tissues of the distal extremities (especially the hand). Multiple small red nodules are often seen grossly. These consist of cavernous vascular spaces between which there is a proliferation of spindle-shaped and plump, round endothelial cells, some of which lie in small compressed vascular spaces (a, b). There is mild to moderate cellular and nuclear pleomorphism and only occasional mitotic activity. Local recurrence is common but metastasis rarely occurs.

Figure 8.69

a

b

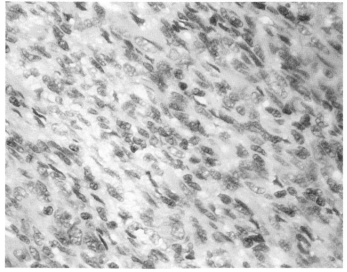

Figure 8.70 Epithelioid haemangioendo-thelioma This is a rare low-grade malignant vascular tumour that may arise in the soft tissues as a solitary lesion or as multiple lesions, some of which may be found in internal organs or bone. Lesions arising in soft tissues are often associated with a medium-sized or large vessel, usually a vein, which may be obstructed by tumour or thrombus. The tumour is poorly defined and shows vascular proliferation (a, b). Numerous ovoid or polygonal tumour cells, arranged in short cords or nests, lie in a mucinous chondroid or hyaline matrix. Tumour cells often appear vacuolated and have intracellular cytoplasmic lumina which gives them a 'signet-ring' cell appearance. Tumour cells are factor VIII positive and show variable cellular and nuclear pleomorphism and mitotic activity. Differential diagnosis include parachordoma, myxoid chondrosarcoma, and secondary mucinous adenocarcinoma. Local recurrence and metastasis, often to regional lymph nodes, may occur.

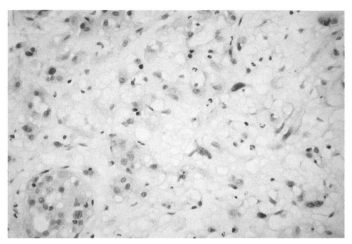

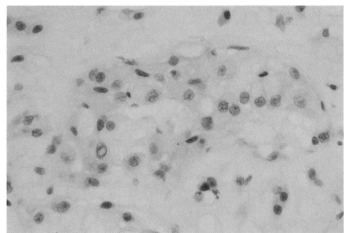

Figure 8.70

a

b

Figure 8.71 Angiosarcoma This term is now used to describe a malignant tumour that arises from endothelial cells lining either blood or lymphatic vessels. The tumour is rare and usually arises in the superficial soft tissues of adults, most commonly in the head and neck region or extremities; it may also rarely occur in internal organs. The tumour consists of diffusely infiltrating, thin-walled, vascular channels lined by plump malignant endothelial cells which show a variable but often high degree of cellular and nuclear pleomorphism (a, b). Solid areas of tumour cell proliferation may be seen where the vascular nature of the tumour is less obvious (c). Mitotic activity is often high but may be variable. The tumour diffusely infiltrates superficial soft tissues, spreading along tissue planes. Tumour cells are factor VIII positive. Chronic lymphoedema, usually in women who have had a radical mastectomy for breast cancer, is strongly associated with the development of an angiosarcoma (formerly termed lymphangiosarcoma). The prognosis is generally poor, widespread metastasis occurring early.

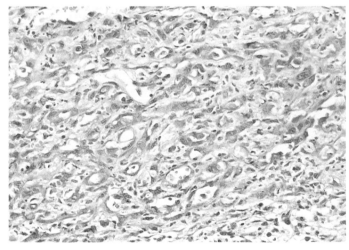

Figure 8.71

a

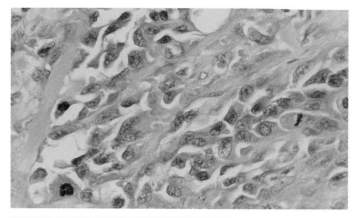

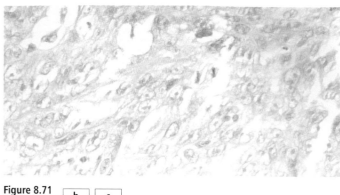

Figure 8.71
continued | b | c |

Figure 8.72 Kaposi's sarcoma This highly vascular tumour is of unknown histogenesis. It most often presents as a cutaneous patch, plaque, or nodule. The classic form is seen in elderly people of Mediterranean or Eastern European descent who present with slow-growing solitary or multiple skin lesions on the distal extremities, especially the foot and lower leg. Kaposi's sarcoma in Africa arises in children and young adults and particularly affects the lymph nodes. Kaposi's sarcoma also arises in organ transplant recipients who receive high doses of immunosuppressive therapy. In addition, approximately one third of patients with acquired immune deficiency syndrome (AIDS) develop nodules of Kaposi's sarcoma, which are often multiple. In all forms of the disease the early lesions are characterized by a granulation-tissue-like proliferation of spindle cells and capillary-sized blood vessels with interstitial inflamma-tion (a, b). In the later nodular phase, numer-ous small capillary-sized or larger dilated vascular channels and proliferating spindle cells are also seen. In addition, there are slit-like spaces, without an obvious endothelial lining, which contain extravasated red cells (long arrow) (b, c). Haemosiderin deposition may also be present. There is moderate cellu-lar and nuclear pleomorphism and a variable degree of mitotic activity (short arrow).

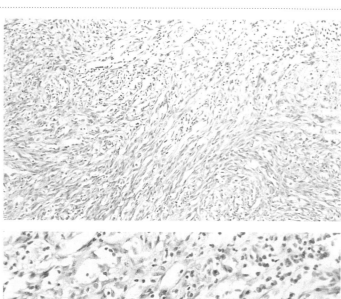

Figure 8.72

| a |
| b |
| c |

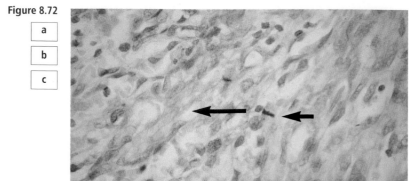

Figure 8.73 **Lymphangioma** Like haemangiomas, most lymphangiomas arise during infancy and childhood. They occur predominantly in the skin; they are usually solitary but may also be multiple. Most cases are probably developmental defects. They are much less common than haemangiomas with which they may sometimes be associated. Cutaneous lymphangiomas are often cavernous in type with fluid-containing spaces lined by a flattened endothelium (a). Cavernous lymphangiomas or capillary lymphangiomas with dilated channels may also be found in deep fibrous tissue within muscle (b). A cystic lymphangioma (cystic hygroma) is a multiloculated swelling composed of numerous cystic spaces lined by a flattened endothelium (c). The lymphatic spaces are separated by a variable amount of fibrous tissue amongst which are found scattered chronic inflammatory cells and lymphoid aggregates. The lesions may recur after excision but do not undergo malignant change.

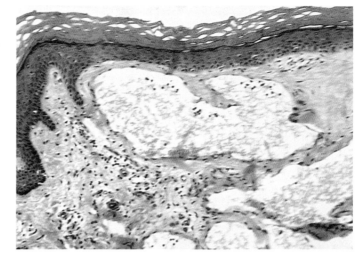

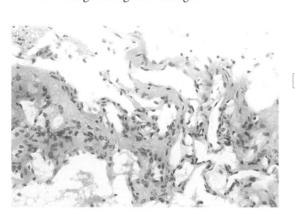

Figure 8.73

	a
b	c

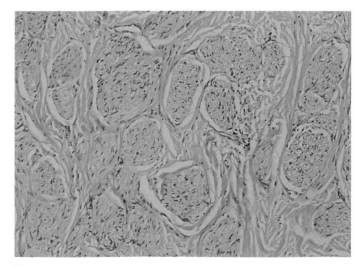

Tumours of neural origin

Figure 8.74 **Traumatic (amputation) neuroma** Following traumatic injury to a peripheral nerve, there is fibroblast and Schwann cell proliferation and growth of axons from the proximal end of the severed nerve fibre. If the proximal and distal ends of the nerve are not correctly apposed, disordered proliferation of these cells results in the formation of a mass termed a neuroma. This is composed of nerve bundles of variable size surrounded and disrupted by fibrous tissue (a, b). There is proliferation of Schwann cells and collagenous fibrous tissue; regenerating axons may be seen with special stains. The lesion is usually solitary. Local recurrence does not occur.

Figure 8.74

a

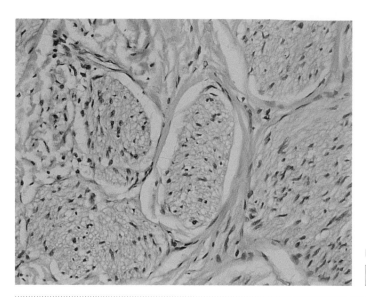

Figure 8.74 continued

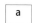

Figure 8.75 **Morton's neuroma (metatar-salgia)** This reactive lesion is due to thickening of one of the interdigital nerves of the foot, usually that between the head of the third and fourth, or the second and third metatarsals. It chiefly presents in females and is generally unilateral. The lesion is poorly defined and shows endoneurial and perineurial fibrosis of nerve bundles in which there is also oedema, loss of myelinated fibres, and occasionally mucinous change (a). In addition, the surrounding connective tissue shows variable oedema, fibrosis, hyalinization and mucinous degeneration, bursa formation (b), and thickening of blood vessel walls. Repeated minor trauma, possibly related to the wearing of high-heeled or poorly fitting shoes, is thought to be important in the pathogenesis. Local recurrence following excision does not occur.

Figure 8.75

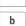

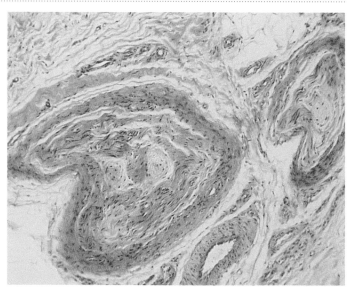

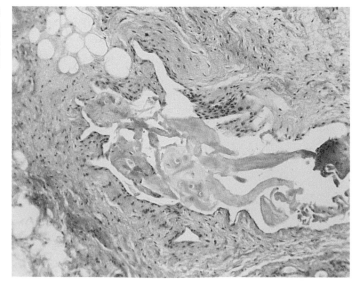

Figure 8.76 **Neurilemmoma (benign schwannoma)** This is a benign periph-eral nerve sheath tumour which usually presents in adult life as a slow-growing swelling in the head and neck region, extremities, mediastinum, or retroperi-toneum. Grossly (a) the lesion is encapsulated, round or fusiform, and usually arises eccentrically from a peripheral nerve. The tumour contains variable amounts of compact cellular Antoni A areas and less cellular Antoni B areas (b). In Antoni A areas spindle cells show nuclear palisading with parallel rows of nuclei and intervening cell processes (Verocay bodies) (c).8.76d shows large-ly an Antoni B area with part of an Antoni A area at one edge. It contains scat-tered spindle-shaped cells with elongated or wavy nuclei lying in a fibrous and mucinous stroma. Foci of xanthoma cells with prominent dilated vessels may also be seen. Schwann cells in neurilemmomas strongly express S-100 protein. Neurilemmomas rarely recur after local excision; malignant change has very rarely been reported.

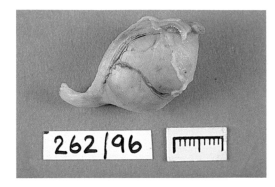

Figure 8.76

a

b c d

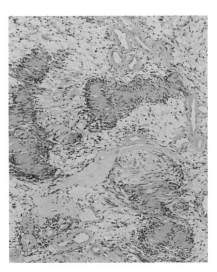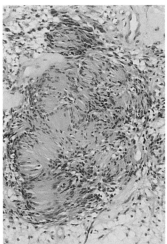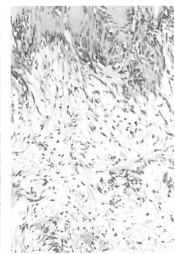

Figure 8.77 **Ancient (degenerate) neurilemmoma** Degener-ative change in a neurilemmoma results in increased prom-inence of Antoni B relative to Antoni A areas. Antoni B areas show hyaline or mucinous degenerative change. There is prominent vascular dilatation or thrombosis (a). Schwann cells show prominent nuclear pleomorphism, hyperchromasia, and occasional multinucleated forms with cytoplasmic vacuolation (b). Mitoses are not usually seen. This lesion is benign and should not be confused histologically with a pleomorphic sarcoma.

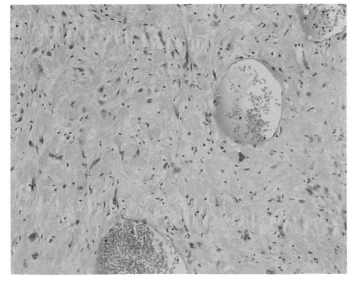

Figure 8.77

a

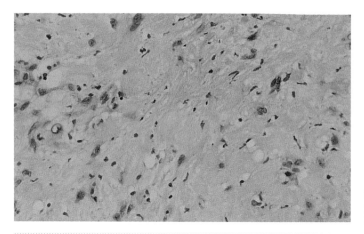

Figure 8.77 continued

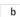

Figure 8.78 Neurofibroma This is a benign peripheral nerve sheath tumour which is usually localized and solitary. It may be multiple in up to 10 per cent of patients of whom a significant proportion have neurofibromatosis (NF-1). Solitary localized neurofibroma usually arises in the superficial soft tissues of young or middle-aged adults. Solitary neurofibromas may also be found in deep soft tissue in relation to a peripheral nerve. The lesion is poorly defined and composed of a proliferation of Schwann cells and fibroblasts (a). There are fascicles and whorls of spindle-shaped cells with indistinct cytoplasm and wavy, serpentine nuclei (b). These lie in a variably collagenous stroma, which may occasionally show hyaline or myxoid change. There is variable expression of S-100 protein in these tumours. Localized solitary neurofibroma rarely recurs or undergoes malignant change. Malignant change is more commonly seen in those patients with NF-1 or in lesions which are located in deep soft tissue.

Figure 8.78

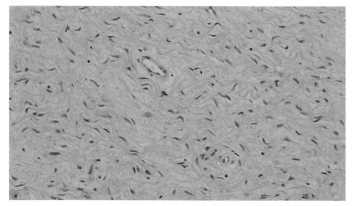

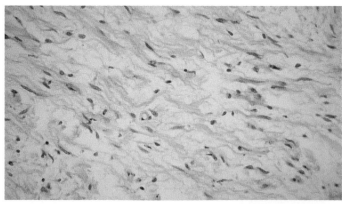

Figure 8.79 Diffuse neurofibroma This uncommon variant of neurofibroma produces a poorly defined, often large swelling in the superficial soft tissues of children and young adults. It occurs most commonly in the trunk or head and neck region. There is a strong association with neurofibromatosis. The dermis and subcutaneous tissue show extensive infiltration of neurofibromatous tissue with proliferation of Schwann cells, fibroblasts, and collagen formation (a). Focally, structures resembling Wagner–Meissner corpuscles are seen (b). There may also be enlargement of nerve trunks.

Figure 8.79

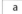

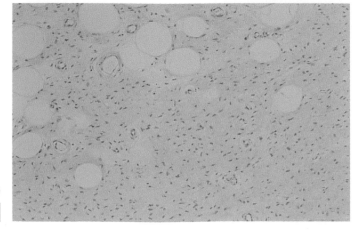

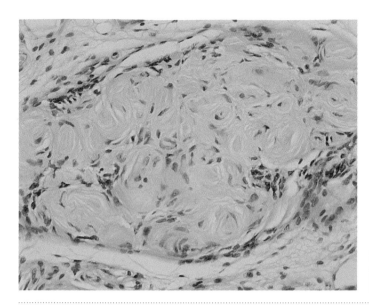

Figure 8.79 continued

b

Figure 8.80 **Plexiform neurofibroma** This variant is seen in association with neurofibromatosis and may arise in superficial or deep soft tissues. If large it causes body disfigurement (elephantiasis). It is characterized by extensive proliferation of Schwann cells and fibroblasts predominantly within the confines of the nerve trunk, but this proliferation may also sometimes extend into the surrounding epineurial tissues. This results in the formation of large discrete nodules of neurofibromatous tissue within the enlarged nerve bundles (a, b). These lesions have a small risk of undergoing malignant change.

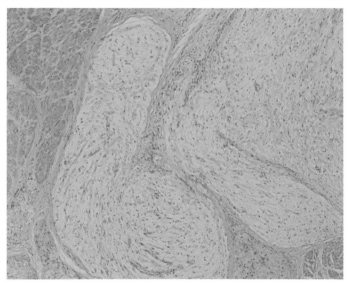

Figure 8.80

a

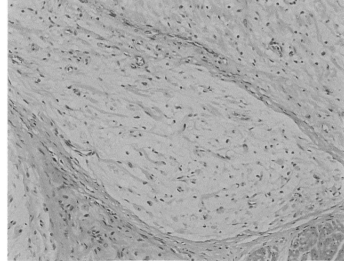

b

Figure 8.81 Neurothekeoma (nerve sheath myxoma) This uncommon benign tumour of peripheral nerves occurs most commonly in the head and neck region, upper limb, and upper trunk of children and young adults, chiefly females. The lesion is poorly defined, multilobulated, and lies within the dermis or subcutaneous tissue. It may be associated with a nerve trunk or neurofibroma. Fibrous bands divide the tumour into lobules composed of stellate or spindle-shaped cells lying in an abundant myxoid matrix (a, b). There is little or no nuclear pleomorphism or mitotic activity. The lesion rarely recurs.

Figure 8.81

a b

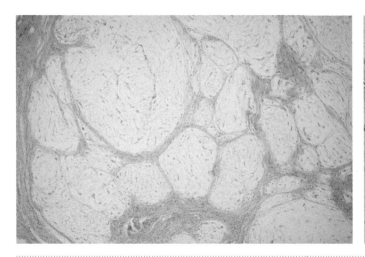 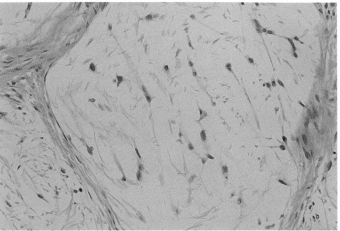

Figure 8.82 Granular cell tumour This tumour was formerly termed granular cell myoblastoma but is now known to be of nerve sheath rather than myoblast origin. It is a relatively common benign tumour of young or middle-aged adults, predominantly females. It presents as a painless, solitary nodule in the dermis or subcutaneous tissue of the extremities and trunk, but may also arise in the tongue and other sites. The lesion is poorly defined and composed of sheets, nests, or cords of large round or polygonal cells with a well defined cell membrane, abundant granular eosinophilic cytoplasm, and small round nucleus (a). The cytoplasm is PAS positive (diastase-resistant) (b). Cells are also positive for S-100 protein. Most granular cell tumours are benign. Malignant granular cell tumours are very rare and may show features identical to those of benign granular cell tumours. Some, however, show more evidence of cellular and nuclear pleomorphism and occasional mitotic activity (c).

Figure 8.82

a b c

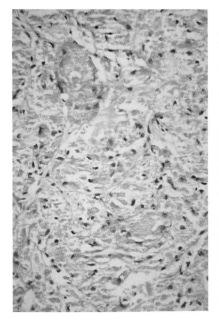 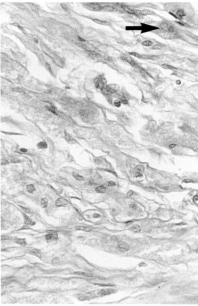 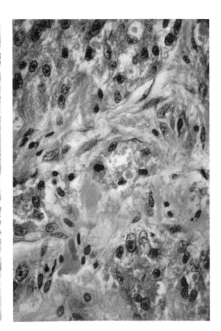

Figure 8.83 **Malignant peripheral nerve sheath tumour (MPNST; malignant schwannoma; neurofibrosarcoma)** This is a relatively uncommon soft tissue sarcoma which most frequently arises in patients with neurofibromatosis. It usually presents as a deep soft-tissue mass in the proximal extremities or trunk of middle-aged or older adults. Malignant change occurs at a younger age and is seen more commonly in males with neurofibromatosis. The tumour often shows rapid enlargement and may be painful. Grossly, the tumour often appears well defined, has a fleshy cut surface, and lies in relation to a major peripheral nerve.

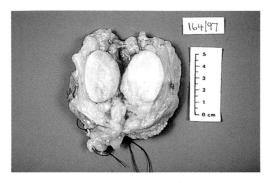

Figure 8.83

Figure 8.84 **Malignant peripheral nerve sheath tumour** Histological appearances are highly variable but generally show densely cellular fascicles composed of spindle-shaped tumour cells with poorly defined cytoplasm and wavy nuclei (a, b). There may be a suggestion of nuclear palisading and nuclear pleomorphism; hyperchromatic figures may be prominent (c). Other areas may show more uniform spindle-shaped cells with elongated cigar-shaped nuclei (d). Mitotic activity (arrow) is often prominent. Some tumours show a nodular or whorled arrangement of spindle cells suggestive of rudimentary tactoid structures (e). Tumour cells are S-100 positive in most cases (f). MPNST is a tumour of poor prognosis; it commonly recurs and produces metastases.

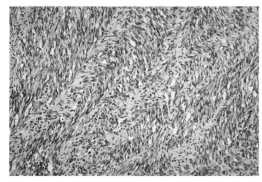

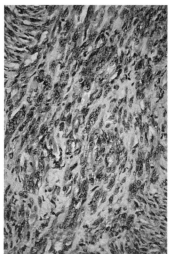
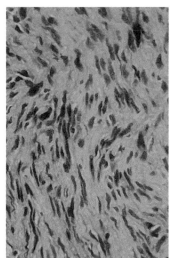
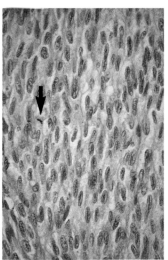
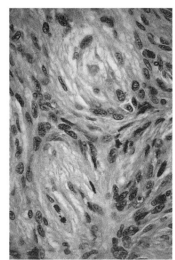

Figure 8.84

	a	
b	c	d	e
	f	

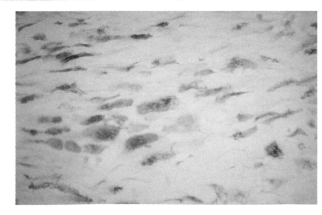

Figure 8.85 **Epithelioid malignant peripheral nerve sheath tumour** This variant of MPNST contains cords or nests of epithelioid tumour cells which may be closely packed or lie in a loose, partly mucinous connective tissue stroma (a, b). These tumours need to be distinguished from melanoma and carcinoma. In other variants of MPNST, heterologous elements such as cartilage, bone, epithelial, or skeletal muscle elements are seen; the latter is termed a malignant Triton tumour and is seen mainly in neurofibromatosis.

Figure 8.85

| a | b |

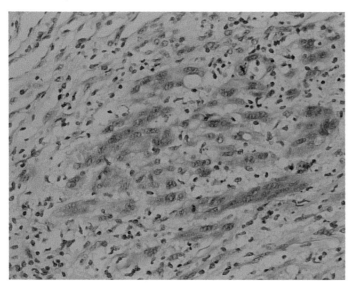
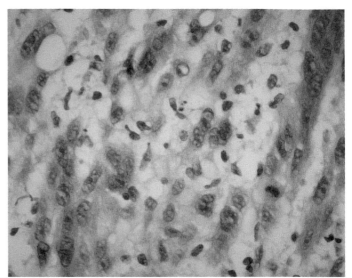

Figure 8.86 **Primitive neuroectodermal tumour (PNET; peripheral neuroepithelioma)** This rare tumour is due to a proliferation of cells of neuroectodermal origin, specifically cells which have migrated from the neural crest. PNET usually presents as a rapidly enlarging, painful mass in the limbs, trunk, or chest wall (Askin tumour) of adolescents and young adults. The tumour may arise in association with a major peripheral nerve trunk. It is composed of sheets, nodules, or nests of cells with scanty indistinct cytoplasm and round or oval hyperchromatic nuclei (a, b). Mitotic activity is frequent. Homer–Wright rosette formation is seen with tumour cells arranged around a central area of neurofibrillary material (c). Like Ewing's sarcoma, which may also arise primarily in soft tissues (see 8.108), tumour cells contain glycogen, express the *MIC-2* gene product and exhibit the reciprocal translocation of chromosomes 11 and 22; stromal reticulin is also not prominent. Unlike Ewing's sarcoma, however, PNET usually shows expression of neural markers such as neurone-specific enolase (NSE). PNET is distinguished from neuroblastoma by its occurrence in an older patient population, the absence of increased urinary catecholamines, and absence of the characteristic 1p deletion seen in most neuroblastomas. PNET is highly aggressive and produces early and widespread metastases.

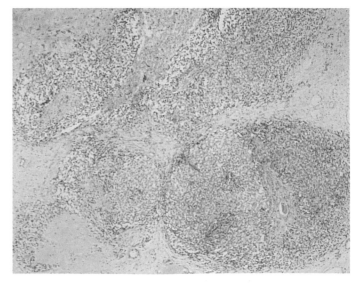

Figure 8.86

| a |

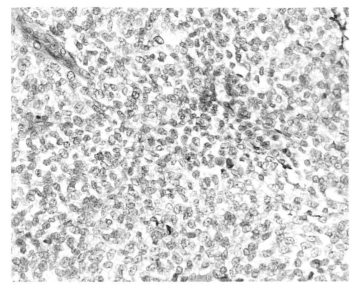

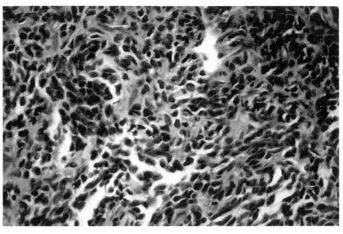

Figure 8.86 continued

b   c

Figure 8.87 **Ganglioneuroma** This is a rare benign tumour of neural elements of the sympathetic nervous system. It most commonly arises in adolescents and young adults and usually presents as a posterior mediastinal or retroperitoneal mass. It is composed of a neurofibroma-like proliferation of Schwann cells and fibroblasts amongst which are found scattered mature ganglion cells with abundant eosinophilic cytoplasm and one or more small round nuclei (a, b). The lesion is usually encapsulated, well defined, and does not undergo malignant change.

Figure 8.87

a

b

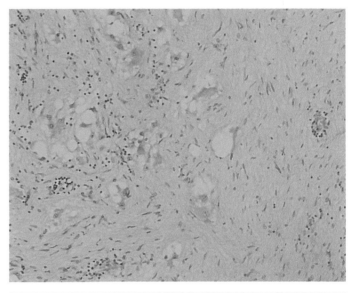

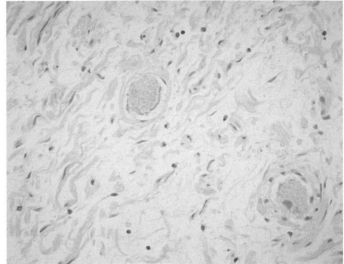

Figure 8.88 **Neuroblastoma and ganglioneuroblastoma**
Neuroblastoma is the least differentiated of the tumours of the sympathetic nervous system. It is a rare tumour but is the third most common solid malignancy of childhood. It mainly presents in the first year of life and is uncommon after the first decade. It arises most commonly in the adrenal medulla and the sympathetic ganglia of the retroperitoneum, mediastinum, and head and neck region; tumours may present as metastases in skin, soft tissue, or bone (see 7.39). Most cases exhibit elevated urinary or serum levels of catecholamine metabolites. Neuroblastomas are composed of a lobular or sheet-like proliferation of small round cells with round or oval nuclei and scanty, ill-defined cytoplasm (a, b). There is rosette formation in better differentiated tumours. Focal areas of maturation of neuroblasts to ganglion cells may be seen in some tumours. Where this is not prominent (i.e. less than 5 per cent of tumour cells) the tumour is termed a ganglioneuroblastoma (c, d). Neuroblastoma cells are positive for neural markers such as NSE, neurofilaments, and Leu-7; S-100 protein is not normally expressed. Neuroblastomas, unlike PNET and Ewing's sarcoma, are negative for the *MIC-2* gene product. Approximately 20 per cent of neuroblastomas are associated with a germline mutation which is transmitted autosomal dominant. The most consistent cytogenetic abnormality is a partial deletion of the short arm of chromosome 1. These tumours also show amplification of the N-*myc* oncogene. Neuroblastomas are highly aggressive tumours which develop early and show widespread metastases. Ganglioneuroblastoma runs a less aggressive course.

Figure 8.88

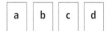

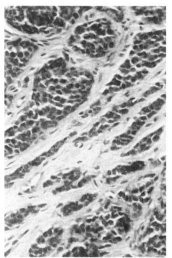 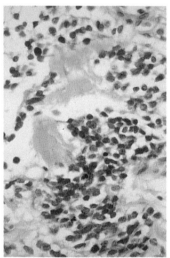 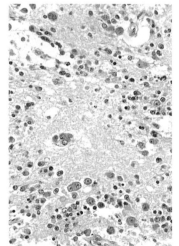 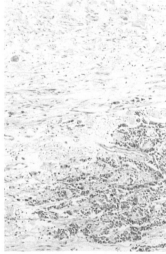

Figure 8.89 **Pigmented neuroectodermal tumour of infancy (retinal anlage tumour)**
This very rare tumour typically presents in the upper or lower jaw as a destructive radiolucent lesion but may also develop in the soft tissues of the head and neck and very rarely elsewhere. It usually arises in infancy. It consists of cords or clusters of small round tumour cells with scanty cytoplasm and round neuroblast-like nuclei (a, b); these tumour cells are mixed with pigmented (melanin-containing) cells. A pseudoglandular pattern may be present and the cells often

Figure 8.89

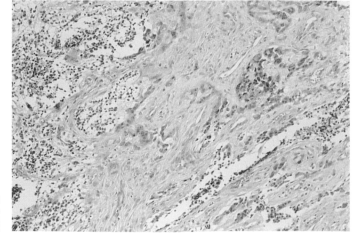

line distinct spaces. Tumour cells lie within a dense fibrous stroma. Most cases are benign but local recurrence is seen in up to 15 per cent of cases. Metastasis may rarely occur.

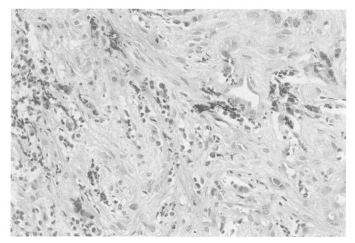

Figure 8.89

b

Figure 8.90 **Paraganglioma** Paragangliomas are very rare tumours that arise in paraganglia, small collections of neuroendocrine cells of neural crest origin that are found throughout the body in association with sympathetic and parasympathetic nervous system structures. Outside the adrenal medulla, these structures include the chemoreceptors of the carotid and aortic bodies, the vagal body, and mediastinal, retroperitoneal, intra-abdominal, and other ganglia. Clinical and histological features vary depending upon the origin of the tumour. The carotid body is the most common site of origin of an extra-adrenal paraganglioma. The tumour is usually small and arises at the bifurcation of the common carotid artery. It is composed of nests (*zellballen*) of plump, pale-staining cells which are surrounded by fibrous tissue (a, b). There is a rich sinusoidal vascular network within the fibrous trabeculae. There is a variable degree of cellular and nuclear pleomorphism and there may be occasional mitotic activity. Most paragangliomas are non-functioning tumours but functioning paragangliomas, particularly those arising in the retroperitoneum, may show more cellular pleomorphism and features somewhat resembling those of an adrenal phaeochromocytoma (c). Most paragangliomas are chromaffin negative; tumour cells are usually argyrophil or argentaffin positive and stain positively for S-100 protein, NSE, and chromogranin. Histological distinction between benign and malignant paragangliomas is not usually possible. Most paragangliomas arising in the branchiomeric paraganglion of the head and neck and upper mediastinum are benign tumours which may recur locally if incompletely excised. Intra-abdominal and retroperitoneal paragangliomas show the highest incidence of malignancy. Metastases may not appear until many years after the diagnosis.

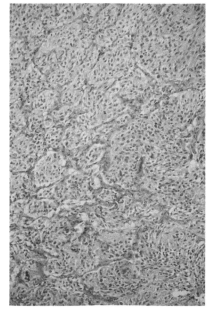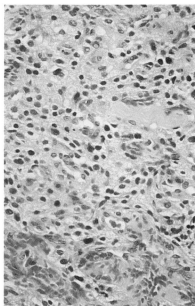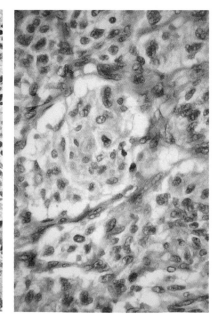

Figure 8.90

a b c

Figure 8.91 **Extracranial meningioma**
Meningiomas may very rarely be found in the soft tissues of the scalp, head and neck region, or along the vertebral axis. They mostly arise from ectopic arachnoid cells in the skin of children or young adults, or less frequently in deeper soft tissue with secondary involvement of skin. They consist of collections of meningiothelial cells which may contain psammoma bodies (arrow).

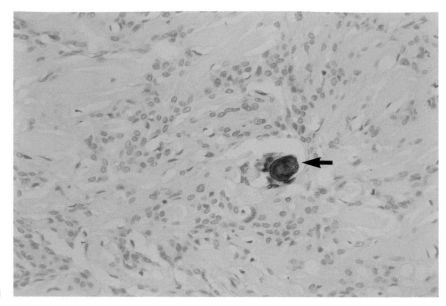

Figure 8.91

Figure 8.92 **Ectopic ependymoma and glioma** Ectopic ependymomas may uncommonly be found in the subcutaneous tissue of the sacrococcygeal area. They most probably arise from neural tube remnants and may be seen in association with spina bifida. Lesions are usually encapsulated and are papillary with fibrovascular cores and cuboidal or columnar lining cells (a). Lesions are often partly cystic. Metastasis has been reported in a number of these rare cases. Ectopic glial tissue ('glioma') may be found in skin and subcutaneous tissue most commonly in the bridge of the nose of infants, but rarely other sites. 8.92b shows glial tissue lying within the respiratory submucosa.

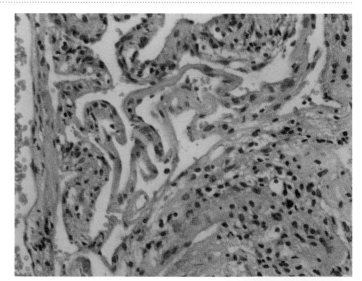

Figure 8.92

 a

b

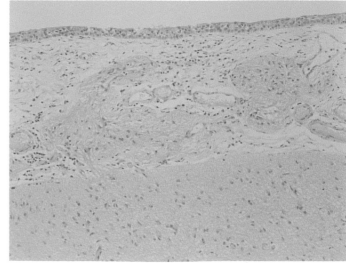

Figure 8.93 **Clear cell sarcoma (malignant melanoma of soft parts)** This uncommon malignant tumour, now known to be of neuroectodermal origin, arises chiefly in relation to tendons or aponeuroses of young adults, predominantly females. The tumour is slow-growing and located in the distal extremities, especially the foot and ankle. It is composed of nests or fascicles of closely packed round or polygonal tumour cells with clear (glycogen-containing) cytoplasm (a). Reticulin staining accentuates the nest-like arrangement of the tumour cells (b). Nuclei of tumours are rounded, vesicular, and contain prominent nucleoli (c). Melanin is usually demonstrable with special stains. Tumour cells express neural markers including NSE, S-100 protein, Leu-7, and melanoma-associated antigen.

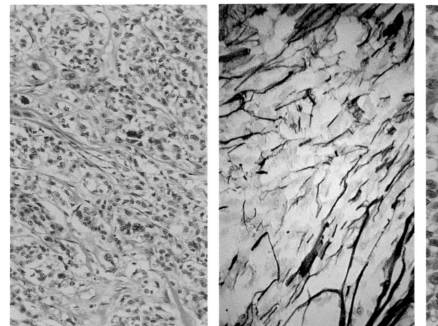

Figure 8.93

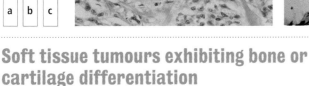

a | b | c

Soft tissue tumours exhibiting bone or cartilage differentiation

Figure 8.94 **Soft tissue chondroma** This uncommon benign tumour usually presents in adults as a solitary, slowly enlarging swelling of the distal extremities, particularly the fingers. The tumour is often closely associated with a nearby tendon sheath or a joint capsule. Radiologically, the lesion lies outside the bone and often contains focal areas of calcification. It is composed of lobules of hyaline cartilage showing variable cellularity (a); occasional binucleated cells (arrow) may be seen (b); calcification may be seen in areas of matrix degeneration. A heavy infiltrate of macrophages and giant cells in a pattern somewhat reminiscent of a giant cell tumour of tendon sheath may be present (c). These tumours rarely recur after excision and do not appear to undergo malignant change. They should be distinguished from synovial chondromatosis and cartilage tumours and tumour-like lesions that may arise in the digits.

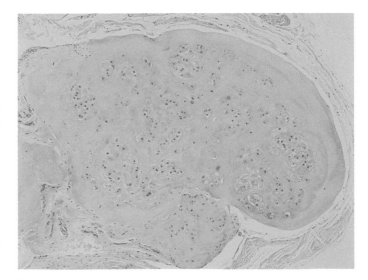

Figure 8.94

a

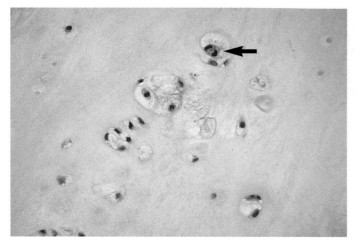

Figure 8.94 continued

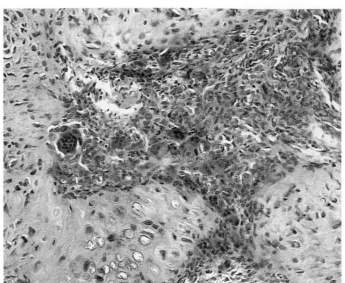

Figure 8.95 **Extraskeletal myxoid chondrosarcoma (chordoid sarcoma)** This rare sarcoma arises in the deep soft tissues of the extremities of adults. It is more common in males. It is a slow-growing lesion which usually has a fibrous capsule and is divided into lobules by fibrous septa. The lobules contain abundant hyaluronidase-resistant mucinous matrix in which there are nests and cords of small, round or polygonal tumour cells with indistinct, glycogen-containing cytoplasm and hyperchromatic nuclei (a, b). There is variable mitotic activity. Tumour cells are usually positive for vimentin and S-100 protein. A non-random reciprocal translocation between chromosomes 9 and 22 has been noted. This is a low-grade sarcoma which frequently recurs and eventually metastasizes if not adequately treated.

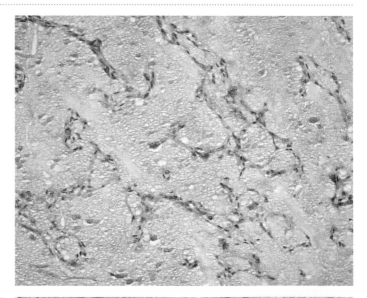

Figure 8.95

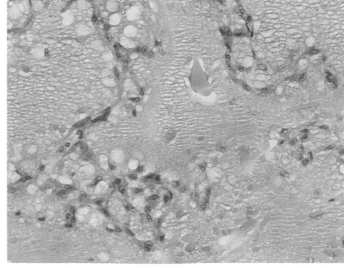

Figure 8.96 Extraskeletal mesenchymal chondrosarcoma This tumour arises more commonly in bone but may also originate in soft tissues, especially of the head and neck region and lower extremities (most commonly the thigh). As in bone, it arises predominantly in adolescents and young adults, and is composed of sheets or cords of round or spindle-shaped tumour cells amongst which are scattered nodules of usually low-grade malignant tumour cartilage (arrow). A prominent haemangiopericytoma-like vascular pattern is usually present. This tumour often grows rapidly, frequently recurs, and metastasizes.

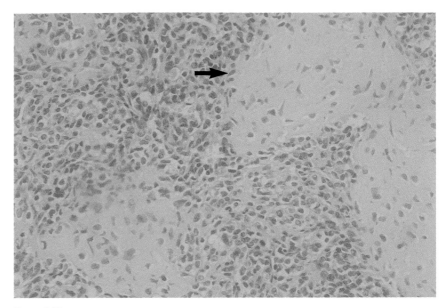

Figure 8.96

Figure 8.97 Extraskeletal osteosarcoma Osteosarcoma rarely arises outside the bone or periosteum. Unlike osteosarcomas of bone origin, soft tissue osteosarcoma arises chiefly in middle-aged and elderly adults; it is more common in males than females. Some cases are associated with previous irradiation. Most lesions are identical to those arising in bone and are characterized by the presence of malignant tumour cells forming osteoid or bone (a). A variable number of osteoclast-like giant cells may be noted (b). These tumours are highly aggressive and often metastasize early. Some forms of giant-cell-rich MFH arising in deep soft tissues show prominent bone or osteoid formation by tumour cells of malignant appearance and are considered by some observers to represent a giant-cell-rich variant of soft tissue osteosarcoma.

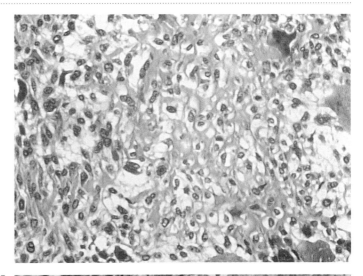

Figure 8.97

a

b

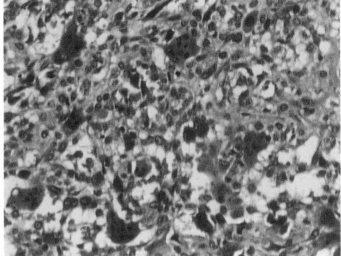

Figure 8.98 **Malignant mesenchymoma** A mesenchymoma is a tumour containing two or more neoplastic mesenchymal components. Many benign mesenchymomas are thought to be hamartomas or developmental abnormalities or to represent areas of metaplasia within a particular soft tissue tumour (e.g. chondroid or osseous metaplasia in a lipoma). A malignant mesenchymoma is generally defined as a tumour showing two or more distinct, unrelated sarcoma elements; by convention, fibrosarcoma, malignant fibrous histiocytoma, and haemangiopericytoma are excluded. These tumours are very rare and usually arise in older patients, most commonly in the deep soft tissue of the thigh or the retroperitoneum. Not uncommonly there is a combination of poorly differentiated liposarcoma (a) and another sarcoma such as osteosarcoma (b). The prognosis depends on the nature and grade of the constituent mesenchymal tumours.

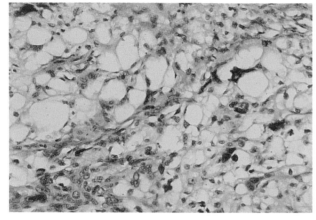
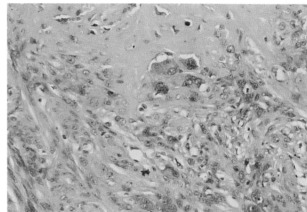

Figure 8.98

a b

Benign soft tissue tumours of uncertain origin

Figure 8.99 **Tumoral calcinosis** This uncommon condition is characterized by the formation of large, painless calcified nodules in periarticular soft tissues, especially along extensor surfaces. The hip, shoulder, and elbow are most commonly affected and the knee, hands, and feet usually spared. Lesions are often multiple and usually present in the first two decades of life. Tumoral calcinosis is more common in blacks than whites. It is often familial and inherited autosomal dominant or recessive. Serum calcium is usually normal but many patients show hyperphosphataemia and some have elevated 1,25-dihydroxyvitamin D_3 levels. Radiographs show a large, dense radio-opaque mass in soft tissue (a). Grossly, these are composed of nodules of hard, white material within subcutaneous tissue (b). Histologically there are large deposits of amorphous calcified material surrounded by dense collagenous connective tissue (c). In active lesions, calcified areas are surrounded by numerous osteoclasts and macrophages (d). Most lesions are asymptomatic but larger lesions may lead to skin ulceration. In chronic renal failure morphologically similar lesions may be seen in soft tissue when there is metastatic calcification.

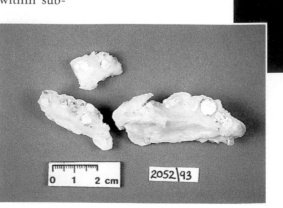

Figure 8.99

a

b

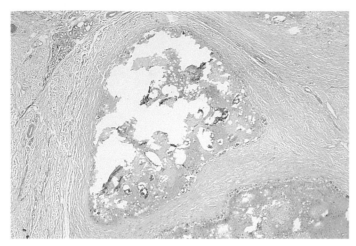

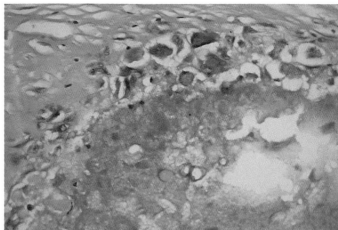

Figure 8.99 continued

c   d

Figure 8.100 Intramuscular myxoma A myxoma is a benign lesion which may arise within muscle (intramuscular), skin (cutaneous), or around joints (juxta-articular). Intramuscular myxoma usually presents in middle-aged or elderly adults, predominantly females, as a slow-growing painless swelling within large muscles of the thigh, shoulder, and buttocks. The tumour has a glairy, mucoid cut surface (a). Most intramuscular myxomas are solitary; multiple lesions may be associated with fibrous dysplasia. Myxomatous tissue surrounds small groups of atrophic muscle fibres and extends between individual muscle cells, particularly at the edges of the tumour (b). The lesion is hypocellular and contains scattered stellate or spindle-shaped cells lying in an abundant hyaluronidase acid-rich mucopolysaccharide matrix in which few or no blood vessels are evident (c). Lesions are benign and rarely recur after excision.

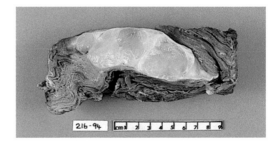

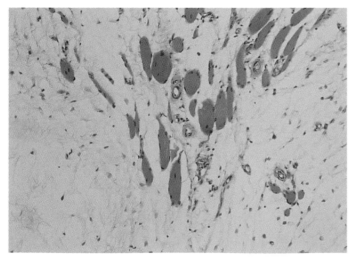

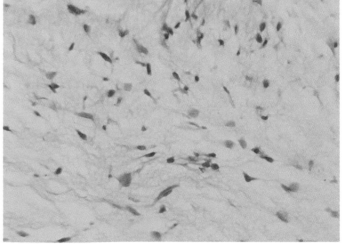

Figure 8.100

a

b   c

Figure 8.101 **Ossifying fibromyxoid tumour of soft tissue**
This very rare soft tissue tumour usually presents as a small, painless lesion in the deep subcutaneous tissue of the upper and lower extremities of adults. The lesion is surrounded by fibrous tissue containing focal areas of metaplastic woven bone formation (arrow) (a, b) and consists of cords of uniform cells with polygonal nuclei and indistinct cytoplasm. Cells lie within a fibromyxoid or collagenous fibrous tissue matrix. Cells are usually positive for S-100 and vimentin. Most tumours are benign but local recurrence occurs in one third of cases and metastasis has rarely been reported.

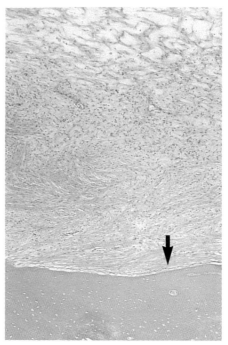

Figure 8.101

a

b

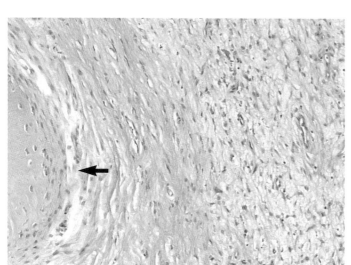

Malignant soft tissue tumours of uncertain origin

Figure 8.102 **Synovial sarcoma** Despite its designation this tumour does not arise from synovial cells and rarely involves the joint. It is a relatively common soft tissue sarcoma. It usually presents as a painful or non-tender deep soft-tissue mass arising in the extremities often near a large joint, most commonly the knee. It also uncommonly arises in the head and neck region, chest, and abdomen. It occurs predominantly in adolescents and young adults and is more common in males. Tumours are often large, multilobular, and show cystic degeneration (a). Focal areas of calcification (arrow) may be seen within the tumour radiologically (b). Synovial sarcoma is thought to arise from a multipotential mesenchymal stem cell which is capable not only of mesenchymal but also epithelial differentiation. Synovial sarcoma commonly recurs and produces metastases via lymphatic and vascular spread. These tumours commonly have a translocation between chromosomes X and 18.

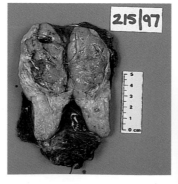
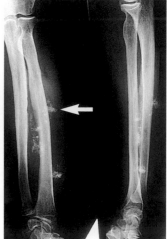

Figure 8.102

a b

Figure 8.103 **Biphasic synovial sarcoma** This tumour contains a proliferation of spindle-shaped tumour cells as well as scattered epithelial elements, usually small glands (a, b) or nests or cords of epithelial cells (c). Proliferating spindle cells are arranged in sheets or broad fascicles and are generally plump and have round or oval vesicular nuclei and indistinct cytoplasm. Mitoses are seen in both the epithelial and spindle cell components. A rare monophasic epithelial synovial sarcoma has also been described.

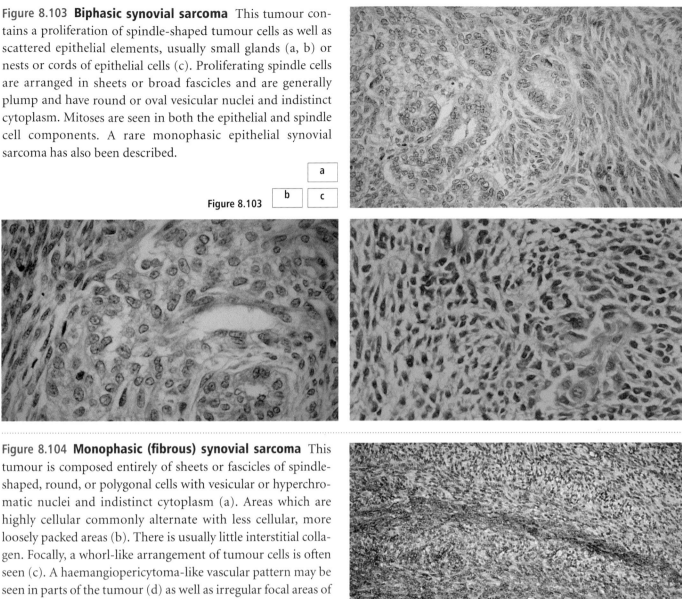

Figure 8.103 | a | b | c |

Figure 8.104 **Monophasic (fibrous) synovial sarcoma** This tumour is composed entirely of sheets or fascicles of spindle-shaped, round, or polygonal cells with vesicular or hyperchromatic nuclei and indistinct cytoplasm (a). Areas which are highly cellular commonly alternate with less cellular, more loosely packed areas (b). There is usually little interstitial collagen. Focally, a whorl-like arrangement of tumour cells is often seen (c). A haemangiopericytoma-like vascular pattern may be seen in parts of the tumour (d) as well as irregular focal areas of calcification (arrow) (e). Scattered spindle cells positive for cytokeratin and other epithelial markers are present (f).

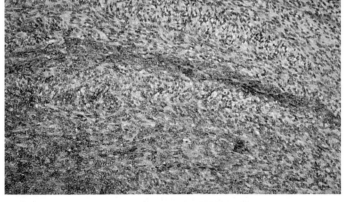

Figure 8.104 | a | b | c |

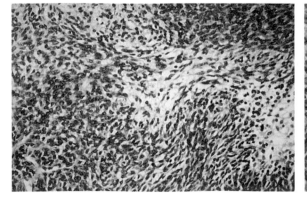

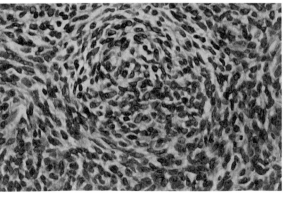

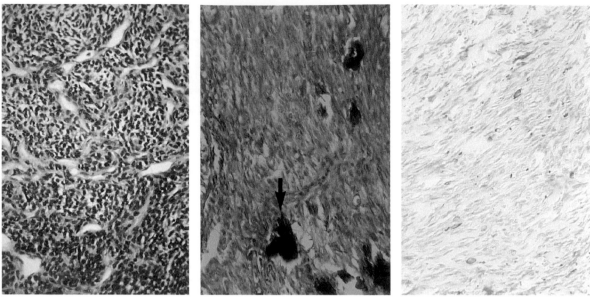

Figure 8.104 continued

d e f

Figure 8.105 **Alveolar soft part sarcoma** This is an uncommon malignant soft tissue tumour which is now thought to be of muscle origin. It mainly arises in adolescents and young adults, usually in the deep soft tissues of the lower limbs. The head and neck regions, particularly the orbit and tongue, are often affected in children. The tumour is painless, large, and slow-growing. It is composed of large round or polygonal cells with granular eosinophilic or sometimes clear cytoplasm and uniform, large vesicular or hyperchromatic nuclei (a, b). Separation of the cells centrally gives these nests a pseudo-alveolar pattern. These cells are arranged in small nests, giving the lesion a prominent organoid growth pattern. The nests are clearly outlined by reticulin stains (c). Prominent fibrous septa traverse the tumour. Tumour cells contain PAS-positive (diastase-resistant) granules or crystals (arrow) (d). Tumour cells express desmin, muscle-specific actin, and the MyoD1 protein. The tumour commonly recurs and frequently metastasizes.

Figure 8.105

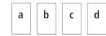

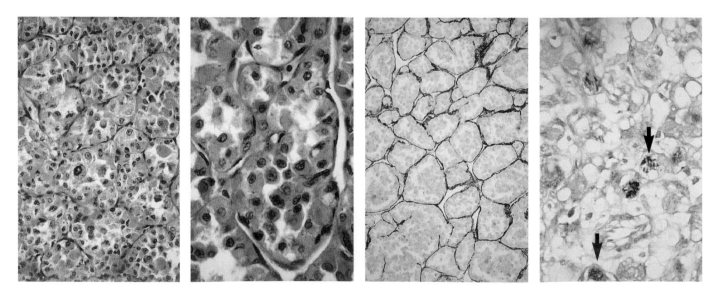

Figure 8.106 Epithelioid sarcoma This rare malignant soft tissue sarcoma usually arises in the dermal or subcutaneous tissue of the distal extremities of young adults. Tumours are usually multinodular. The nodules are separated by fibrous tissue and may exhibit central necrosis or degeneration (a). The nodules are composed of masses of large polygonal cells with abundant eosinophilic cytoplasm and large vesicular or hyperchromatic nuclei which show pleomorphism and occasional mitotic activity (b, c). Positive staining for vimentin and cytokeratin is usually observed. The lesion commonly recurs and eventually metastasizes in most cases.

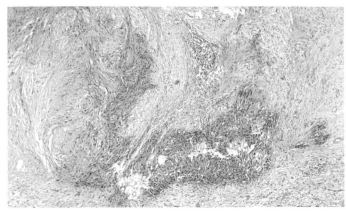

Figure 8.106

a

b | c

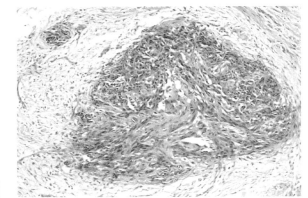

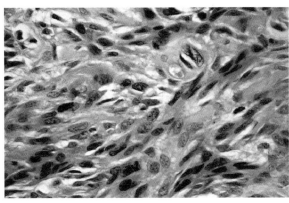

Figure 8.107 Desmoplastic small cell tumour of childhood This rare malignant soft tissue tumour usually presents as a well-defined tumour in the abdomen and pelvis of adolescents and young adults. It is composed of small and large collections of tumour cells which are surrounded by a cellular fibrous stroma (a, b). Small nests of tumour cells may resemble tumour glands. The tumour cells are relatively uniform with scanty cytoplasm and vesicular or hyperchromatic nuclei which show increased mitotic activity (arrow) (c). Tumour cells are positive for cytokeratin, epithelial membrane antigen, desmin, and NSE. These tumours exhibit a reciprocal translocation involving chromosomes 11 and 22, suggesting a relationship with PNET and Ewing's sarcoma. This tumour behaves aggressively, producing early and widespread metastases.

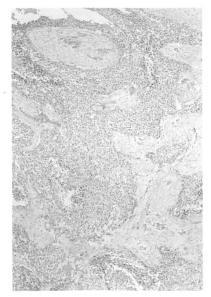

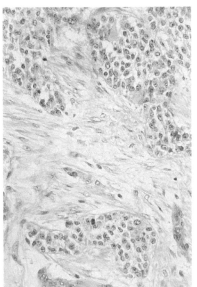

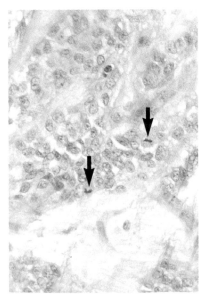

Figure 8.107

a | b | c

Figure 8.108 Extraskeletal Ewing's sarcoma
This is a rare tumour which has many clinical, pathological, and cytogenetic characteristics in common with PNET. It consists of closely packed cells with round or ovoid vesicular nucleus and scanty cytoplasm (a). Tumour cells are arranged in sheets or lobules. Reticulin is scanty or absent between individual tumour cells (b). Tumour cells contain glycogen and are positive for the *MIC-2* gene product. Mitotic activity is variable. Ewing's sarcoma is distinguished from PNET by the absence or relative paucity of rosette formation and lack of expression of NSE and other neural markers. This tumour needs to be distinguished from other round cell tumours that can arise in soft tissue (e.g. embryonal rhabdomyosarcoma, neuroblastoma, malignant lymphoma).

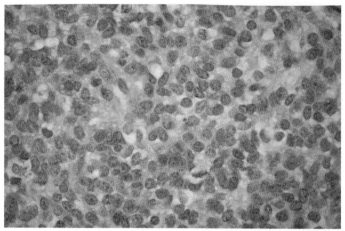

Figure 8.108

a

b

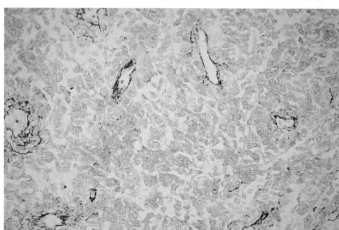

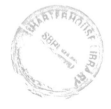

Bibliography

Chapter 1: Normal skeletal structure and development

Athanasou, N. A. (1996). Cellular biology of bone-resorbing cells. *Journal of Bone and Joint Surgery* **78A**, 1096–112.

Bilezikian, J. P., Raisz, L. A., and Rodan, G. A. (eds) (1996). *Principles of bone biology.* Academic Press, San Diego.

Brighton, C. T., Frielander, G., and Lane, J. N. (eds) (1994). *Bone formation and repair.* AAOS, Rosemont IL.

Freeman, M. A. R. (ed.) (1979). *Adult articular cartilage.* Pitman, London.

Ham, A. W. and Cormack, D. H. (1979). *Histophysiology of cartilage, bone and joints.* J. B. Lippincott, Philadelphia.

Schmorl, G. and Junghanns, H. (1971). *The human spine in health and disease,* 2nd edn. Grune and Stratton, New York.

Chapter 2: Repair, necrosis, and reactive changes in skeletal tissues

Davidson, J. K. (ed.) (1976). *Aseptic necrosis of bone.* Excerpta Medica, Amsterdam.

Glimcher, M. J. and Kenzora, J. E. (1979). The biology of osteonecrosis of the human femoral head and its clinical implications III. Discussion of the aetiology and genesis of the pathological sequelae: comments on treatment. *Clinical Orthopaedics and Related Research* **140**, 273–312.

Rosen, V. and Scott Thies, R. (1995). *The cellular and molecular basis of bone formation and repair.* R. G. Landes, Austin.

Salisbury, J. R., Woods, C. G., and Byers, P. D. (eds) (1994). *Diseases of bone and joints: cell biology, mechanisms, pathology.* Chapman and Hall, London.

Sevitt, S. (1981). *Bone repair and fracture healing in man.* Churchill Livingstone, Edinburgh.

Chapter 3: Infections of bone and joint

Gillespie, W. F. and Nade, S. (1987). *Musculoskeletal infections.* Blackwell, Melbourne.

Green, N. E. and Edwards, K. (1987). Bone and joint infections in children. *Orthopaedic Clinics of North America* **18**, 555–76.

Gustilo, R. B., *et al.* (eds) (1989). *Orthopaedic infection: diagnosis and treatment.* W. B. Saunders, Philadelphia.

Jaureguile, L. E. (ed.) (1995). *Diagnosis and management of bone infections.* Marcel Dekker, New York.

Martini, M. (ed.) (1988). *Tuberculosis of the bones and joints.* Springer, Berlin.

Schlossberg, D. (1988). *Orthopaedic infection.* Springer, New York.

Chapter 4: Disorders of skeletal development

Beighton, P. (1988). *Inherited disorders of the skeleton.* Churchill Livingstone, Edinburgh.

Beighton, P., *et al.* (1992). International classification of the osteochondrodysplasias. *American Journal of Medical Genetics* **44**, 223–9.

Dietz, F. R. and Mathews, K. D. (1996). Update on the genetic basis of disorders with orthopaedic manifestations. *Journal of Bone and Joint Surgery* **78A**, 1583–98.

Kaplan, F. S. (ed.) (1997). Symposium: fibrodysplasia ossificans progressiva. *Clinical Orthopaedics and Related Research* **346**, 2–140.

Sillence, D. O., *et al.* (1979). Morphologic studies in the skeletal dysplasias. *American Journal of Pathology* **96**, 813–60.

Wynne-Davies, R., *et al.* (1985). *Atlas of skeletal dysplasias.* Churchill Livingstone, Edinburgh.

Chapter 5: Metabolic and endocrine disorders of the skeleton

Avioli, L. V. and Krane, S. M. (eds) (1998). *Metabolic bone disease and clinically related disorders.* W. B. Saunders, Philadelphia.

Erikson, E. S., Axelrod, D. W., and Melson, F. (1994). *Bone histomorphometry.* Raven Press, New York.

Favus, M. J. (ed.) (1993). *Primer on the metabolic bone diseases and disorders of mineral metabolism,* 3rd edn. Raven Press, New York.

Revell, P. A. (1986). *Pathology of bone.* Springer, Berlin.

Stevenson, J. C. (ed.) (1991). *New techniques in metabolic bone disease.* Wright, London.

Chapter 6: Diseases of joints and periarticular tissues

Eulderink, F. (1982). The synovial biopsy. In *Bone and joint disease* (ed. C. L. Berry), Current Topics in Pathology, Vol. 71, pp. 26–72.

Gardner, D. L. (1992). *Pathological basis of connective tissue diseases.* Edward Arnold, London.

Jaffe, H. L. (1972). *Metabolic, degenerative and inflammatory diseases of bones and joints.* Lea and Febiger, Philadelphia.

Koopman, W. F. (ed.) (1997). *Arthritis and allied conditions.* Lea and Febiger, Philadelphia.

Revell, P. A. (1982). Tissue reactions to joint prostheses and the products of wear and corrosion. In *Bone and joint disease* (ed. C. L. Berry), Current Topics in Pathology, Vol. 71, pp. 73–101.

Freemont, A. J. and Denton, J. (1991). *Atlas of synovial fluid cytopathology.* Kluwer, Dordrecht.

Chapter 7: Bone tumours and tumour-like lesions

Dorfman, H. D. and Czerniak, B. (1998). *Bone tumors.* Mosby, St Louis.

Fechner, R. E. and Mills, S. E. (1992). *Tumors of the bones and joints* (3rd series: Fascicle 8). Armed Forces Institute of Pathology, Washington, DC.

Huvos, A. G. (1991). *Bone tumors: diagnosis, treatment and prognosis.* W. B. Saunders, Philadelphia.

Jaffe, H. L. (1958). *Tumors and tumorous conditions of the bones and joints.* Lea and Febiger, Philadelphia.

Mirra, J. M. (1989). *Bone tumors: clinical, radiologic and pathologic correlations.* Lea and Febiger, Philadelphia.

Schajowicz, F. (ed.) (1993). *Histological typing of bone tumours: World Health Organization international histological classification of tumours,* 2nd edn. Springer, Berlin.

Schajowicz, F. (1995). *Tumors and tumor-like lesions of bone and joints,* 2nd edn. Springer, New York.

Unni, K. K. (1996). *Dahlin's bone tumors.* Raven Press, Philadelphia.

Chapter 8: Soft tissue tumours and tumour-like lesions

Coffin, C., Dener, L. P., and O'Shea, P. A. (1997). *Paediatric soft tissue tumors: a clinical, pathological and therapeutic approach.* Williams and Wilkins, Baltimore.

Dass Gupta, P. K. and Chaudhuri, P. K. (1998). *Tumors of the soft tissues.* Appleton Lange, Stamford.

Enzinger, F. M. and Weiss, S. W. (1995). *Soft tissue tumors,* 3rd edn. Mosby, St Louis.

Fletcher, C. D. M. (1991). Recent advances in the pathology of soft tissue tumours. *Diagnostic Oncology* 1, 5–11.

Ninfo, V., Chung, E. B., and Cavazzana, A. O. (eds) (1991). *Tumors and tumor-like lesions of soft tissue.* Churchill Livingstone, New York.

Weiss, S. W. (ed.) (1994). *Histological typing of soft tissue tumours.* World Health Organization international histological classification of tumours. Springer, Berlin.

Index

abscess
Brodie's 42
in pyogenic osteomyelitis 40
achondrogenesis 56
achondroplasia 54–5
acid-fast bacilli 46
acquired immune deficiency
syndrome 208
actin 197, 198, 228
Actinomyces israelii 48
actinomycosis 48
adamantinoma
age at presentation 116
intraosseous location 117
long bones 151
relationship with osteofibrous
dysplasia 159
adenoma, parathyroid 72
adipocytes 2
adolescent coxa vara 70
age
at presentation of bone tumours
and tumour-like lesions 116
at presentation of soft tissue
tumours 166
AIDS 208
alkaptonuria 95
alcoholism 24
alkaline phosphatase 72
deficiency 78
in FIO 84
in Paget's disease 83
Albright's syndrome 68
aluminium bone disease 79
amyloid arthropathy 95–6
amyloidosis 43
primary 95, 96, 162
secondary 162
amyloid tumour of bone 162
anaemia, leucoerythroblastic 63
angiofibroma, juvenile
(nasopharyngeal) 174
angioleiomyoma 196
angiolipoma 189
angiolymphoid hyperplasia with
eosinophilia 203
angiomatosis, skeletal 143
angiosarcoma
bone 145
soft tissue 166, 207–8
ankylosing hyperostosis 102, 107
ankylosing spondylitis 102
ankylosis in rheumatoid arthritis
100
antacid excess 79
appendicular skeleton 2

arthritis
infective 43
pyogenic 44–5
reactive 103
tuberculous 46
see also osteoarthritis; rheumatoid
arthritis
AS 102
Askin tumour 216
asphyxiating thoracic dwarfism 58
atypical decubital fibroplasia 172
autoimmune disorders, arthritis
associated 104–5
avulsion exostosis 31
axial skeleton 2

basic calcium phosphate crystal
deposition 94
Behçet's disease 104
β2–microglobulin amyloid 95,
162
bisphosphonates 84
bizarre parosteal
osteochondromatous proliferation
117, 160–1
blood dyscrasias 23, 96
BMU 11
bone
autografts 29
cancellous 2, 5, 11
cells 6–8
composition 2
cortex 2
cortical 2, 4, 11
creeping substitution 26, 29
development, see ossification
grafting / transplantation 29
gross structure 2
homografts 29
infarction 23, 24, 25, 26, 27, 116
lamellar 3, 4, 8
longitudinal growth 10
metastatic carcinoma 22
necrosis, see osteonecrosis
radiation effects 32
reaction to internal fixation
devices 29–30
remodelling 6, 11
structure 2–6
subperiosteal formation 28
trabeculae 5
tumours and tumour-like lesions
116–63
woven 3–4, 8, 9, 10, 20
bone island 118
bone lining cells 6–7

bone multicellular unit 11
bony spur 31
Borrelia burgdorferi 50
Brodie's abscess 42
brown tumour 74, 137
brucellosis 47
bursa 34
in rheumatoid arthritis 98
button phenomenon 81

Caisson disease 24, 27
calcific tendinitis 35, 94
calcium hydroxyapatite 2, 35
calcium oxalate 86
calcium pyrophosphate dihydrate
93–4, 95
calcospherites 158
callus
external 19, 20
internal 19, 20
primary 19, 20, 21
secondary 21
cambium 5
Camurati–Engelmann disease 64
carbon-reinforced polyethylene
implants 111
carotid body 219
carpal tunnel syndrome 35
cartilage 2, 10
abnormalities in skeletal dysplasias
54–9
articular 12–13
in haemophilia 96
in ochronosis 95
in osteoarthritis 89
in rheumatoid arthritis 99
traumatic injury 33
epiphyseal 13
formation following bone fracture
20
hyaline 12
tumours 127–35
cartilage oligomeric matrix protein
gene abnormalities 56, 57
CDH 70
cement lines 6, 11, 62
in Erdheim–Chester disease 157
in FIO 84
in osteogenesis imperfecta 62
Charcot joint 91
Chlamydia trachomatis 103
cholesterol clefts 182
chondroblastoma 130–1
age at presentation 116
intraosseous location 117
chondrocalcinosis 93, 106, 110

chondrocytes 10, 12, 20, 33
in bizarre parosteal
osteochondromatous
proliferation 160, 161
in osteochondroma 129, 130
in primary synovial
chondromatosis 113
chondroitin sulphate 12
chondrolysis 70
chondroma 221
periosteal (juxtacortical) 116,
128–9
chondromalacia patellae 91
chondrosarcoma 113, 132–3
age at presentation 116, 166
central 132
clear cell 134–5
age at presentation 116
intraosseous location 117
dedifferentiated 133
extraskeletal mesenchymal 223
extraskeletal myxoid 222
intraosseous location 117
juxtacortical (periosteal) 135
mesenchymal 134
age at presentation 116, 166
skeletal location 117
peripheral 132
secondary 132
skeletal location 117
chordoma 116, 117, 150–1
chondroid 150
chromatin 138, 142
chronic renal failure 74, 79, 86, 94,
224
cleft palate 57
cloacae 41
collagen 3, 5, 13, 15
type I 2, 60, 62
type II 12, 56, 57
type IV 197
type IX 57
type X 57
collagen diseases 94
COMP gene abnormalities 56, 57
congenital dislocation of the hip 70
continuous ambulatory peritoneal
dialysis 95
corticosteroid therapy 24, 44, 82
coxa vara, adolescent 70
CPPD 93–4, 95
cranial fasciitis 170
creeping substitution 26, 29
CREST syndrome 105
Crohn's disease 103
Cushing's disease 24, 82

cystic hygroma 209
cysts
    bone
        aneurysmal 116, 117, 153
        ganglion / juxta-articular
            154–5
        solitary / simple 116, 117, 152
    epidermal 117
    epidermoid inclusion 154
    hydatid 51
    meniscal 33
    subchondral 89, 154
cytokeratin 197, 229

degenerative joint disease, see
    osteoarthritis
densitometry 81
dentinogenesis imperfecta 60, 61,
    62
DeQuervain's disease 35
dermatan sulphate 65
dermatofibrosarcoma protuberans
    182
desmin 197, 198, 228
desmoid tumour 117, 177
desmoplastic small cell tumour of
    childhood 229
DFSP 182
diabetes mellitus 43, 44, 82
diaphyseal aclasis 59
diaphysis 2, 10
diffuse idiopathic skeletal
    hyperostosis 107
disappearing bone disease 144
discitis 43
DISH 107
drug misuse 38, 43
Dupuytren's disease / contracture
    175
dwarfism 66
dyschondroplasia, see
    enchondromatosis
dysplasia epiphysialis hemimelica 59

Echinococcus granulosus 51
elastofibroma 168
elephantiasis 213
enchondroma 58, 127–8
    age at presentation 116
    intraosseous location 117
    skeletal location 117
enchondromatosis (Ollier's disease)
    58, 128, 132
endosteum 5
enostosis 118
enthesopathy 102, 103
eosinophilia 105
eosinophilic fasciitis 105
ependymoma, ectopic 220
epiphysis 2, 9, 10
Erdheim–Chester disease 157
erythema chronicum migrans 50
Escherichia coli 38

Ewing's sarcoma 138–9, 216
    age at presentation 116
    atypical 138–9
    extraskeletal 230
    intraosseous location 117
    skeletal location 117

familial retinoblastoma 116
Fanconi's syndrome 78
fat, tumours of 188–95
FGFR3 gene abnormalities 54, 55
fibrin 34
fibrin bodies 98, 99
fibroblast growth factor receptor-3
    gene abnormalities 54, 55
fibroblastoma, giant cell 169
fibroblasts 15
fibrocartilage 12, 13, 15
fibrocartilaginous mesenchymoma
    159
fibrodysplasia ossificans progressiva
    67
fibrogenesis imperfecta ossium
    84–5
fibrohistiocytic tumours 179–87
fibrolipoma 188
    neural 191
fibroma
    calcifying (juvenile) aponeurotic
        169
    chondromyxoid 116, 117, 131
    desmoplastic 146–7
    non-ossifying 116, 117, 155
    ossifying 159
    tendon sheath 168
fibromatosis 175
    abdominal 177
    deep 175
    infantile 178
    infantile digital 174
    intra-abdominal 177
    mesenteric 177
    multicentric 176
    musculoaponeurotic (desmoid)
        176
    palmar 175
    plantar 176
    superficial 175
fibromatosis colli 178
fibro-osseous tumour of digits 160
fibrosarcoma
    bone 32, 116, 117, 147, 148
    infantile 179
    soft tissue 166, 179
fibrous cortical defect (non-ossifying
    fibroma) 116, 117, 155
fibrous dysplasia 116, 117, 151, 158
    polyostotic 68–9, 158
fibroxanthoma, atypical 182–3
fibula, stress fracture 22
FIO 84–5
floret cells 190
fluorosis 63, 85

FOP 67
foreign body synovitis 97
Forestier's disease 107
fracture
    fatigue / stress 18, 22
    healing 18
        early reparative changes 19
        initial response 18
        morphological changes 18
        primary callus 19, 20
        secondary callus 21
    histological features 18
    march 22
    non-union 21
    open / compound 18
    pathological 18, 22, 43
    pseudarthrosis 21
    simple / closed 18
    subchondral 24
Freiberg's disease 28

ganglion 34
    intraosseous 154–5
ganglioneuroblastoma 218
ganglioneuroma 217
Gardner's syndrome 118, 177
gargoylism 65
Gaucher's cells 66–7
Gaucher's disease 24, 27, 38, 66–7
genu valgum 66
giant cell arteritis 106
giant cell fibroblastoma 169
giant cell granuloma of small bones
    137
giant cell reparative granuloma
    117, 136–7
giant cell-rich malignant fibrous
    histiocytoma 186, 223
giant cell-rich osteosarcoma 123
giant cells 106
    aneurysmal bone cyst 153
    fibrocartilaginous
        mesenchymoma 159
    non-ossifying fibroma 155
    osteoclastic: differential diagnosis
        in bone tumours 136
    pleomorphic lipoma 190
    pleomorphic liposarcoma 195
    Touton 181
giant cell tumour 74
    bone 116, 117, 135–6
    tendon sheath 78, 112
glioma 220
glomangioma 205
glomus tumour 143, 205
glucocerebrosidase deficiency 66
glycogen 138
glycosaminoglycans 2, 12, 65
golfer's elbow 35
gonococcal infection 44
Gorham's disease 144
gout 34, 92–3
gouty tophi 92

Gram-negative bacilli 38, 43, 44
granular cell tumour 214
granulocytopenia 63
granuloma
    in atypical Mycobacterium
        infection 47
    eosinophilic 116, 117, 156–7
    giant cell reparative (central giant
        cell) 117, 136–7
    giant cell of small bones 137
    gingival in pregnancy 203
    pyogenic 203
    in sarcoidosis 48
    tuberculoid 46
growth plate 2, 9, 10
    effects of osteomyelitis 43
    in rickets 75
    in slipped capital femoral
        epiphysis 70
    in thanatophoric dysplasia 55
    in type II osteogenesis imperfecta
        61

haemangioendothelioma
    epithelioid 145, 207
    spindle cell 206
haemangioma 143–4
    age at presentation 116
    arteriovenous 202
    capillary 201
    cavernous 202
    epithelioid 203
    histiocytoid 143
    intramuscular 204
    intraosseous location 117
    sclerosing 180
    skeletal location 117
    synovial 96, 114
haemangiopericytoma 78, 166,
    205–6
haematoma
    in bone fracture 18
    encysted 23
haematopoietic stem cell 6
haematopoietic tissue 2
haemodialysis 79, 95
haemophilia 23, 96–7
Haemophilus influenzae 44
haemosiderin
    in aneurysmal bone cyst 153
    in benign fibrous histiocytoma
        180
    in fibrous dysplasia 158
    in haemophilia 96
    in joint injury 33
    in Kaposi's sarcoma 208
    in non-ossifying fibroma 155
    in PVNS 112
    in siderotic synovitis 96
hamartoma 224
    fibrolipomatous of nerve 191
    fibrous of infancy 172–3
    infantile cartilaginous of rib 161

Hand–Schüller–Christian disease 156
HAP crystal deposition 94
Haversian canals 4
Haversian systems 4
heavy metal poisoning 63
Heberden's nodes 88
heparan sulphate 65
hereditary multiple exostoses 59, 129, 132
hibernoma 190
histiocytoma 27, 112
 benign fibrous 155, 179–80
 malignant fibrous 133
histiocytosis X 156, 181
histomorphometric analysis 72
Hodgkin's disease 141
 metastatic 162
Homer–Wright rosettes 216
homogentisic acid oxidase deficiency 95
housemaid's knee 34
Howship's lacunae 7, 83
hyaluronic acid 12
hydatid cyst 51
hydrocephalus 54
hydroxyapatite crystal deposition 94
hypercalcaemia 72
hypergammaglobulinaemia 105
hyperlipidaemia 182
hyperparathyroidism 22, 74
 primary 72–3
 secondary 74–5, 79, 86
hypertrophic pulmonary osteoarthropathy 28
hyperuricaemia 92
hypogonadism 82
hypophosphataemia 72, 78
hypophosphatasia 78

infantile cartilaginous hamartoma of rib 161
infantile cortical hyperostosis 28
infantile digital fibromatosis 174
infantile fibromatosis 178
infantile fibrosarcoma 179
infantile myofibromatosis 173
infection
 non-pyogenic 45–51
 pyogenic 38–45
internal fixation devices, bone reaction to 29–30
intervertebral disc disease 106
intestinal disease, arthritis associated 103
intravascular fasciitis 170
involucrum 40, 41
ischaemic fasciitis 172
ivory exostosis 118
Ixodes ricinus 50

jaw
 fibro-osseous lesions 117

giant cell reparative granuloma 117, 136–7
joint capsule 12
joints
 diarthrodial (synovial) 12
 disorders 88–114
 non-diarthrodial 12
 structure 12
 traumatic injury 33
juvenile angiofibroma 174
juvenile aponeurotic fibroma 169
juvenile osteoporosis 80
juvenile rheumatoid arthritis 101
juvenile xanthogranuloma 181

Kaposi's sarcoma 208
Kasabach–Merritt syndrome 202
keloid 167
keratan sulphate 12, 66
keratoderma blennorrhagica 103
Kienböck's disease 28
Kimura's disease 203
knee
 osteoarthritis 88
 pigmented villonodular synovitis 112
knuckle pads 175
Köhler's disease 28
kyphoscoliosis 57, 66
kyphosis 45, 76

laminin 197
Langerhans cell granulomatosis 156
Langerhans cells 156, 157
leiomyoblastoma 198
leiomyoma
 cutaneous 195
 deep soft tissue 196
 genital 195
 superficial 195
leiomyosarcoma
 bone 148–9
 epithelioid 198
 soft tissue 166, 197
leprosy 47
Letterer–Siwe disease 156
leucoerythroblastic anaemia 63
leukaemia 78, 92, 141
ligaments 5, 15
 degenerative changes 35
 injury 35
lipoblastoma 191
lipoblastomatosis 191
lipoblasts 192, 193, 194
lipoma 146, 188
 intramuscular 188
 perineurial 191
 pleomorphic 190
 spindle cell 189, 190
lipomatosis, synovial 114
liposarcoma 166, 192
 dedifferentiated 192
 myxoid 193–4

pleomorphic 195
 round cell 194
 well-differentiated 192–3
Looser's zones 76
Lyme disease 50
lymphangioma 143, 209
lymphangiosarcoma 207
lymphoedema following mastectomy 207
lymphoma 116, 117, 140

macrodactyly 191
macrophage colony-stimulating factor 63
maduromycosis 49
Mafucci's syndrome 58, 202
malignant fibrous histiocytoma (MFH)
 angiomatoid 166, 187
 bone 116, 117, 148
 giant cell-rich 186, 223
 inflammatory 186–7
 myxoid 185–6
 soft tissue 166, 184–7, 192
 storiform-pleomorphic 185
malignant melanoma
 metastatic 163
 of soft parts 221
malignant peripheral nerve sheath tumour 215
 epithelioid 216
Marfan's syndrome 62
Marjolin's ulcer 43
Masson's tumour 204
mastocytoma 86
mastocytosis 86
melanin 221
melon-seed bodies 46
melorheostosis 64
meningioma, extracranial 220
menisci
 cystic degeneration 33
 injury 33
mesenchymoma
 fibrocartilaginous 159
 malignant 224
mesothelioma 166
metabolic and endocrine disorders 65–7, 72–86
metaphyseal chondrodysplasia / dysostosis 57
metaphyseal fibrous defect 155
metaphysis 2, 10
metastatic tumours in bone 63, 116, 117, 162–3
metatarsalgia 210
MFH, see malignant fibrous histiocytoma
MIC-2 gene product 138, 216, 218, 230
Milwaukee shoulder syndrome 94
monosodium urate 92
Morquio's syndrome 66

moth-eaten appearance 140, 147, 148
MPNST 215, 216
mucopolysaccharidoses (MPS) 65–6
multicentric reticulohistiocytosis 181
multiple endocrine neoplasia type I 72
multiple epiphyseal dysplasia 57
muscle tumours
 smooth muscle 195–8
 striated muscle 198–201
mycetoma 49
Mycobacterium avium 47
Mycobacterium kansasii 47
Mycobacterium leprae 47
Mycobacterium marinum 47
Mycobacterium tuberculosis 45
myeloma 22, 78, 142–3
 age at presentation 116
 intraosseous location 117
 multiple 142, 162
 skeletal location 117
 solitary 142
myelomatosis 142
myoblastoma, granular cell 214
MyoD1 protein 228
myofibroma, infantile 173
myofibromatosis, infantile 173
myoglobin 198
myositis, proliferative 171
myositis ossificans 31
myositis ossificans progressiva 67
myxoma 149
 intramuscular 225
 juxta-articular 114
 nerve sheath 214

naevoxanthoendothelioma 181
neonatal osteomyelitis 43
nephrolithiasis 86
nerve sheath myxoma 214
neurilemmoma 150, 211
 ancient (degenerate) 211–12
neuroblastoma
 bone 116, 139–40
 soft tissue 166, 218
neuroectodermal tumour
 bone 139
 primitive 139
neurofibroma 212
 diffuse 212–13
 plexiform 213
neurofibromatosis 69, 116, 212
neurofibrosarcoma 215, 216
neuroma
 Morton's 210
 traumatic (amputation) 209–10
neurone-specific enolase 216, 218
neuropathic arthropathy 91
neurothekeoma 214
neutrophil polymorphs 39, 41, 45

N-*myc* oncogene 218
nodular fasciitis 170
nodular tenosynovitis 112
NSE 216, 218

OA, see osteoarthritis
ochronosis 95
OI, see osteogenesis imperfecta
Ollier's disease (enchondromatosis)
    58, 128, 132
Osgood–Schlatter's disease 28
ossification
    endochondral 9, 10, 129, 130,
        159
    heterotopic 32, 67–8
    intramembranous 8–9
ossifying fasciitis 170
ossifying fibromyxoid tumour of soft
    tissue 226
osteoarthritis (OA) 88–90
    primary 88
    secondary 24, 70, 88
    spine 107
osteoblastoma 120
    age at presentation 116
    aggressive 120
    intraosseous location 117
    skeletal location 117
osteoblasts 5, 6, 7, 8, 9, 10, 11
    in bone grafts 29
    in fracture healing 20, 21
    in infarct healing 25, 26
    in osteoblastoma 120
    in osteoid osteoma 119
    in Paget's disease 83
osteocalcin 2
osteochondritis dissecans 27
osteochondritis juvenilis 28
osteochondroma 59, 129–30
    age at presentation 116
    intraosseous location 117
    skeletal location 117
osteoclasts 6, 7–8, 11, 21
    in bone grafts 29
    in osteoid osteoma 119
    in osteopetrosis 63
    in Paget's disease 83
    in primary hyperparathyroidism 73
osteocytes 3, 6, 7
    in osteonecrosis 23
    in type IV osteogenesis imperfecta
        62
osteofibrous dysplasia 159
osteogenesis imperfecta (OI) 22,
    60, 116
    type I 60
    type II 61
    type III 61, 62
    type IV 62
osteoid 2, 8, 9, 10, 20
    in osteomalacia 76
    in osteoporosis 82
    in Paget's disease 83

in primary hyperparathyroidism
    73
in rickets 75
in secondary hyperparathyroidism
    74
osteoid osteoma 119
    age at presentation 116
    intraosseous location 117
    skeletal location 117
osteolysis
    massive 144
    prosthetic joint replacement 108
osteoma 116, 117, 118
osteomalacia 22, 72, 74, 75
    in chronic renal failure 79
    following bisphosphonate-treated
        Paget's disease 84
    hypophosphataemic 78
    oncogenic 78
    vitamin D deficiency 76
    vitamin D-dependent 77
osteomyelitis 63
    in actinomycosis 48
    acute 38, 39, 40
    chronic 41–2, 116
    chronic recurrent multifocal 44
    complications 43
    neonatal 43
    pyogenic 38, 39, 40, 41
    radiation-induced 32
    tuberculous 46
    vertebral 43–4, 48
osteon 11
    osteonecrosis 23, 63
        conditions associated 24
        idiopathic avascular 24
        medullary 27
        subchondral avascular 24, 25,
            26, 38
    osteonectin 2
osteons 4
osteopaenia 60, 61, 62, 86
    in chronic renal failure 79
    in rheumatoid arthritis 99
osteopetrosis 63
osteophytes 88, 90, 107
osteopoikilosis 64–5, 118
osteopontin 2
osteoporosis 22, 72, 80–1
    high-turnover 82
    juvenile 80
    low-turnover 81
    mastocytosis in 86
    post-menopausal / type I 80, 81
    primary 80
    secondary 80, 82
    senile / age-related / type II 80, 81
    steroid-induced 82
osteoprogenitor cells 5, 6, 7, 8, 25
osteosarcoma 63, 121–3
    age at presentaion 116, 166
    chondroblastic 122
    extraskeletal 116, 223

fibroblastic 122
giant cell-rich 123
high-grade surface 126
intraosseous location 117
low-grade intramedullary 125
osteoblastic 122
parosteal 116, 125
periosteal 126
sclerosing 122
skeletal location 117
small (round) cell 124
soft tissue 166
telangiectatic 124
osteosclerosis 63, 157, 162
oxalosis 86

Paget's disease of bone 63, 72, 76,
    83–4, 116
    mastocytosis in 86
    osteomalacia following treatment
        84
Paget's sarcoma 116, 127
pannus 99, 100
papillary endothelial hyperplasia
    204
paraganglioma 166, 219
paraproteinaemia 84
parathyroid
    carcinoma 72
    hyperplasia 72, 74
parathyroid hormone (PTH) 74
    ectopic production 72
patella, subluxation 91
perichondrium 9
periosteal (juxtacortical) chondroma
    116, 128–9
periosteum 2, 5, 9, 12
periostitis, florid reactive 160
periostitis ossificans 160
peripheral neuroepithelioma
    (primitive neuroectodermal
    tumour) 166, 216–17
Perthes' disease 28
phantom bone disease 144
phosphaturia 78
pigmented neuroectodermal tumour
    of infancy 218–19
pigmented villonodular synovitis
    96, 112
plasmacytoma 142
platyspondyly 57
plexiform fibrohistiocytic tumours
    184
PNET 166, 216–17
POH 68
polyarteritis nodosa 28
polymeric biomaterials, reactions to
    111
polymyalgia rheumatica 106
popcorn calcification 61
primary centres of ossification 9
primary synovial chondromatosis
    113

primitive neuroectodermal tumour
    166, 216–17
progressive diaphyseal dysplasia 64
progressive osseous heteroplasia 68
proliferative fasciitis 170–1
proliferative myositis 171
prostatic carcinoma, metastatic
    162, 163
prosthetic joint replacement
    aseptic loosening 108–10
    metallic wear particles 110
    polymethylmethacrylate (PMMA)
        wear particles 108–9
    septic loosening 111
    ultra-high molecular weight
        polyethylene (UHMWP) wear
        particles 109
proteoglycans 12
psammoma bodies 220
PSC 113
pseudarthrosis 21
    congenital 69
pseudoachondroplasia 56
pseudocysts, subchondral 88, 89
pseudogout 93, 94
pseudomembrane, prosthetic joints
    108
Pseudomonas aeruginosa 38, 43
pseudotumour
    haemophiliac 96, 97
    lytic 111
psoriasis 92
psoriatic arthropathy 104
PTH, see parathyroid hormone
punched out appearance 142
PVNS 96, 112
pyrophosphate arthropathy 93–4

RA, see rheumatoid arthritis
radiation, effects on bone 32, 116
Reiter's syndrome 103
renal cell carcinoma, metastatic 163
renal osteodystrophy 79
reticulin 205, 206
reticulohistiocytoma 181
retinal anlage tumour 218–19
retinoblastoma, familial 116
reversal lines 6
rhabdomyoma 198
rhabdomyosarcoma 198–9
    alveolar 166, 200
    embryonal 166, 199
    pleomorphic 166, 200–1
rheumatoid arthritis (RA) 34, 44,
    98–100
    juvenile 101
rheumatoid factor 98, 101
rheumatoid nodules 100–1
rib, infantile cartilaginous
    hamartoma 161
rickets 75
    vitamin D deficiency 75
    vitamin D-dependent 77

X-linked hypophosphataemic 77
ring of Ranvier 10
Russell bodies 98, 99

Salmonella 38, 103
sarcoidosis 47, 48
sarcoma
    alveolar soft part 166, 228
    bone 116
    chordoid 222
    clear cell 166, 221
    epithelioid 166, 229
    radiation-induced 32, 116
    synovial 114, 166, 226
        biphasic 227
        monophasic epithelial 227
        monophasic fibrous 227–8
scar, hypertrophic 167
Schmorl's node 106
schwannoma
    benign 211
    malignant 166, 215
scleroderma 104–5
scurvy 80
sea urchin spine injuries 97
secondary centres of ossification 9
secondary osteochondromatosis 113
SEDC 57
septicaemia 43
sequestrum 40, 41
seronegative inflammatory
    arthropathies 102–6
Sever's disease 28
Shigella flexneri 103
sickle cell disease 24, 27, 38
signet-ring appearance 207
silicone rubber (Silastic) implants
    111
Sinding–Larsen disease 28
skeletal dysplasias 54
    with abnormal bone formation
        60–2
    with abnormal cartilage
        development 54–9
    sclerosing 63–5

slipped capital femoral epiphysis 70
sodium etidronate 84
soft tissue tumours and tumour-like
    lesions 166–230
solar elastosis 182
spine
    amyloid arthropathy 95
    ankylosing spondylitis 102
    bamboo 102
    cord compression 54
    disc prolapse 54
    in FIO 84
    joint disease 106–7
    ochronosis 95
    osteoarthritis 107
    osteoporosis 81
    rugger jersey 63
spondylosis 107
spondyloepiphyseal dysplasia
    congenita 57
spondylosis, spine 107
spongiosa
    primary 10
    secondary 10
stag-horn spaces 205
Staphylococcus aureus 38, 44
Sternberg–Reed cells 141
Still's disease 101
strawberry naevus 201
streptococci 38, 44
subchondral pseudocysts 88, 89
subchondral sclerosis 88, 89
subungual exostosis 30, 117, 160
sucked candy appearance 144
sulphur granules 48
symphysis 12
synchondrosis 12
syndesmosis 12
synovial fluid in gout 92
synovial intima 14
synovial lining cells 15
    type A 14
    type B 14
synovial membrane 14
    in haemophilia 96

in osteoarthritis 90
in pyrophosphate arthropathy
    94
in rheumatoid arthritis 98–9
tumours and tumour-like
    conditions 112–14
synovial osteochondromatosis 113
synovitis
    detritic 91
    foreign body 97
    granulomatous 47
    pigmented villonodular 96, 112
    siderotic 33, 96
syphilis 49
systemic lupus erythematosus 104
systemic sclerosis 104–5

talipes equinovarus 57
temporal artery in giant cell arteritis
    106
tendinitis, calcific 35, 94
tendons 5, 15
    degenerative changes 35
    injury 35
tendon sheath 15
    fibroma 168
    giant cell tumour 78, 112
    in rheumatoid arthritis 98
tennis elbow 35
tenosynovitis, nodular 112
tetracycline labelling
    osteomalacia 76
    osteoporosis 81
    primary hyperparathyroidism
        73
    renal osteodystrophy 79
    secondary hyperparathyroidism
        74
thanatophoric dysplasia 55
thorn injuries 97
thyrotoxicosis 82
tophi, gouty 92
torticollis 178
total parenteral nutrition 79
traction exostosis 31

Treponema pallidum 49
Treponema pertenue 50
Trevor's disease 59
trigger finger 35
Triton tumour 216
tuberculosis 34, 45
tumoral calcinosis 94, 224–5

ulcer, Marjolin's 43
ulcerative colitis 103
Ureaplasma urealyticum 103
urinary tract infection 38, 43
urticaria pigmentosa 86

vanishing bone disease 144
varicose veins 28
vasculitis
    in giant cell arteritis 106
    in rheumatoid arthritis 101
VDDR 77
Verocay bodies 150, 211
vertebral osteomyelitis 43–4, 48
vimentin 229
vitamin A excess 63
vitamin C deficiency 80
vitamin D
    deficiency 75, 76
    excess 63
    vitamin D-dependent rickets 77

Waldenstrom's macroglobulinaemia
    142
Whipple's disease 103
window-frame appearance 83
Wolff's law 11

xanthelasma 182
xanthogranuloma, juvenile 181
xanthoma 181, 182

yaws 50
Yersinia enterocolitica 103

zellballen 219
Ziehl–Neelsen stain 46

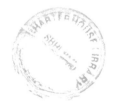

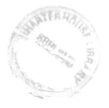